Clinical Pharmacy and Pharmaceutical Science

Clinical Pharmacy and Pharmaceutical Science

Edited by **Sean Boyd**

Callisto Reference
New York

Published by Callisto Reference,
106 Park Avenue, Suite 200,
New York, NY 10016, USA
www.callistoreference.com

Clinical Pharmacy and Pharmaceutical Science
Edited by Sean Boyd

International Standard Book Number: 978-1-63239-716-4 (Hardback)

Printed in China.

Contents

Preface

Every book is initially just a concept; it takes months of research and hard work to give it the final shape in which the readers receive it. In its early stages, this book also went through rigorous reviewing. The notable contributions made by experts from across the globe were first molded into patterned chapters and then arranged in a sensibly sequential manner to bring out the best results.

Clinical Pharmacy refers to a branch of medicinal science which works to provide better and optimum use of drugs to ensure health, wellness of the patients and also works towards disease prevention. Clinical Pharmacy depends on pharmaceutical science for the formation of drugs which is done by using the principles of chemistry, biology, statistics, mathematics, physics, etc. This book will trace the progresses made in this field and highlight some of its key concepts and applications in a multidisciplinary approach. It will elucidate the new concepts and prospective developments made in clinical pharmacy. Those with an interest in this topic will find this book extremely helpful as it provides researches from across the globe. Coherent flow of topics, reader-friendly language and extensive use of examples make this book an invaluable source of knowledge.

It has been my immense pleasure to be a part of this project and to contribute my years of learning in such a meaningful form. I would like to take this opportunity to thank all the people who have been associated with the completion of this book at any step.

Editor

1

Use of Cumulative Assessments in U.S. Schools and Colleges of Pharmacy

Deepti Vyas †,*, Jenana Halilovic †, Myo-Kyoung Kim †, Marcus C. Ravnan †, Edward L. Rogan † and Suzanne M. Galal †

University of the Pacific, Thomas J. Long School of Pharmacy and Health Sciences, 751 Brookside Road Stockton, CA 95207, USA; E-Mails: jmaker@pacific.edu (J.H.); mkim@pacific.edu (M.K.K.); mravnan@pacific.edu (M.C.R.); erogan@pacific.edu (E.L.R.); sgalal@pacific.edu (S.M.G.)

† These authors contributed equally to this work.

* Author to whom correspondence should be addressed; E-Mail: vyasd80@gmail.com

Academic Editor: Keith Wilson

Abstract: The Accreditation Council of Pharmacy Education (ACPE) has taken a strong stance on assessment in pharmacy education. One available assessment tool is cumulative assessments, which may be administered at various points in the curriculum. This article presents the results of a survey of U.S. schools of pharmacy regarding the use of cumulative assessments within their curriculum. A 20-question survey tool was emailed to 125 schools of pharmacy. A total of 105 out of 125 schools participated (response rate 84%). Of these, 52 schools currently have a cumulative assessment program; 18 have one cumulative exam prior to advanced pharmacy practice experiences (APPEs); 19 have a cumulative exam every didactic year; and seven have accumulative exams every semester, except during APPEs ($n = 44$). Increased faculty workload emerged as the top challenge faced by schools that have implemented a cumulative assessment program. Eighteen schools indicated that no outcomes are measured to determine the utility of the cumulative assessment. From these results, it appears that almost half of participating U.S. schools have implemented a cumulative assessment plan. However, it is apparent that more research needs to be done to determine which outcomes are expected to improve with the implementation of such an assessment plan.

Keywords: comprehensive assessment; cumulative assessment; milestone examination; progress assessment

1. Introduction

The Accreditation Council of Pharmacy Education (ACPE) has taken a strong stance on assessment within the pharmacy curriculum [1]. Current accreditation guidelines (Guideline 15.1) state that "In general, the college or school's evaluation of student learning should: incorporate periodic, psychometrically sound, comprehensive, knowledge-based, and performance-based formative and summative assessments, including nationally standardized assessments (in addition to graduates' performance on licensure examinations) that allow comparisons and benchmarks with all accredited and college or school-determined peer institutions." The recent 2016 draft guidelines have expanded this edict by including language that assessment should evaluate student readiness to: (1) enter advanced pharmacy practice experiences (APPE); (2) provide direct patient care; and (3) contribute as a member of an interprofessional team [2]. This draft also makes reference to the use of the Pharmacy Curriculum Outcomes Assessment (PCOA), an optional, standardized, multiple choice exam developed by the National Association of the Boards of Pharmacy to measure student knowledge in different content areas. These draft ACPE guidelines clearly indicate that assessment of student achievement and readiness is an integral part of ensuring the quality of our pharmacy graduates. In making reference to PCOA, these guidelines also direct attention to the fact that a cumulative assessment tool is needed to assess student performance and to determine and document readiness for entrance into the APPE curriculum.

When considering assessment, there are several techniques that can assess student readiness and achievement of learning. These may include: "Written tests, oral examinations, student reflections, instructor evaluations, and performance in simulated settings." [3]. However, most of these assessments are done within individual courses or course blocks. On the other hand, cumulative assessments or progression examinations are generally defined as assessments administered across the curriculum with the goal of measuring student acquisition and retention of knowledge that is based on a defined set of curricular outcomes [4–14]. Cumulative assessments are not linked to any one course, but instead measure the achievement of global curricular outcomes. These cumulative assessments may be used to: (1) identify students who may benefit from remediation exercises; (2) determine minimal competency to allow progression through the curriculum; (3) help ascertain retention of previous coursework; and (4) evaluate the overall curriculum by identifying curricular deficiencies. Data obtained from these assessments may also be used for benchmarking across various institutions. However, utilization of data for benchmarking may be difficult due to inherent differences in curricular sequencing across institutions [14].

Although extensive data are limited, some schools have instituted cumulative assessments at various points in their curriculum [4–13]. At the University of Houston, Sansgiry *et al.* published an article outlining their case-based written Milemarker exam, which is formative for the first two years and then summative in the third year, with the goal of ensuring student readiness for APPEs [4,5]. To ascertain student accountability, students are informed that failing the last part of Milemarker exam could result in delayed progression to APPEs [5]. Another paper written by Alston *et al.* described a cumulative assessment plan comprised of multiple choice questions designed to measure the acquisition of skills [6]. As part of this assessment plan, faculty have in place a rigorous process for assessing the reliability and validity of the cumulative exam, stressing that this is an important step in developing and implementing a cumulative assessment strategy. A more comprehensive plan was described by Me´sza´ros at Touro University-California, where a knowledge-based and objective-structured clinical exam (OSCE) is administered on an annual basis. Exam validity is ascertained by comparing exam results to APPE preceptor evaluations [7]. At the University of Kansas, Ragan and colleagues described a longitudinal OSCE administered annually to determine student competence for entrance into APPEs [9]. While most of these studies describe assessments that have been developed in-house, Scott and colleagues described the use of PCOA at Palm Beach Atlantic University [10]. The paper contended that the PCOA has great utility in identifying student and curricular deficiency, especially against national benchmarks. However, Scott also mentioned current limitations in using PCOA as a benchmarking tool. Scott argued that not only is participation across pharmacy schools limited, but student accountability varies across schools, making direct program comparison difficult and perhaps inaccurate.

Cumulative assessment utility has also been recommended in the literature by expert opinion and position papers, which further add support to their use in higher education [14,15]. Plaza published a paper recommending that schools use multiple types of cumulative assessments. When strategically placed after the establishment of knowledge and skill domains, these cumulative assessments afford institutions the opportunity to systematically measure students' overall competence [14]. Plaza further argued that knowledge-based assessments may overly emphasize rote memorization of material; therefore, Plaza recommended the use of both knowledge and skill evaluations. Plaza opined that OSCEs would generate a clearer and more robust picture of individual student competence. When taking a composite of the literature reports and expert opinions, one common theme prevails: that cumulative assessments are opportunities to gain insight only when the assessment plans are founded on sound reliability and validity measures [6,7,14,15].

The last comprehensive evaluation and documentation of cumulative assessment utility in U.S. schools and colleges of pharmacy occurred in 1998 [16]. Data from that survey revealed that 19.6% (nine out of 77) of pharmacy programs administered cumulative assessments [16]. These results lack program representation considering that the number of pharmacy schools and colleges has nearly doubled since the study was conducted. Consequently, as evidence and literature bolsters the implementation of cumulative assessment in higher education, it is important to continue to collect data and document the progress of U.S. schools in implementing cumulative assessments within the pharmacy curriculum. To address recent dynamic changes within pharmacy education, we sought to survey all U.S. schools and colleges of pharmacy in order to gain insight about their experiences towards cumulative assessments. These data will provide valuable information to schools looking to develop or strengthen their existing assessment programs.

2. Experimental Section

A 20-question survey instrument consisting of 3 distinct evaluation sections was developed. Of the three sections, questions in Section 1 targeted school demographics and cumulative assessment utilization. Section 2 contained survey questions, which would aid in determining barriers to instituting cumulative assessments and the challenges faced by those schools that currently incorporate these assessments in their curriculum. Upon completing Sections 1 and 2, only schools and colleges that have a cumulative assessment plan were asked to complete Section 3. Section 3 of the survey contained items designed to address assessment format, assessed topics, personnel responsible for plan development, validation methods utilized and, finally, outcome measurement.

The respondent pool for the survey instrument was identified through the American Association of Colleges of Pharmacy (AACP) faculty database, which included 125 partially- and fully-accredited U.S. colleges and schools of pharmacy. Inclusion criteria were individuals listed as chairs of the pharmacy practice department and/or individuals responsible for assessment. Schools that were identified as having pre-candidate status by ACPE were excluded from this study. The survey instrument was electronically administered through SurveyMonkey® in April 2014 [17]. All data collected were input and collated in Microsoft Excel® and analyzed using descriptive statistics. Participant consent was obtained at the beginning of the online survey. This study is approved by the University of the Pacific Institutional Review Board (Protocol No. 13-48).

3. Results and Discussion

3.1. Results

A total of 105 out of 125 schools participated in the study, a response rate of 84% (survey available as an Appendix). Respondent demographics are summarized in Table 1. Of the respondents, 53 (50.5%) reported not having or utilizing cumulative assessments; however, 13 of these (12.4%) reported that they are in the process of developing a cumulative assessment program. Of the 40 (38.1%) respondent programs without a cumulative assessment program, the most common reasons cited for "not" instituting such an assessment included "lack of resources" and that "knowledge assessed in individual courses is adequate" (Table 2).

Table 1. Demographics of respondent schools.

	Specification	Have a Cumulative Assessment Plan?		
		Yes (n = 52)	**No (n = 40)**	**In Development (n = 13)**
Private School	Student Enrollment 100 or less	16 (30.7%)	8 (20%)	5 (38%)
	Student Enrollment >100	11 (21%)	10 (25%)	4 (30.7%)
Public School	Student Enrollment 100 or less	14 (27%)	11 (27.5%)	2 (15%)
	Student Enrollment >100	11 (21%)	11 (27.5%)	2 (15%)

Table 2. Reasons cited for "not" having a cumulative assessment plan.

Reason (Respondents Could Select More Than One)	n = 40
Lack of resources (faculty time, financial constraints, *etc.*)	23 (57.5%)
Knowledge is already assessed in individual courses	20 (50%)
Unconvinced it would add value to the current education program	17 (42.5%)
Unsure of what to do with the results	9 (22.5%)
Lack of evidence in the literature supporting its use	8 (20%)
Faculty have never considered it	5 (12.5%)

Of the fifty two (49.5%) schools that indicated having a cumulative assessment program within their curriculum, 19 (36.5%) have had cumulative assessments in place for more than five years. The most common reasons cited for implementing cumulative assessments included; "to ensure minimal competency in core educational outcomes" (77%), "help students identify deficiencies" (75%) and "ensure student accountability for developing a cumulative knowledge and skill set" (60%) (Table 3).

Table 3. Purpose of a cumulative assessment plan within the curriculum.

	Purpose	***n*** **= 52**
Student specific	Help students self-identify educational and learning deficiencies	39 (75%)
	Provide feedback to students affording them developmental opportunities	36 (69%)
	Ensure student accountability for developing a cumulative knowledge and skill set	31 (60%)
Program specific	Ensure minimal competency in meeting core educational outcomes	40 (77%)
	Identify curricular gaps and or deficiencies	32 (61.5%)
	Ensure a level of competence that is expected before student progresses in the program	30 (57.7%)

With regard to development of the cumulative assessment program, 31 schools involve all faculty members responsible for the delivery of content and material being tested, while 10 have a specific and dedicated cumulative assessment committee. For the remaining 12 schools, it is the assessment committee that is responsible for developing the cumulative assessment program. An overwhelming majority of schools (38 of 52) have an in-house assessment, whereas the remaining 14 have purchased a commercial question bank. As a composite, schools indicated that their assessments generally test knowledge/skills related to a variety of topic areas (Table 4).

Table 4. Areas assessed in the cumulative assessment plan.

Topic (Respondents Could Select More Than One)	***n*** **= 52**
Therapeutics	43
Patient assessment	41
Pharmacy calculations	41
Medication counseling	41
Drug information and literature search	41
Kinetics	38
Pharmacology	37
Physiology	37
Medicinal chemistry	33
Law	32

As far as the timing and placement of the cumulative assessment plan, 18 schools only have one exam prior to APPEs; 19 schools have an exam every didactic year; and seven schools have a cumulative assessment every semester, excluding APPEs ($n = 44$, eight schools skipped this question). The format also varied, with 15 schools having both a written and oral exam, 29 having only a written exam and six having only an oral exam ($n = 50$, two schools skipped this question). Of the schools with an oral exam or oral exam portions, 14 use OSCEs to assess student performance; 14 assess patient interview/counselling skills; eight use simulations; and nine use an oral question and answer session (some schools use multiple formats). For those with a written exam or written exam component, 37 schools have a multiple choice exam question format; 18 utilize a case-based exam; while nine have a short answer/essay type exam, again with some schools using multiple formats.

With regard to the summative *vs.* formative nature of the assessments, 18 schools have both a low and high-stakes component; 19 have only a low-stakes exam with no consequence; and 10 schools have only high-stakes summative assessments in their curriculum ($n = 47$, five schools skipped this question). Of those with a high-stakes component, 11 schools indicated that students are given opportunities for remediation, but progression is halted if a student fails despite remediation efforts; four indicated that they offered unlimited remediation opportunities; and one indicated that failing the assessment results in a halt in progression without opportunity for remediation ($n = 16$, 12 skipped this question).

When asked about challenges to instituting a cumulative assessment plan, the majority cited "increased faculty workload" and "lack of evidence that these assessments actually improve long-term retention of knowledge" (Table 5). When asked about exam validation, 28 reported having no formal validation measures or standards in place. Of those claiming validation, seven validate by comparing performance on cumulative assessments with cumulative GPA, seven with national board exam pass rates, and 10 schools use validated package exams, such as the PCOA. When asked about outcome measurement since implementing the assessment, 18 schools indicated that no specific outcomes are measured. Of those who have measured outcomes, the most common responses were "improvements in board exam pass rates" ($n = 5$) and "performance on APPEs" ($n = 5$).

Table 5. Challenges faced by schools having a cumulative assessment plan within their curriculum.

Challenge (Respondents Could Select More Than One)	$n = 52$
Increased faculty workload	30 (57.6%)
Lack of evidence that progress exams actually improve long-term retention of knowledge	25 (48%)
Lack of exam validation	25 (48%)
Difficulty figuring out what to do with deficient students	24 (46%)
Inadequate remediation strategies	23 (44%)
Lack of student buy-in	15 (28.8%)
Lack of faculty buy-in	13 (25%)
No challenges faced	4 (7.7%)

3.2. Discussion

This study provides insight into the utilization of cumulative assessments in U.S. schools and colleges of pharmacy. Our results indicate that almost 50% of the surveyed schools have cumulative assessment in place, and an additional 12% are planning implementation. These numbers are substantially higher than the 19.6% reported in 2000 and may be reflective of the growing emphasis placed on learning as it relates to the achievement of curricular outcomes [16]. Nevertheless, it should be noted that the majority of schools with cumulative assessment plans have a low-stakes emphasis (no impact to progression). While low-stakes examinations avoid student stress and need for remediation, Szilagyi reported that the pass rate of the first Milemarker exam increased to 68.6% to 85.7% from 7% to 23.9% when the school added rewards and punishments to their formative assessment plan [11]. Therefore, when taken into consideration, low student effort and motivation can negatively impact performance, decreasing the validity of exam results [18]. To then find the right balance, it may be that a combination of both formative and summative assessments should be utilized as a means of assessing both student learning and curricular effectiveness [14].

In addition, based on one expert's opinion, cumulative assessments should include both knowledge and skill assessments, so as to truly evaluate a student's overall competence [14]. Despite these recommendations, very few schools (15) have implemented a plan that includes both of these components.

As the current 2007 ACPE standards do not provide guidance on the specific format for cumulative assessments, our results indicate that the schools have developed a variety of assessments administered at different time points in the curriculum. The advantage of this approach is that it gives schools the ability to develop assessments tailored towards their own curriculum, resource availability and knowledge domain acquisition timing. On the other hand, having each school devise individual cumulative assessments results in increased faculty work load and inability to benchmark and compare results across different programs. From the data collected, 10 schools indicated that their institutions have adopted PCOA. Published experience from other schools of pharmacy indicates that PCOA scores highly correlate with student GPA and may be a better measure of student knowledge than student perceptions of their own knowledge [10,12]. While the PCOA has the potential to provide meaningful information, there are also several current limitations associated with its use [10].

Although the majority of schools with a cumulative assessment plan reported several challenges associated with implementation, faculty workload was chosen as the leading challenge. Faculty engagement is needed for the plan to be successful, but the burden on faculty should be carefully balanced to avoid burn-out. Certainly, faculty involvement is substantial, as it involves plan development, implementation and maintenance, as well as ongoing effort and attention to question writing, grading/evaluation and remediation.

In addition to the assessment itself, another challenge faced by the schools is how to find an effective way to remediate students who "fail" the cumulative assessment or who show significant deficiencies in core content areas. The current health sciences literature indicates that early detection, development of an individualized remediation plan and assessment of the effectiveness of remediation can all be important pieces of the overall remediation strategy [19]. Additionally, the cumulative assessment plan itself can and should be part of the early detection system to identify and correct student deficiencies. In answering the "how to best remediate" question, our research was unable to identify any literature on the assessment of remediation strategies specifically related to cumulative assessments. Generally, the policies on academic progression vary widely among different schools, and there is little literature on the remediation strategies in pharmacy education [19].

With regard to impact on long-term retention, studies in the medical literature indicate that repeated testing results in repeated retrieval of memories and increases long-term retention [21–23]. Interestingly, almost half of the programs with cumulative assessment plans questioned both its validity and utility in improving long-term retention among students. As noted earlier, only a few schools have published validity (and reliability) findings of their cumulative assessments, and we were unable to identify studies that specifically evaluated long-term retention pre- and post-implementation of a cumulative assessment plan within pharmacy education.

Finally, student buy-in must be factored in as it can have a major impact on performance. As noted in the literature, students' passing scores increase considerably in formative exams if a high-stakes incentive or punishment is in place [5,11]. In the article described by Sansgiry, the most productive incentive was carryover points towards a high-stakes exam [5]. One limitation of our study is that we did not specifically survey schools regarding incentive mechanisms currently in place. Surveying schools regarding incentive mechanisms would have provided valuable information for other programs looking to develop or improve their cumulative assessment plans.

4. Conclusions

Data gathered from this study show that almost half of U.S. schools and colleges of pharmacy have implemented cumulative assessment plans. However, these plans vary greatly in format and student accountability. Additionally, based on feedback, these assessment plans are fraught with challenges, including a lack of exam validity, a lack of student accountability and a lack of evidence demonstrating improved long-term retention. Unfortunately, the majority of schools do not attest that their use of cumulative assessments is tied to improvement in measured learning outcomes. Further study is needed to wholly justify the ongoing use of energy and resources that cumulative assessments require. Further study is also needed to determine the optimal format and sequencing of cumulative assessments so that minimal competency and student readiness for pharmacy practice is truly measured.

Author Contributions

Deepti Vyas, Jenana Halilovic, Myo Kyoung Kim, Edward Rogan, Marcus Ravnan and Suzanne Galal all contributed to the study and survey design. Deepti Vyas was responsible for the write up of the Introduction and Results sections. Marcus Ravnan and Edward Rogan worked on the Experimental Section. Jenana Halilovic and Myo Kyoung Kim worked on the Discussion Section. Suzanne Galal worked on the Conclusions Section.

Conflicts of Interest

The authors declare no conflict of interest.

Appendix

Survey Questions

1. What is the name of your program?
2. Please provide the most accurate description of your school/college.
    a. Private University system
    b. Public University
    c. Private standalone
3. How many students do you enroll per class year?
4. Does your school/institution have or utilize comprehensive learning assessment(s)?
    a. Yes
    b. No
    c. In development
5. Please click on the reason(s) your program does not use a comprehensive learning assessment. Check all that apply.
    a. Lack of evidence in the literature supporting its use

   b. Knowledge is already assessed in individual courses
   c. Faculty have never considered it
   d. Unsure of what to do with the results
   e. Lack of resources (faculty time, financial constraints, etc)
   f. Unconvinced it would add value to the current education program
   g. Other

6. How long have you utilized a comprehensive learning assessment at your institution?
   a. 1-2 years
   b. 3-5 yeas
   c. More than 5 years
7. What is the purpose of the comprehensive learning assessment? check all that apply
   a. Ensure minimal competency in meeting core educational outcomes
   b. Ensure student accountability for developing a cumulative knowledge and skill set
   c. Help students self-identify education and learning deficiencies
   d. Ensure a level of competence that is expected before student progresses in the program
   e. Identify curricular gaps and or deficiencies
   f. Provide feedback to students affording them developmental opportunities
   g. Other
8. How many assessments do you have during the duration of your curriculum?
   a. 1 per academic year
   b. 1 per academic year except during APPEs
   c. 1 per semester
   d. 1 per semester except during APPEs
   e. 1 exam only, prior progression to APPEs
9. Please describe the exam delivery style
   a. Oral exam
   b. Written exam
   c. Both oral and written exam
10. If applicable, please describe the oral exam format. Check all that apply
    a. Oral questions/answer session
    b. Patient interview/counselling
    c. Objective Structured Clinical Exam (OSCE)
    d. Simulations
    e. Not applicable
11. If applicable, please describe the written exam format. Check all that apply.
    a. Short answer/essay
    b. Multiple choice
    c. Case based/Problem based solution (Progress note/SOAP note case, Drug information)
12. Who develops the comprehensive learning assessment every year?
    a. All faculty involved in teaching that material
    b. Comprehensive learning assessment faculty committee
    c. Preceptors/practitioners
    d. Administration
    e. Assessment committee
    f. Other

13. Which of the following best describes the goal of the comprehensive learning assessment?
    a. High stakes summative assessment
    b. Low stakes formative assessment
    c. Both high and low stakes assessment
14. Which of the following best describes the consequence to those students who do not pass the exam? Check all that apply
    a. Remediation one time then stop progression
    b. Unlimited remediation
    c. Stop progression
    d. No consequence
15. Which of the following topics do you assess in the comprehensive learning assessment?
    a. Therapeutics/clinical pharmacology
    b. Kinetics
    c. Pharmacology
    d. Physiology/pathophysiology
    e. Medicinal chemistry
    f. Pharmacy calculations
    g. Medication counselling
    h. Drug information and literature research
    i. Patient assessment
    j. Law and regulation
16. What challenges have you faced with incorporating a comprehensive learning assessment into your curriculum? Check all that apply.
    a. Increased faculty workload
    b. Difficulty figuring out what to do with deficient students
    c. Lack of exam validation
    d. Lack of student buy-in
    e. Lack of faculty buy-in
    f. Inadequate remediation strategies
    g. Lack of evidence that progress exams actually improve long term retention
    h. No challenges faced
    i. Other
17. Do you have a formal process to ensure validity of the assessment
    a. Yes
    b. No
18. If yes, what method do you use to validate the assessment?
    a. Correlation with cumulative GPA
    b. Correlation with board exam pass rate
    c. Correlation with time to graduation
    d. We use a question bank with validated questions
19. Where do you acquire questions for the exam? Check all that apply
    a. Faculty provide questions
    b. Use a pre-bought question bank
    c. They are prior exam that have been recycled

20. Have you measured any outcomes since you instituted the comprehensive learning assessment?
    a. Yes
    b. No
    c. If yes, please describe.

References

1. Accreditation Council of Pharmacy Education. *Accreditation Standards and Guidelines for the Professional Program in Pharmacy Leading to the Doctor of Pharmacy Degree*. Accreditation Council for Pharmacy Education: Chicago, IL, USA, 2011. Available online: https://www.acpe-accredit.org/pdf/FinalS2007Guidelines2.0.pdf (accessed on 22 August 2014).
2. Accreditation Council of Pharmacy Education. *Accreditation Standards and Guidelines for the Professional Program in Pharmacy Leading to the Doctor of Pharmacy Degree*. Accreditation Council for Pharmacy Education: Chicago, IL, USA, 2011; Draft Standards, 2016 (Released 2/3/2014). Available online: https://www.acpe-accredit.org/deans/StandardsRevision.asp (accessed on 22 August 2014).
3. Kirschenbaum, H.L.; Brown, M.E.; Kalis, M.M. Programmatic curricular outcomes assessment at colleges and schools of pharmacy in the United States and Puerto Rico. *Am. J. Pharm. Educ.* **2006**, *70*, article 8.
4. Sansgiry, S.S.; Nadkarni, A.; Lemke, T. Perceptions of PharmD students towards a cumulative examination: The *Milemarker* process. *Am. J. Pharm. Educ.* **2004**, *68*, article 93.
5. Sansgiry, S.S.; Chanda, S.; Lemke, D.; Szilagyi, J.E. Effect of incentives on student performance on *Milemarker* Examinations. *Am. J. Pharm. Educ.* **2006**, *70*, article 103.
6. Alston, G.L.; Love, B.L. Development of a reliable, valid annual skills mastery assessment examination. *Am. J. Pharm. Educ.* **2010**, *74*, article 80.
7. Me´sza´ros, K.; Barnett, M.J.; McDonald, K.; Wehring, H.; Evans, D.J.; Sasaki-Hill, D.; Goldsmith, P.C.; Knapp, K.K. Progress examination for assessing students' readiness for Advanced Pharmacy Practice Experiences. *Am. J. Pharm. Educ.* **2009**, *73*, article 109.
8. Kelley, K.A.; Beatty, S.J.; Legg, J.E.; McAuley, J.W. A progress assessment to evaluate pharmacy students' knowledge prior to beginning advanced pharmacy practice experiences. *Am. J. Pharm. Educ.* **2008**, *72*, article 88.
9. Ragan, R.E.; Virtue, D.W.; Chi, S.J. An assessment program using standardized clients to determine student readiness for clinical practice. *Am. J. Pharm. Educ.* **2013**, *77*, article 14.
10. Scott, D.M.; Bennett, L.L.; Ferrill, M.J.; Brown, D.L. Pharmacy curriculum outcomes assessment for individual student assessment and curricular evaluation. *Am. J. Pharm. Educ.* **2010**, *74*, article 183.
11. Szilagyi, J.E. Curricular progress assessments: The Milemarker. *Am. J. Pharm. Educ.* **2008**, *72*, article 101.
12. Naughton, C.A.; Freisner, D.L. Comparison of pharmacy students' perceived and actual knowledge using the pharmacy curricular outcomes assessment. *Am. J. Pharm. Educ.* **2012**, *76*, article 63.

13. Medina, M.S.; Britton, M.L.; Letassy, N.A.; Dennis, V.; Draugalis, J.R. Incremental development of an integrated assessment method for the professional curriculum. *Am. J. Pharm. Educ.* **2013**, *77*, article 122.
14. Plaza, C.M. Progress examinations in pharmacy education. *Am. J. Pharm. Educ.* **2007**, *71*, article 66.
15. Winslade, N. A system to assess the achievement of doctor of pharmacy students. *Am. J. Pharm. Educ.* **2001**, *65*, 363–392.
16. Ryan, G.J.; Nykamp, D. Use of cumulative examinations at US schools of pharmacy. *Am. J. Pharm. Educ.* **2000**, *64*, 409–412.
17. SurveyMonkey, Palo Alto, CA, USA. Available online: http://www.surveymonkey.com (accessed on 1 April 2014).
18. Wise, S.L.; DeMars, C.E. Low examinee effort in low-stakes assessment: Problems and potential solutions. *Educ. Assess.* **2005**, *10*, 1–17.
19. Maize, D.F.; Fuller, S.H.; Hritcko, P.M.; Matsumoto, R.R.; Soltis, D.A.; Taheri, R.R.; Duncan, W. A review of remediation programs in pharmacy and other health professions. *Am. J. Pharm. Educ.* **2010**, *74*, article 25.
20. Poirier, T.I.; Kerr, T.M.; Phelps, S.J. Academic progression and retention policies of colleges and schools of pharmacy. *Am. J. Pharm. Educ.* **2013**, *77*, article 25.
21. Larsen, D.P.; Butler, A.C.; Roedger, H.L., III. Comparative effects of test-enhanced learning and self-explanation on long-term retention. *Med. Educ.* **2013**, *47*, 674–682.
22. Larsen, D.P.; Butler, A.C.; Roedger, H.L., III. Repeated testing improves long-term retention relative to repeated study: A randomised controlled trial. *Med. Educ.* **2009**, *43*, 1174–1181.
23. Keresztes, A.; Kaiser, D.; Kovács, G.; Racsmány, M. Testing Promotes Long-Term Learning via Stabilizing Activation Patterns in a Large Network of Brain Areas. *Cereb. Cortex* **2014**, *24*, 3025–3035.

2

Perceived Stress, Stressors, and Coping Mechanisms among Doctor of Pharmacy Students

Jennifer W. Beall, Renee M. DeHart *, Robert M. Riggs, and John Hensley

McWhorter School of Pharmacy, Samford University, 800 Lakeshore Drive, Birmingham, AL 35229, USA; E-Mails: jwbeall@samford.edu (J.W.B.); rmriggs@samford.edu (R.M.R.); jhensley@samford.edu (J.H.)

* Author to whom correspondence should be addressed; E-Mail: rmdehart@samford.edu

Academic Editor: Maree Donna Simpson

Abstract: The primary purpose of this study was to examine perceived stress in doctor of pharmacy students during their first, second, and third years of their program in a fully implemented new curriculum. The secondary objectives were to determine if there is a relationship between perceived stress and certain demographic variables, to compare student pharmacist perceived stress to the perceived stress in the general population, and to examine student reported stressors during pharmacy school and coping strategies employed for those stressors. A previously validated survey (Perceived Stress Scale-10) was given to first, second, and third year student pharmacists. Females exhibited higher mean stress scores than males. The under 22 years and over 32 years age categories exhibited higher mean stress scores than the 22 to 26 year old student population. There was no significant difference in perceived stress scores between classes of the program. Only a portion of the variation in stress scores was predicted by gender, age, marital status, race, and year in curriculum. Stress scores among these student pharmacists are higher overall than those in previously published probability samples in the general population. Class assignments and completing electronic portfolios were the top stressors reported. Spending time with family and friends was the most frequent coping mechanism reported. Programming related to stress reduction (particularly among female and nontraditional age students) appears warranted.

Keywords: perceived stress; stressors; coping mechanisms; student pharmacists

---

1. Introduction

Stress can be thought of as a state resulting from an "imbalance between demands and resources" or as occurring when "pressure exceeds one's perceived ability to cope" [1]. While stress is often associated with negative events or problems in a person's life, it can also result from positive life occurrences, such as enrolling in professional programs to start/advance one's career. Stress in college students can be triggered from a variety of issues including relationships, academics, and financial concerns [2]. Stress in student pharmacists is significant, because a correlation between increased stress and decreased health-related quality of life has been observed in at least one study of student pharmacists [2].

Accreditation Council for Pharmacy Education (ACPE) accreditation standards and guidelines specifically contain guidance for Standard 24.e regarding student stress: "Colleges and schools are encouraged to assess and correct underlying causes of ineffective learning experiences. Such assessments consider the amount of student effort, the quality of faculty teaching, and the appropriateness of learning assessments used within the courses. In this regard, these assessments include measurements of perceived stress in faculty, staff, and students and an evaluation of stress' potential for a negative impact on programmatic outcomes and morale." [3]. While these accreditation standards have been updated for 2016, student affairs' professionals still work regularly to improve/enhance student wellness during pharmacy school. Management of non-academic issues like stress is important for academic success [4].

Despite ACPE recommendation and several tools being available, little literature is actually published examining stress levels in student pharmacists [2,4–11]. Two studies that have examined student pharmacist stress verses other health professional students stress yielded conflicting results [7,9]. Henning *et al.*'s research demonstrated student pharmacists' stress level on average was higher than medical students [7], while Abhay's *et al.*'s research demonstrated the opposite [9]. There is also conflicting data on whether female student pharmacists experience more stress than their male counterparts [2,4] and whether certain years of the pharmacy school experience are more stressful than others [4,10].

A variety of assessment tools are available and have been used to examine stress in student pharmacists [2,4–15]. These tools include the Perceived Stress Scale (PSS), the Student-Life Stress Inventory, the Beck Stress Inventory, the Derogatis Stress Profile, and a survey adapted from a nurse practitioner tool [2,4–8]. The most commonly used tool for assessing student pharmacist stress to date is the Perceived Stress Scale (PSS). The PSS is available as a 10 (PSS-10) or 14 (PSS-14) question tool [12]. At least five investigator groups have used the PSS to assess stress among student pharmacists [2,9–11,14]. The one study to date using the PSS-10 revealed that women reported higher stress than men and that year in program correlated negatively with stress levels. This study yielded a mean PSS-10 score in female students of 19.0 and of 17.26 in male students [14]. These prior studies (particularly those of Cohen and Votta) provide initial data for other programs to benchmark to moving forward as they assess student stress. This current study will be the second study published to date that uses the PSS-10 in U.S. student pharmacists. Based on previous studies (gender) and faculty perceptions (age of student), subgroup comparisons were made in this study to examine differences in student stress based on gender and age. Since the school's curriculum was changed in 2009 to include the use of horizontal integration of course content (integration of course content within the same year) and the use of e-portfolios, examining these areas, and their contribution to student stress were also of particular interest to the investigators. Information from this study will also help provide a benchmark for other pharmacy programs' student affairs professionals who may be evaluating which stress assessment tool to use in practice.

The primary purpose of this study was to examine perceived stress in student pharmacists during their first, second, and third years of the doctor of pharmacy program in a fully implemented new curriculum. In 2009, the school implemented an integrated curriculum model that included intentional sequencing of content in the pharmaceutical sciences and pharmacotherapy courses, weekly integrated pharmacy application laboratories, introductory pharmacy practice experiences (IPPEs) starting in week five of the first professional year, and electronic portfolios. We wanted to explore which, if any of these, significantly contributed to stress among students. We also wanted to determine if intentional sequencing of course content across multiple courses in our new curriculum led to differing or similar levels of perceived stress across years in the didactic curriculum. Additional secondary objectives of this study were to determine if there is relationship between perceived stress and certain demographic variables (gender, year in curriculum, and age), to compare student pharmacist perceived stress to the perceived stress in the general population (as reported in previously published literature), and to examine student reported triggers for stress during pharmacy school and coping strategies employed for those stressors.

2. Methods

2.1. Materials

This study was approved by Samford University's Institutional Review Board. First, second, and third year student pharmacists at one private university were asked to complete a survey during a class meeting during the spring semester 2012. The survey included demographic information and the 10 item PSS. The PSS is available as a 10 (PSS-10) or 14 (PSS-14) question tool [12]. The PSS-10 is a validated stress instrument and does not lose any psychometric quality when compared with the longer version but is shorter and takes less time to complete [13]. Additionally, the PSS-10 has been used in large probability samples, allowing for the comparison of pharmacy students to a more general, non-pharmacy based population [13].

2.2. Procedures

Participation was voluntary and anonymous. Participants received information about the survey at the time of survey completion in accordance with usual Institutional Review Board (IRB) expectations at the institution. Participants were not compensated or incentivized in any way for their participation. The paper survey included the 10 item PSS, demographic questions, and questions concerning stressors and relievers (derived from the study by Marshall *et al.*) [2]. Based on previous studies showing higher stress scores in female pharmacy students [2], it was decided prospective to compare female and male stress scores to each other. Likewise, the study was prospectively designed to examine stress scores based on age (due to faculty perceptions of higher stress among younger students at the institution). For stress, trigger and alleviator questions responses of "very often", "fairly often" or "sometimes" were considered a "yes" response to the question.

2.3. Data Analyses

All data were entered and analyzed in Microsoft Excel 2010. Chi square tests were used when comparing nominal data. *T*-tests were used for comparisons of continuous data between two groups (gender) and ANOVA tests were used when comparing three or more groups (year in the curriculum, age groups).

3. Results

Two hundred and forty two students completed the survey (response rate 68.4%). Demographics can be seen in Table 1. The composition of the sample is very similar to the entire student body in regards to gender, age, race, and marital status. PSS score by class, age, and year in curriculum can be seen in Table 2. Due to similarities in the stress score results of the age 22 to 26 and 27–31 groups, as well as similarities in the stress score results for the age 31–36 and 37 and over groups, these groups are combined in our results section. Further examination of the age range categories revealed a bimodal distribution in terms of mean PSS scores. The under 22 years of age and over age 32 categories exhibited higher mean perceived stress scores than those students aged 22–32 ($p = 0.01$). While *t*-test results showed female students reporting higher levels of perceived stress (Table 3) compared to their male counterpart ($p = 0.0001$), there was no statistical difference in perceived stress between Caucasian, African American, Hispanic, Asian, and Native American students. There was no statistical difference in perceived stress between the P1, P2 and P3 classes (Table 3; $p = 0.123$). The perceived stress scale (PSS) questionnaire results of the overall group can be seen in Table 2.

Multiple linear regression including include age, race, pharmacy year, marital status, dependent status, previous education level, and gender (as independent variables) was conducted to explore associations with stress level. Using these variables in the regression model yielded an R-squared of 0.13, indicating these variables only predict a small amount of the variation of stress scores among students.

Table 1. Demographics for survey participants ($n = 242$).

Characteristic	**No. (%)**
Sex	
Male	72 (29.8)
Female	170 (70.2)
Marital Status	
Single and not in a committed relationship	90 (37.2)
In a committed relationship	94 (38.8)
Married	58 (24.0)
Divorced or separated	0 (0)
Have Children [a]	
Yes	23 (9.6)
No	217 (90.4)
Highest completed Education Level [b]	
No degree	69 (28.6)
Bachelor's degree	64 (26.6)
Master's degree	102 (42.3)
Doctoral degree	6 (2.5)

Table 1. *Cont.*

Characteristic	No. (%)
Age	
< 22	23 (9.5)
22–26	173 (71.5)
27–31	33 (13.6)
> 32	13 (5.4)
School Class[c]	
P1	20.24 (6.72)
P2	18.1 (6.91)
P3	18.1 (6.37)
Race[d]	
Caucasian	213 (88.0)
African American	17 (7.0)
Hispanic	3 (1.2)
Asian	12 (5.0)
Native American	3 (1.2)

[a] Two responders did not answer this question; [b] One responder did not answer this question; [c] $p = 0.123$ for comparison among classes; [d] Total is greater than 100% because four responders indicated multiple race.

Table 2. Perceived Stress Scale[12] Results ($n = 242$).

	Never N (%)	**Almost Never N (%)**	**Sometimes N (%)**	**Fairly Often N (%)**	**Very Often N (%)**	**Overall Response Score [Range 0–4] Mean (SD)**
In the last month, how often have you been upset because of something that happened unexpectedly?	18 (7.4)	65 (26.8)	100 (41.3)	38 (15.7)	21 (8.7)	1.91 (1.03)
In the last month, how often have you felt that you were unable to control the important things in your life?	23 (9.5)	71 (29.3)	80 (33.1)	51 (21.1)	17 (7.0)	1.87 (1.07)
In the last month, how often have you felt nervous and "stressed"?	2 (0.8)	14 (5.8)	66 (27.8)	79 (32.6)	81 (33.4)	2.92 (0.95)
In the last month, how often have you felt confident about your ability to handle your personal problems?	1 (0.4)	8 (3.3)	77 (31.8)	99 (40.9)	57 (23.6)	1.61 (0.84)
In the last month, how often have you felt that things were going your way?	1 (0.4)	26 (10.7)	107 (44.2)	89 (36.8)	19 (7.9)	1.59 (0.80)
In the last month, how often have you found that you could not cope with all the things that you had to do?	32 (13.2)	84 (34.7)	68 (28.1)	45 (18.6)	13 (5.4)	1.68 (1.08)
In the last month, how often have you been able to control irritations in your life?	4 (1.7)	28 (11.6)	100 (41.3)	92 (38.0)	18 (7.4)	1.62 (0.85)

Table 2. *Cont.*

	Never N (%)	Almost Never N (%)	Sometimes N (%)	Fairly Often N (%)	Very Often N (%)	Overall Response Score [Range 0–4] Mean (SD)
In the last month, how often have you felt that you were on top of things?	11 (4.5)	52 (21.5)	101 (41.7)	64 (26.4)	13 (5.4)	1.93 (0.94)
In the last month, how often have you been angered because of things that were outside of your control?	16 (6.6)	65 (26.9)	93 (38.4)	48 (19.8)	20 (8.3)	1.96 (1.03)
In the last month, have you felt difficulties were piling up so high that you could not overcome them?	29 (12.0)	70 (28.9)	75 (31.0)	43 (17.8)	25 (10.3)	1.86 (1.16)

Table 3. PSS-10 Score results [a].

	No. (%)	Overall Mean	SD
Male	72 (29.8%)	16.1	6.74
Female	170 (71.2)	19.6	6.29
Under 22 years of age	23 (9.5%)	21.4	6.54
22–31 years of age	206 (85.1%)	18.0	6.54
32 years of age and over	13 (5.4%)	21.9	6.71

[a]: Possible range of scores: 0–40; $p = 0.123$ (for comparison among year in pharmacy school); PSS: Perceived Stress Scale; SD: Standard Deviation.

3.1. Stressors

Class assignments and completing electronic portfolios were the top stressors reported among our student pharmacists. There was a higher percentage of female participants that selected the items in the survey as stressors compared to males in all surveyed stress trigger items but one. Males had a higher percentage of stress than females concerning completing survey(s) from faculty or administration. A majority of students perceived IPPEs as a major stressor. Tables 4 and 5 illustrate the stressors analyzed between genders and among age groups, respectively.

Table 4. Results [a] for stress triggers.

Survey Item	Male (n = 72)		Female (n = 170)		Total
	No. (%)	SD	No. (%)	SD	No. (%)
1. Class assignments	60 (83.3)	0.95	154 (90.6)	0.88	214 (88.4)
2. Completing electronic portfolios	48 (66.7)	1.2	143 (84.1)	1.01	191 (78.9)
3. Financial concerns	46 (63.9)	1.22	114 (67.1)	1.3	160 (66.1)
4. Introductory pharmacy practice experiences (IPPEs)	43 (59.7)	1.38	114 (67.1)	1.41	157 (64.9)
5. Family and relationships	35 (48.6)	1.12	111 (65.3)	1.12	146 (60.3)
6. Health or maintaining health	36 (50.0)	1.15	103 (60.6)	1.15	139 (57.4)
7. Academic competition	30 (41.7)	1.23	105 (61.8)	1.58	135 (55.8)
8. Extracurricular employment	37 (51.4)	1.26	92 (54.1)	1.27	129 (53.3)
9. Daily commute	25 (34.7)	1.29	81 (47.6)	1.32	106 (43.8)
10. Completing survey from faculty or administration	28 (38.9)	1.18	55 (32.4)	1.06	83 (34.3)

Table 4. *Cont.*

Survey Item	Male (n = 72)		Female (n = 170)		Total
	No. (%)	SD	No. (%)	SD	No. (%)
11. Completing capstone student surveys	12 (16.7)	0.88	49 (28.8)	1.05	61 (25.2)
12. Other	1 (1.4)	1.07	2 (1.2)	1	3 (1.2)

[a] Results include surveys marked with response of the listed trigger very often, fairly often or sometimes causing stress.

Table 5. Results for stress triggers.

	< 22 [N = 23] (%)	22–31 [N = 206] (%)	32 & over [N = 13] (%)
1. Class assignments	21 (91.3)	179 (86.9)	13 (100)
2. Completing electronic portfolios	20 (86.9)	160 (77.7)	11 (84.6)
3. Financial concerns	15 (65.2)	134 (65.0)	11 (84.6)
4. Introductory pharmacy practice experiences (IPPEs)	18 (78.3)	129 (62.6)	10 (76.9)
5. Family and relationships	16 (69.6)	120 (58.3)	10 (76.9)
6. Health or maintaining health	13 (55.5)	115 (55.8)	11 (84.6)
7. Academic competition	16 (69.6)	111 (53.9)	8 (61.5)
8. Extracurricular employment	12 (52.2)	107 (51.9)	10 (76.9)
9. Daily commute	8 (34.8)	91 (44.2)	7 (53.8)
10. Completing survey from faculty or administration	7 (30.4)	71 (34.5)	5 (38.5)
11. Completing capstone student surveys	5 (21.7)	53 (25.7)	3 (23.1)
12. Other	0 (0)	3 (1.5)	0 (0)

3.2. Coping Mechanisms

Participants reported that spending time with family and friends as the best way to alleviate stress. Table 6 is an all-inclusive list of the surveyed coping mechanisms. Females had a higher percentage of participants that preferred shopping, sleeping/taking naps and/or eating as a means to improve stress levels. Playing video or online games, drinking alcohol and exercising were significantly higher in males as a means to relieve stress compared to females.

Table 6. Results[a] for stress alleviators.

	Male (n = 72)	Female (n = 170)	Total (n = 242)
Stress Alleviator	No. (%)	No. (%)	No. (%)
1. Spending time with family and friends	62 (86.1)	162 (95.3)	224 (92.6)
2. Personal time alone	54 (75.0)	147 (86.5)	201 (83.1)
3. Eating	52 (72.2)	140 (82.4)	192 (79.3)
4. Exercising or playing sports	60 (83.3)	127 (74.7)	187 (77.3)
5. Sleeping or taking naps	46 (63.9)	131 (77.1)	177 (73.1)
6. Watching television	52 (72.2)	122 (71.8)	174 (71.9)
7. Shopping	14 (19.4)	105 (61.8)	119 (49.2)
8. Drinking alcohol	36 (50.0)	63 (37.1)	99 (40.9)
9. Study group	26 (36.1)	56 (32.9)	82 (33.9)
10. Reading at leisure	20 (27.8)	42 (24.7)	62 (25.6)

Table 6. *Cont.*

	Male ($n = 72$)	Female (n = 170)	Total (n = 242)
11. Playing video or online games	35 (48.6)	20 (11.8)	55 (22.7)
12. Nonprescription, herbal anti-anxiety or sleep aid meds	6 (8.3)	23 (13.5)	29 (12.0)
13. Prescription anti-anxiety medications or sleep aids	5 (6.9)	18 (10.6)	23 (9.5)
14. Other	6 (8.3)	17 (10.0)	23 (9.5)
15. Smoking cigarettes or use of other tobacco products	10 (13.9)	7 (4.1)	17 (7.0)

[a] Results include surveys marked with response of the listed trigger very often, fairly often or sometimes causing stress.

4. Discussion

Our current study yielded a trend of females reporting higher stress, similar to the findings of Votta. Unlike the study by Votta, however, our study did not yield a negative correlation between year in the curriculum and stress score. Compared to Votta and Benau, it might be that our curriculum integration has led to less stress among students overall and equally rigorous years throughout the curriculum.

Marshall and colleagues reported mean PSS-14 scores for females and males were significantly different (28.1 *vs.* 22.4, respectively; $p < 0.002$) [2]. The authors also reported stressors and alleviators, with family and relationships ranking highest as a trigger and exercising ranking highest as an alleviator. Similarly, our current study found female students reporting higher levels of stress than their male counterparts. Strikingly different, however, we found the highest overall trigger in our current study was class assignments and the highest overall alleviator was spending time with family and friends. The timing of the survey in the Marshall study fell during the third week of a four-week pharmacotherapy block. It may be that differences in curriculum structure (blocks *versus* horizontal integration) resulted in differences in the degree to which class assignments precipitate stress among students. Our program horizontally integrates content within the same semester (*i.e.*, pharmaceutical sciences, pharmacotherapy, and integrated pharmacy laboratory course content are sequenced very intentionally to cover the same content around the same timeframe within a semester).

Gupchup and colleagues investigated the association between stress and health-related quality of life in first-, second-, and third-year student pharmacists [4]. Those authors also reported significantly higher stress scores for third-year students than for first-year students (148.60 *vs.* 133.43, respectively; $p = 0.006$). Our study findings were not consistent with Gupchup in this regard.

Dutta and colleagues studied stress in second-year student pharmacists in four different institutions [8]. The Derogatis Stress Profile (DSP) was used to measure stress in this study. The DSP associates scores above 63 to be experiencing psychiatric levels of distress. Scoring for the PSS-10 does not include excessive stress levels like the DSP. Therefore, our current study cannot determine those students who could experience stress at possible psychiatric levels.

Cohen and Janicki-Deverts reported psychological stress in a general population probability sample from 2009 using the PSS-10 (the same tool used in the current study) [13]. Men in this sample reported similar stress scores to those in our current study (15.52 *vs.* 15.9, respectively). However, women in Cohen's study reported a lower stress score than the women in our study (16.14 *vs.* 19.6, respectively). Although age categories are divided into slightly different ranges between this previous study and our study (making exact comparisons difficult), there was lower stress reported by those less than 25 years of age in the Cohen study compared to our students in this study less than 22 years of age and our students 22 to 31 years of age (16.78 *vs.* 21.43 and 18.0, respectively). The difference in age categories between the two studies make comparisons difficult, yet the highest stress scores reported overall in the Cohen study was 17.46 by those ages 25–34 years. Our highest stress scores were for students ages 32 and averaged 21.92. Looking at this data overall, it does appear that student pharmacists report higher levels of perceived stress compared to the probability sample in the general population.

As a result of our findings, several initiatives have been taken at our institution. First, programming on student wellness and self-care delivered by the university's social work faculty has been added to co-curricular programming during the first year of pharmacy school. Second, a focus group of nontraditional students was conducted to identify their unique needs. As a result of our study and the focus group results, a nontraditional student group has been formed and programming (networking, balancing multiple priorities) has been developed to help the nontraditional student and their families make the pharmacy school transition successfully. Third, because class assignments were identified as a key stressor, programming on time management as it relates to class assignments has been added to Orientation. Fourth, because finances were an important stressor, an information session on budgeting/financial planning (delivered by students for students) has been added to first year pharmacy student Orientation. Also related to finances, an "Applying for Financial Aid 101" booklet been developed for incoming students. Lastly, our methods for collecting and reviewing portfolio information are currently being re-evaluated by the school's assessment personnel.

Limitations of this study include the fact that this study was performed at one private, church-based institution in the southeastern U. S. Therefore, the generalizability to other institutions may be limited and activities such as drinking alcohol may have been underreported. Additionally, our overall response rate was high at 68.4%; however, this ranges from 47.4% from the first-year class to 96.7% of the third-year class. The third-year response rate was due primarily to administration of the survey during an IPPE and, therefore, mandatory attendance. This IPPE activity was a one afternoon simulation activity on the university campus during what is otherwise a didactic semester. After explaining the study and the voluntary nature of participation, students' anonymous responses were collected by non-faculty members. Additionally, the survey being administered in a large classroom environment could have led to students being able to view each other's answers on the Scantron sheets used to collect the data. Another limitation is that the surveys were not administered at the same time. There were approximately 3–4 weeks between administration times for the three classes. In addition, when comparing the data to probability samples reported by Cohen and colleagues, different age categories were used [13]. This difference in age categories makes direct comparisons more challenging. Lastly, this study did not examine quality of life and, therefore, conclusions regarding stress and association with impact on quality of life cannot be made. Future study in that area may be warranted.

5. Conclusions

First-year female students reported the highest levels of stress than any other group in this study while second-year males reported the lowest levels of stress. Females in general perceived more stress than males, and the youngest and oldest age categories reported higher levels of stress. Given the results of our linear regression, additional variables not examined in this study (finances, health of students, *etc.*) may contribute to student stress and further study is warranted. Spending time with family and friends ranked highest as a stress alleviator and class assignments ranked highest as a stress trigger. Programming on stress reduction (particularly among female and nontraditional age students) appears warranted. Further study is needed to determine is such programming has an impact on stress levels after full implementation.

Author Contributions

Jennifer Beall and Renee DeHart conceived and designed the study. Jennifer Beall and Renee DeHart performed the experiment/study. Robert Riggs, John Hensley, and Renee DeHart analyzed the data. Jennifer Beall and Renee DeHart wrote the paper.

Conflicts of Interest

The authors declare no conflict of interest.

References

1. Folkman, S. Personal control and stress and coping processes: A theoretical analysis. *Pers. Soc. Psychol.* **1984**, *46*, 839–852.
2. Marshall, L.L.; Allison, A; Nykamp, D; Lanke, S. Perceived stress and quality of life among doctor of pharmacy students. *Am. J. Pharm. Educ.* **2008**, *72*, 1–8.
3. Accreditation council for Pharmacy Education. "Guidance for the accreditation standards and key elements for the professional program in pharmacy leading to the doctor of pharmacy degree." 25 January 2015. Available online: https://www.acpe-accredit.org/pdf/GuidanceforStandards2016 FINAL.pdf (accessed on 12 October 2015).
4. Gupchup, G.V.; Borrego, M.E.; Konduri, N. The impact of student life stress on health related quality of life among doctor of pharmacy students. *Coll. Stud. J.* **2004**, *38*, 292–301.
5. Beck, D.L.; Hackett, M.B.; Srivastava, R.; McKim, E.; Rockwell, B. Perceived level and sources of stress in university professional schools. *J. Nurs. Educ.* **1997**, *36*, 180–186.
6. Canales-Gonzales, P.L.; Kranz, P.L. Perceived stress by students in a pharmacy curriculum. *Education* **2008**, *129*, 139–146.
7. Henning, K.; Ey, S.; Shaw, D. Perfectionism, the imposter phenomenon and psychological adjustment in medical, dental, nursing, and pharmacy students. *Med. Educ.* **1998**, *32*, 456–464.
8. Dutta, A.P.; Pyles, M.A.; Miederhoff, P. Measuring and understanding stress in pharmacy students. In *Stress and Mental Health*; Landow, M.V., Ed; Nova Sciences Publishers, Inc: Hauppauge, NY, USA, 2006; pp. 1–28.
9. Abhay, M.; Krishnakumar, M.K.; Niranjan, P.C.; Hiremath, S.G. Differences in perceived stress and its correlates among students in professional courses. *J. Clin. Diagn. Res.* **2011**, *5*, 1228–1233.
10. Maynor, L.M.; Baugh, G.C. Perceived stress, academic self-concept, and coping strategies of pharmacy students. *Int. J. Pharm. Ed. Pract.* **2012**, *9*, 1–9.
11. Frick, L.J.; Frick, J.L.; Coffman, R.E.; Dey, S. Student stress in a three-year doctor of pharmacy program using a mastery learning educational model. *Am. J. Pharm. Educ.* **2011**, *75*, 1–6.
12. Perceived Stress Scale. Available online: http://www.psy.cmu.edu/~scohen/scales.html (accessed on 10 December 2014).

13. Cohen, S.; Janicki-Deverts, D. Who's Stressed? Distributions of psychological stress in the United States in probability samples from 1983, 2006, and 2009. *J. Appl. Soc. Psychol.* **2012**, *42*, 1320–1334.
14. Votta, R.J.; Benau, E.M. Predictors of stress in doctor of pharmacy students: Results from a nationwide survey. *Curr. Pharm. Teach. Learn.* **2013**, *5*, 365–372.
15. Hirsch, J.D.; Do, A.H.; Hollenbach, K.A.; Manoguerra, A.S.; Adler, D.S. Students' health-related quality of life across the preclinical pharmacy curriculum. *Am. J. Pharm. Educ.* **2009**, *73*, 1–6.

3

Self-Reported Digital Literacy of the Pharmacy Workforce in North East Scotland

Katie MacLure †,* and Derek Stewart †

School of Pharmacy and Life Sciences, Robert Gordon University, Aberdeen AB10 7GJ, UK;
E-Mail: d.stewart@rgu.ac.uk

† These authors contributed equally to this work.

* Author to whom correspondence should be addressed; E-Mail: k.m.maclure@rgu.ac.uk

Academic Editor: Keith A. Wilson

Abstract: In their day-to-day practice, pharmacists, graduate (pre-registration) pharmacists, pharmacy technicians, dispensing assistants and medicines counter assistants use widely available office, retail and management information systems alongside dedicated pharmacy management and electronic health (ehealth) applications. The ability of pharmacy staff to use these applications at home and at work, also known as digital literacy or digital competence or e-skills, depends on personal experience and related education and training. The aim of this research was to gain insight into the self-reported digital literacy of the pharmacy workforce in the North East of Scotland. A purposive case sample survey was conducted across NHS Grampian in the NE of Scotland. Data collection was based on five items: sex, age band, role, pharmacy experience plus a final question about self-reported digital literacy. The study was conducted between August 2012 and March 2013 in 17 community and two hospital pharmacies. With few exceptions, pharmacy staff perceived their own digital literacy to be at a basic level. Secondary outcome measures of role, age, gender and work experience were not found to be clear determinants of digital literacy. Pharmacy staff need to be more digitally literate to harness technologies in pharmacy practice more effectively and efficiently.

Keywords: digital literacy; pharmacy workforce; pharmacy technology; ehealth; change management; Scotland

---

1. Introduction

Pharmacy staff across all practice settings are increasingly reliant on information technology [1–4]. Pharmacists, graduate (pre-registration) pharmacists, pharmacy technicians, dispensing assistants and medicines counter assistants use widely available office, retail and management information systems alongside dedicated pharmacy management and electronic health (ehealth) applications in a range of community, hospital and other pharmacy settings. The abilities of pharmacy staff to use these applications at home and at work, also known as digital literacy or digital competence or e-skills, depends on personal experience and related education and training [5,6].

The British Computer Society defines digital literacy as, "being able to make use of technologies to participate in and contribute to modern social, cultural, political and economic life" [7]. A similar definition of digital literacy is adopted in the United States (U.S.), "the ability to use information and communication technologies to find, evaluate, create, and communicate information; it requires both technical and cognitive skills" [8]. Both definitions are grounded in historical and conceptual definitions of digital literacies [9]. United Nations Educational Scientific and Cultural Organisation (UNESCO) identifies digital literacy as both a "life skill" and "gate skill" because "it targets all areas of contemporary existence" [10]. The European Commission Information Society (ECIS) promotes and tracks citizens' and member states' digital engagement [11]. Similarly, the European Parliament promotes digital literacy for lifelong learning along with a recommendation for "better identification of occupational needs" [12].

A government commissioned report into digital literacy in Australia concluded that "both citizen and worker will need to be digitally literate for the digital economy to work effectively" while a report from New Zealand argues "that technology can change the nature of work faster than people can change their skills" [13,14]. In the United Kingdom (UK), a range of strategic principles, national competency frameworks for training, core skills and digital literacies for the general public, and recently more specific targets for the health sector, have been developed by government, advisory and healthcare related professional bodies [15–17].

Healthcare in the UK is politically devolved to its national parliaments. The Scottish Government's policy driven National Health Service (NHS) is regionalised to 14 local Health Boards. Each Board manages the delivery of pharmacy services within hospitals and contracts community pharmacies to offer a range of core services most of which are technology based. In Scotland, community and hospital pharmacies are sited in remote and rural or urban settings with a diverse level of technology implemented, from the minimum required to facilitate electronic transfer of prescriptions (ETP) starting from a broadband networked single computer with linked printer and barcode reader through to advanced robotic medicines management systems [18].

The regulatory body for the pharmacy profession in the UK, which also sets standards for education and training, is the General Pharmaceutical Council (GPhC) [19]. Unlike the U.S., where the Accreditation Council for Pharmacy Education (ACPE) added health informatics in 2007, digital skills are not explicitly identified in pharmacy curricula in the UK [20].

However, the way ahead for the pharmacy workforce is a central issue in the most recent "Review of NHS Pharmaceutical Care of Patients in the Community in Scotland" [21]. It recommended, "developing and using the skills of the whole pharmacy team" to inform and support the "Prescription for Excellence" through person-centred, pharmaceutical care [22]. The main policy driver is the promotion of patient safety through upskilling and development of roles within the pharmacy workforce supported and facilitated by technology. The Scottish Government and NHS in Scotland envisage, "making more and better use of technology and facilities to increase access to services and improve efficiency," also promising to ensure that everyone working within the integrated health and social care sector "is supported to make the best use of new technology" [23,24]. Policy and strategy drivers aim to change the role of pharmacy practice, upskilling the role of each member of the pharmacy team, within the integrated health and social care team, releasing the pharmacist for a more clinical, patient-facing role [25]. The policy driven intention is to support role development with technology therefore pharmacy needs a digitally literate workforce.

The aim of this research was to gain insight into the self-reported digital literacy of the pharmacy workforce in the North East (NE) of Scotland.

2. Experimental Section

2.1. Design

A purposive case sample survey was conducted across NHS Grampian in the NE of Scotland as part of a larger study.

2.2. Setting

NHS Grampian health board manages eight hospitals (two main in Aberdeen and Elgin) and 131 community pharmacies (51 in Aberdeen City, 53 in Aberdeenshire, 27 in Moray) that serve a population of over half a million across the North East of Scotland [26].

2.3. Sampling of Community and Hospital Pharmacies

Experts from the local health board and practicing academic pharmacists were engaged to assist with stratified purposive sampling taking into account the range of:

- urban, remote and rural geographical settings;
- technology infrastructures;
- pharmacy management systems implemented; and
- hospital pharmacy (community, major) and community pharmacy (small independent through to small, medium or large chain multiples; in the NHS Grampian area there are 23 small independents (single pharmacy), 67 small (1–4 pharmacies) to medium (5–25 pharmacies) chain multiples, and 41 national chain multiples) [26].

2.4. Recruitment of Pharmacy Owners and Managers

Professional networks of academic pharmacists based at Robert Gordon University (RGU), one of two centres offering graduate level pharmacy courses in Scotland, made the initial approach to local area network of pharmacy owners and managers. They outlined the proposed study and those who expressed an interest were emailed an information sheet and consent form by the research team. Management consent included facilitating contact with the wider pharmacy team.

2.5. Recruitment of Pharmacists, Pharmacy Technicians, Dispensing Assistants and Medicines Counter Assistants

Where distance allowed, the researcher arranged a preliminary site visit as a follow up to email contact. This served multiple purposes of introducing the researcher to potential participants, familiarising the researcher with the pharmacy location and layout and for distribution of information sheets and consent forms. It was emphasised that consent was both voluntary and individual. Where the preliminary visit was not possible a study pack was posted to the pharmacy.

2.6. Data Collection

The study was conducted between August 2012 and March 2013 in 17 community and two hospital pharmacies across the NHS Grampian area. Preliminary site vetting during sampling provided data on pharmacy setting (community/hospital), type (from small/medium/large single/independent/chain multiple), rural/urban, high/low technology and pharmacy management system. Categorisation as a "low tech" pharmacy was allocated where the minimum specification necessary to operate was implemented. For example, single or multiple PCs connected to a network server with secure N3 broadband connection, barcode scanner(s), label dispenser(s), printer(s) and, very often, a fax machine. If the pharmacy had robotic medicines management capability it was categorised as "high tech."

During the consent process, participants provided five further items of data: sex, age band, role, pharmacy experience, plus answering a final question, "As a gauge of your current information technology experience which of the following would be the most appropriate challenge for you?", followed by titles of six digital literacy courses listed in order of difficulty (Table 1), which formed the primary outcome measure for this study.

Table 1. Information Technology (IT) course titles descriptions listed in order of difficulty.

Increasing level of difficulty →	Course title	Description
	Computing for the Terrified	If you are new to computing then this is the course for you. This short course gives you the opportunity to explore the basics of using a computer in a friendly and relaxed environment. Overcome your fears of using a computer and learn a new subject.
	Computing for the Quietly Confident	To provide students with a firm understanding of Microsoft Office applications. Learners should finish the course with a good grasp of word processing.
	Computing for the Courageous	Learners should finish the course with a more advanced grasp of word processing, basic spreadsheets, basic databases and basic presentations.
	European Computer Driving Licence (ECDL)	Attaining a European Computer Driving Licence is the best way to ensure you have all the necessary computing qualifications of any workplace. This course covers the first steps of using a computer—IT fundamentals, the internet, email and security.
	ECDL Advanced	Enables the learner to work more effectively with IT. This unit looks at using advanced tools to save time and effort when producing word processed documents, presentations and spread sheets.
	Computing Degree or Diploma	Course content includes: Computer Architecture, Computer Operating Systems 1; Computing: Planning; Computing: Graded Unit; Information Technology: Applications Software 1, Working within a Project Team.

Source of table content: local community learning advertisements placed by Aberdeenshire Council in conjunction with Aberdeen College (now NE Scotland College).

2.7. Data Analysis

The site data was collated and tabulated (Table 2) to show pharmacy types, description, rurality, number of pharmacy staff taking part, volume of dispensing, level of technology and pharmacy management system implemented. Participating pharmacies were described as small independent single or chain multiples (1–4 pharmacies) through large independent chain multiples (5–25 pharmacies), up to large chain multiples (>25 pharmacies) in the community sector plus two of the main hospitals in the area. Data gathered during the consent process were explored using descriptive statistics and presented in graphical form comparing: age, role, pharmacy experience and self-reported perception of digital literacy.

This study was approved by the Ethics Review Panel of Robert Gordon University School of Pharmacy and Life Sciences and deemed service evaluation by the Research & Development office of NHS Grampian.

Table 2. Overview of participating pharmacy demographics.

Case	Setting	chain multiple Type	Rural/Urban	P	PT	DA	MCA	No. of Rx per month	High tech/ Low tech	Pharmacy Management system
1	community	large, independent, chain multiple	R	1	1	0	4	8000	L	Cegidem
2	community	small, independent, chain multiple	U	1	0	1	3	5000	L	ProScript
3	community	small, independent, chain multiple	U	1	1	0	2	7000	L	ProScript
4	community	small, independent, chain multiple	R	1	1	0	1	4000	L	ProScript
5	community	small, independent, chain multiple	R	1	1	0	2	4500	L	Cegidem
6	community	small, independent, chain multiple	R	1	0	1	2	6500	L	Cegidem
7	community	small, independent, chain multiple	R	1	0	1	1	3000	L	Cegidem
8	community	small, independent, chain multiple	R	1	0	0	1	850	L	Cegidem
9	community	small, independent, chain multiple	R	0	0	0	1	1350 items	L	Cegidem
10	community	large, chain multiple	U	1	0	0	1	11,000	L	Nexphase
11	community	small, independent, chain multiple	U	3	2	1	2	Info withheld	H	Positive Solutions
12	community	small, independent, chain multiple	U	1	1	0	1	2500 items	L	ProScript
13	community	large, independent, chain multiple	R	1	1	0	2	3500	L	Cegidem
14	community	large, chain multiple	R	1	1	1	3	11,000	L	ProScript
15	community	small, independent, chain multiple	U	1	1	0	4	Info withheld	H	Positive Solutions
16	community	small, independent, chain multiple	U	3	0	2	2	8000	L	Cegidem
17	community	small, independent, chain multiple	U	2	2	2	2	Info withheld	H	Positive Solutions
18	hospital	medium	U	4	3	1	0	not available	L	JAC
19	hospital	large	U	1	4	5	0	> 800 items per day	H	JAC

Notes: small independent chain multiple (1–4 pharmacies); large independent chain multiple (5–25 pharmacies); large chain multiple (> 25 pharmacies); P = Pharmacist; PT = Pharmacy Technician; DA = Dispensing Assistant; MCA = Medicines Counter Assistant; Rx = prescription.

3. Results and Discussion

3.1. Types of Pharmacy and Settings

Two of the community pharmacies that had expressed an initial interest in taking part in the study withdrew before the consent process due to staff illness and holiday commitments. No potential participants withheld consent or subsequently withdrew from the study. The figures given reflect the number in each role available and willing to participate on the arranged day and time which is not necessarily the number employed at that pharmacy.

Although prescriptions and item quantities dispensed are not directly comparable, it provided an impression of dispensing volume per pharmacy. These ranged from approximately 850 prescriptions per month in a small, rural community pharmacy to over 800 items per day in a large, hospital pharmacy dispensary. Three community pharmacies withheld dispensing volume information citing commercial confidentiality reasons and the information was not available from one of the hospital.

3.2. Hardware and Software Implemented

Fourteen of the community pharmacies and one hospital pharmacy were categorised as "low tech" with three community and one hospital pharmacy deemed "high tech." Neither hospital had introduced HEPMA (hospital electronic prescribing and medicines administration). A range of commercially available pharmacy management software applications were implemented. Two ran the specialist hospital pharmacy software, JAC, while the community pharmacy systems included Cegidem ($n = 8$), Positive Solutions ($n = 3$), ProScript ($n = 5$) and Nexphase ($n = 1$).

3.3. Participant Demographics

There were 94 participants from the 19 pharmacies including:

- 24 pharmacists, two of whom were locums;
- 2 pre-registration pharmacy graduates;
- 19 pharmacy technicians;
- 15 dispensing assistants; and
- 34 medicines counter assistants.

Of the 13 male participants, ten were pharmacists, one was a dispensing assistant and two were medicines counter assistants. While half the pharmacists were aged 29 or younger, other pharmacy staff groups featured a broader age range (Figure 1). The participants' experience working in pharmacy ranged from an MCA with one-month experience to 35 years, also an MCA. The sample population showed similarities in the age range, sex and role to the national demographics [27].

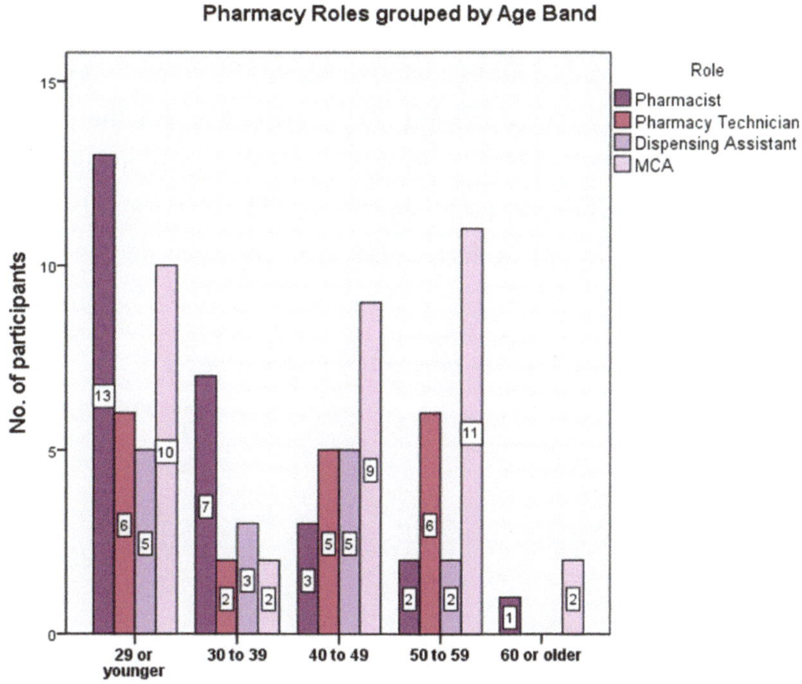

Figure 1. Participant roles grouped by age band.

As previously described, participants self-selected from six IT course titles listed in order of difficulty (Table 1) as a self-reported measure of their digital literacy. The most frequently self-selected IT course across all pharmacy roles (Figure 2) was "Computing for the Quietly Confident" (n = 39) followed by "Computing for the Terrified" (n = 19). These two least difficult courses together accounted for the selections of nearly two-thirds of participants. The remainder selected "European Computer Driving Licence" (ECDL; n = 14), "Computing for the Courageous" (n = 13), "ECDL Advanced" (n = 5) or "Degree or Diploma" (n = 4).

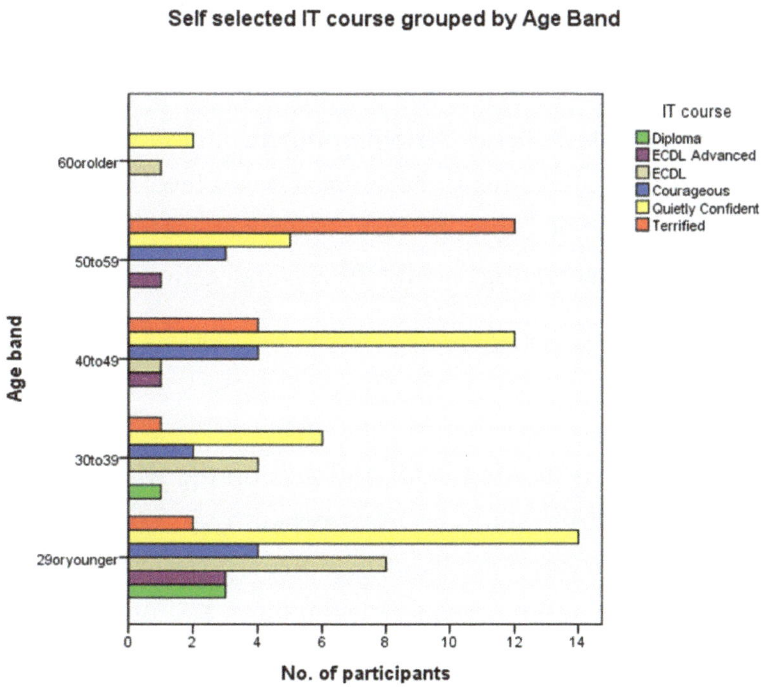

Figure 2. Self-selected IT course by age band.

Similarly, grouping self-selected IT course by age band, showed "Computing for the Quietly Confident" as the most frequently selected in all age bands except "50 to 59" where "Computing for the Terrified" was the predominant option selected (Figure 2). "Computing for the Terrified" featured as a choice for all age bands except the "60 or older." Although one third of pharmacists ($n = 8$) in the "29 or younger" age band self-selected "ECDL" as their appropriate IT challenge, the predominance of the lower level courses, indicative of basic levels of digital literacy, was clear across all roles and age bands (Figure 3).

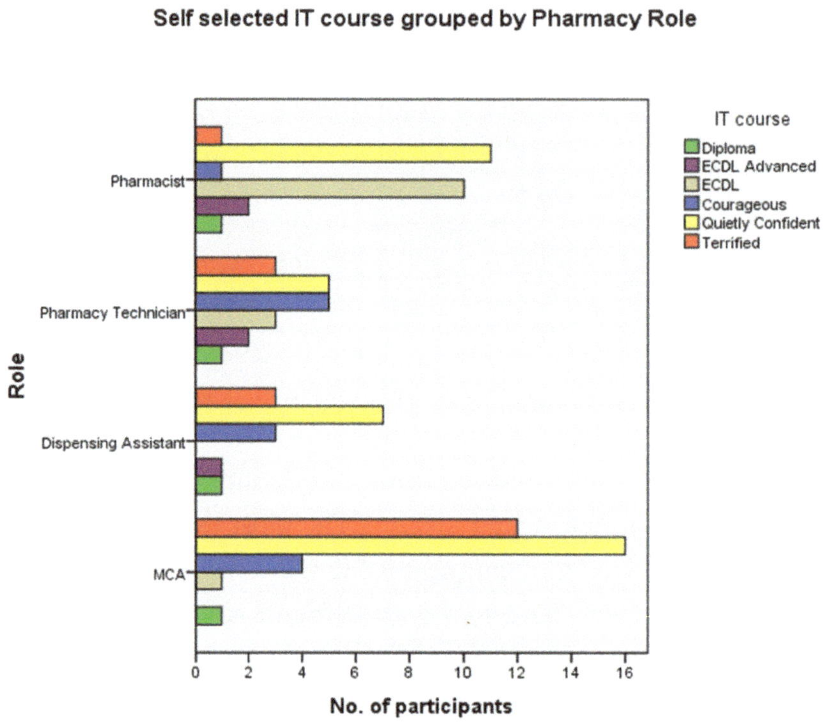

Figure 3. Self-selected IT course by pharmacy role.

3.4. Key Findings

With few exceptions, pharmacy staff in the NHS Grampian area work with minimum levels of technology and perceive their own digital literacy to be at a basic level. Role, age, gender and work experience were not clear determinants of digital literacy. Pharmacy staff need to be trained, supported and mentored to harness pharmacy technologies effectively and efficiently in support of pharmacy practice development.

3.5. Strengths and Weaknesses

To the best of our knowledge, this is the first study to focus on the whole pharmacy team and their digital literacy. The generalisability of the study is strengthened by its stratification of pharmacy staff from all roles, age bands and with varying lengths of pharmacy experience. Sampling had facilitated access to a breadth of pharmacy type, setting, level of technology and pharmacy management system implementation. However, the study is limited by the inherent bias of self-reporting, its geographical focus on a relatively small sample, from one local health board area in the North East of Scotland.

3.6. Interpretation in Context with Existing Literature

Greenhalgh *et al.* explored the diffusion of innovation in health service organisations from several theoretical perspectives including Rogers "Adopter Categories" and "Attributes of Innovation" to account for the complexity of combining socio and technical systems [28,29]. This study identifies socio-technical and political competing forces at play which Lewin described in his Force Field theory as where, "an issue is held in balance by the interaction of two opposing sets of forces—those seeking to promote change (driving forces) and those attempting to maintain the status quo (restraining forces)" [30].

3.7. Driving Forces for Technology in Pharmacy

Clear driving forces for technology in pharmacy to support healthcare have been evidenced nationally by the Scottish Government through the:

- "eHealth Strategy" [2];
- "Better eHealth: Better Care—Citizen eHealth Survey" [31];
- "2020 Vision for Quality" [32];
- "2020 Route Map" [33];
- "Prescription for Excellence" [22]; and
- locally, by NHS Grampian [26]

Technology in pharmacy has been supported jointly by RPS & Royal College of General Practitioners, by the Royal Pharmaceutical Society, the GPhC with further backing from the "Review of Pharmaceutical Care of Patients in the Community", endorsed by Community Pharmacy Scotland [15,16,19,21,34].

Another driving force is the educational support designed for the healthcare workforce to provide the digital literacy skills needed to use technology in pharmacy through the "2020 Workforce Vision", NHS Knowledge & Skills Framework and British Computer Society "Preparing the NHS for an information revolution" to support upskilling of the workforce [23,35,36].

Societal healthcare needs and technological advances have driven the organisational adoption decision in favour of technology but this study demonstrates the need to upskill all members of the pharmacy team to effectively and efficiently harness change.

3.8. Restraining Forces for Technology in Pharmacy

If policy is the driver bringing technology into pharmacy practice, the main restraining forces are the pharmacy team, its leadership and the individuals within the pharmacy team. Findings depict a workforce who self-reported their digital literacy levels as basic. Although a small sample ($n = 94$), the evidence seems to counter the commonly held perception that younger, professional people are more digitally literate. Although there were notable exceptions, most pharmacies had the minimum level of technology implemented with unaddressed usability issues acting as barriers, or additional restraining forces. Changing roles may also lead to the pharmacist spending less time with the pharmacy team depriving the team of the cascading of knowledge. The decisions of individuals to adopt technology may be influenced by their use of technology outside work but Adair and Lewin would also argue that leadership and group acceptance of technology are influential in the change management needed to counter the restraining forces [37,38].

3.9. Conditions for Change

In "Human Relations in Curriculum Change," Lewin outlined the conditions for change, the tensions at play in his Force Field theory and combinations of educational and organisational measures to "change the strength of opposing forces" [30,38]. Lewin considered the power of "social habits and group standards," where there is resistance to change, to be amenable to a three step process of "unfreeze, change, refreeze". Pharmacy worldwide employs a capable and skilled workforce. Providing the opportunity and motivation for behavioural change will be part of the on-going challenge [39].

3.10. Further Work

To the best of our knowledge, this is the only study to consider the digital literacy of the whole pharmacy team in both community and hospital settings. An observational case study is underway which will build on these findings. National surveys of digital literacy amongst not just the pharmacy workforce but also the broader healthcare workforce would provide a benchmark for evaluation of educational interventions and inform curricula design. Evaluation of progress towards implementation of policy around adoption of technology to support role development across the pharmacy team is also indicated.

4. Conclusions

Although this was a local study, the findings hold implications at the national level. Evidence from the findings suggests there is a policy driven intention to support changing roles in pharmacy by increasing and improving the provision of technology and providing the associated education and training of all pharmacy staff. With few exceptions, pharmacy staff in the NHS Grampian area work with minimum levels of technology and self-report their own digital literacy levels as basic. This tends to indicate organisational and social factors may act as restraining factors against the driving forces for technology in pharmacy and associated digital literacy training. Aspirational national and international policies have been shown to need local solutions for adoption to be successful [40]. Grudin's law warns that, "when those who benefit are not those who do the work, the system is doomed to fail" [41]. Engaging and supporting the pharmacy workforce to improve their digital literacy is key to embracing greater access to technology in pharmacy practice and providing the opportunity to "unfreeze, change, refreeze" will be key to its success.

Key Messages

- With few exceptions, pharmacy staff in the NHS Grampian area work with minimum levels of technology and perceive their own digital literacy to be at a basic level.
- Role, age, gender and work experience were not clear determinants of digital literacy.
- Pharmacy staff need to be trained to harness pharmacy technologies effectively and efficiently in support of their role development.

Acknowledgments

The authors wish to thank all the participating pharmacies and pharmacy staff in the NHS Grampian area. Thanks also to Alison Strath for her contribution to the early stages of the study design and academic and NHS experts for assistance in identifying potential participants.

Author Contributions

Katie MacLure drafted the manuscript, which was then revised by Derek Stewart.

Conflicts of Interest

The authors declare no conflict of interest.

References

1. Darzi, A. *High Quality Care for All: NHS Next Stage Review Final Report*; Department of Health: London, UK, 2008. Available online: http://www.dh.gov.uk/en/Publicationsandstatistics/Publications/PublicationsPolicyAndGuidance/DH_085825 (accessed on 12 June 2009).
2. Scottish Government. *eHealth Strategy 2011–2017*. Scottish Government: Edinburgh, Scotland, 2011. Available online: http://www.gov.scot/resource/doc/357616/0120849.pdf (accessed on 12 April 2012).
3. Department of Health. *A Report from the NHS Future Forum: Education and Training*; Department of Health: London, England, 2011. Available online: https://www.gov.uk/government/uploads/system/.../dh_132025.pdf (accessed on 12 June 2012).
4. Crown, J. *Review of Prescribing, Supply & Administration of Medicines. Final Report*; Department of Health: London, England, 1999. Available online: webarchive.nationalarchives.gov.uk/.../http:/.../dh_4077153.pdf (accessed on 1 June 2010).
5. General Pharmaceutical Council. Future Pharmacists: Standards for Initial Education and Training of Pharmacists, 2011. Available online: www.pharmacyregulation.org (accessed on 4 February 2012).
6. Beetham, H.; McGill, L.; Littlejohn, A. Thriving in the 21st Century: The Report of the LLiDA Project (Learning Literacies for the Digital Age): Provision in the UK. 2009. Available online: http://www.jisc.ac.uk/media/documents/projects/llidareportjune2009.pdf (accessed on 23 November 2012).
7. British Computer Society. Digital Literacy for Life Programme. 2013. Available online: http://dlfl.bcs.org/ (accessed on 11 October 2013).
8. American Library Association. Digital Literacy, Libraries, and Public Policy: Report of the Office for Information Technology Policy's Digital Literacy Task Force. 2013. Available online: http://www.districtdispatch.org/wp-ontent/uploads/2013/01/2012_OITP_digilitreport_1_22_13.pdf (accessed on 1 October 2013).
9. Lankshear, C.; Knobel, M. *Digital Literacies: Concepts, Policies and Practices*; Peter Lang: New York, NY, USA, 2008, Volume 30.
10. UNESCO. Institute for Technologies in Education Policy Brief: Digital Literacy in Education. 2011. Available online: http://iite.unesco.org/publications/3214688/ (accessed on 19 November 2012).

11. European Commission. Digital Agenda for Europe. 2012. Available online: http://ec.europa.eu/information_society/digital-agenda/index_en.htm (accessed on 29 February 2013).
12. European Commission. eHealth Action Plan 2012–2020 Public Consultation. 2012. Available online: http://ec.europa.eu/information_society/activities/health/ehealth_ap_consultation/ index_en.htm (accessed on 1 May 2011).
13. Innovation & Business Skills Australia. Scoping Study—Identifying Digital Literacy Skills: Cybercitizen and E-Employee in the 21st Century. 2010. Available online: http://www.ibsa.org.au/Portals/ibsa.org.au/docs/Research%20&%20Discussion%20Papers/IBSA%20%20%20Identifying%20Digital%20Literacy%20Skills%2027%2004%2010%20v1.pdf (accessed on 10 October 2013).
14. New Zealand Ministry of Education. Digital Information Literacy: Supported Development of Capability in Tertiary Environments. 2010. Available online: http://www.educationcounts.govt.nz/__data/assets/pdf_file/0006/80628/Digital-Information-Literacy-Research-Report-FINAL-pdf.pdf (accessed on 10 October 2013).
15. Royal Pharmaceutical Society & Royal College of General Practitioners. *Joint Statement: Breaking down the Barriers—How Community Pharmacists and GPs can Work together to Improve Patient Care*; Royal Pharmaceutical Society & Royal College of General Practitioners (RPS & RCGP): London, England, 2011. Available online: www.rpharms.com/public-affairs-pdfs/RPSRCGPjointstatement.pdf (accessed on 1 October 2012).
16. Royal Pharmaceutical Society. *Empowering Pharmacists to Improve Pharmaceutical Care and Medicines Safety through Information Technology: Information Technology Strategic Principles*; Royal Pharmaceutical Society: Edinburgh, Scotland, 2011. Available online: www.rpharms.com/...pharmacy-pdfs/imt---nov-2012---it-principles.pdf (accessed on 1 October 2012).
17. e-Skills UK. National Occupational Standards for IT Users. 2011. Available online: https://www.e-skills.com/standards-and-qualifications/national-occupational-standards-nos/ (accessed on 20 January 2011).
18. NHS Education for Scotland. ePharmacy Toolkit for Community Pharmacists. NHS Education for Scotland: Glasgow, Scotland, 2008. Available online: www.gov.scot/resource/doc/209438/0055428.pdf (accessed on 1 April 2010).
19. General Pharmaceutical Council. Annual Report 2012/13. 2013. Available online: http://www.pharmacyregulation.org/sites/default/files/Annual%20Report%202013.pdf (accessed on 28 February 2013).
20. Accreditation Council for Pharmacy Education. Available online: https://www.acpe-accredit.org/default.asp (accessed on 23 June 2012).
21. Wilson, H.; Barber, N. Review of NHS Pharmaceutical Care of Patients in the Community in Scotland. 2013. Available online: http://www.scotland.gov.uk/Resource/0043/00430209.pdf (accessed on 15 August 2013).
22. Scottish Government. Prescription for Excellence: A Vision and Action Plan for the Right Pharmaceutical Care through Integrated Partnerships and Innovation. 2013. Available online: http://www.scotland.gov.uk/Resource/0043/00434053.pdf (accessed on 11 November 2013).
23. Scottish Government. Everyone Matters: 2020 Workforce Vision. 2013. Available online: http://www.scotland.gov.uk/Publications/2013/06/5943 (accessed on 11 November 2013).

24. NHS Health Scotland. A Fairer Healthier Scotland: Our Strategy 2012–2017. 2012. Available online: http://www.healthscotland.com/uploads/documents/18922-CorporateStrategy.pdf (accessed on 11 November 2013).
25. Scottish Government. Public Bodies (Joint Working) (Scotland) Bill. 2013. Available online: http://www.scottish.parliament.uk/parliamentarybusiness/Bills/63845.aspx (accessed on 14 August 2013).
26. NHS Grampian. NHS Grampian Annual Review 2012/13. 2013. Available online: http://www.nhsgrampian.co.uk/nhsgrampian/gra_display.jsp;jsessionid=B56539D81BD0E705E5C988111E34A969?pContentID=6997&p_applic=CCC&p_service=Content.show& (accessed on 12 December 2013).
27. Centre for Workforce Intelligence. Annual Review April 2010 to March 2011. 2011. Available online: www.cfwi.org.uk (accessed on 1 October 2011).
28. Greenhalgh, T.; Robert, G.; MacFarlane, F.; Bate, P.; Kyriakidou, O.; Peacock, R. *Storylines of Research in Diffusion of Innovation: A Meta-Narrative Approach to Systematic Review. Soc. Sci. Med.* **2005**, *61*, 417–430.
29. Rogers, E.M. *Diffusion of Innovations*; Free Press: Glencoe, Scotland, 1995.
30. Lewin, K. *Field Theory in Social Science*; Harper & Row: New York, NY, USA, 1947.
31. Scottish Government. Better eHealth: Better Care—Citizen eHealth Survey. 2011. Available online: http://www.ehealth.scot.nhs.uk/?page_id=143 (accessed on 1 November 2011).
32. Scottish Government. Achieving Sustainable Quality in Scotland's Healthcare: A '20:20' Vision. 2011. Available online: http://www.knowledge.scot.nhs.uk/media/CLT/ResourceUploads/4002697/Achieving%20Sustainable%20Quality%20in%20Scotlands%20Healthcare%20-%20A%2020_.doc (accessed on 12 October 2015).
33. Scottish Government. Route Map to the 2020 Vision for Health and Social Care. 2013. Available online: http://www.scotland.gov.uk/Topics/Health/Policy/Quality-Strategy/ routemap2020vision (accessed on 11 July 2013).
34. Community Pharmacy Scotland. Policy Response from Chief Executive to Introduction of "Prescription for Excellence". 2013. Available online: http://www.communitypharmacyscotland.org.uk/news,-policy-and-publications/policy/policy-responses-by-cps-%281%29/policy-responses-by-cps/ (accessed on 12 January 2013).
35. National Health Service Knowledge and Skills Framework. NHS Knowledge and Skills Framework. 2013. Available online: http://www.ksf.scot.nhs.uk/ (accessed on 4 April 2013).
36. British Computer Society. *Preparing the NHS for an Information Revolution: BCS Report on the NHS Information Revolution Consultation Proposal*; British Computer Society: London, England, 2013. Available online: https://www.bcs.org/upload/pdf/liberating-the-nhs.pdf (accessed on 1 December 2014).
37. Adair, J.E. *Action-Centred Leadership*; McGraw-Hill: London, England, 1973.
38. Muntyan, K.D.; Benne, B. *Human Relations in Curriculum Change*. Available online: http://www.channelingreality.com/Niwa/Documents/Social_Engineering/1951_HRCC_Benne_122710.pdf (accessed on 12 October 2015).

39. Michie, S.; van Stralen, M.M.; West, R. The behaviour change wheel: A new method for characterising and designing behaviour change interventions. *Implemen. Sci.* **2011**, *6,* 42. Available online: http://www.implementationscience.com/content/6/1/42 (accessed on 5 July 2012).
40. Eason, K.; Waterson, P. The implications of e-health system delivery strategies for integrated healthcare: Lessons from England. *Int. J. Med. Inform.* **2012**, *82*, 96–106. Available online: www.ncbi.nlm.nih.gov/pubmed/23266062 (accessed on 5 July 2013).
41. Patterson, E.S. Technology support of the handover: Promoting observability, flexibility and efficiency. *BMJ Qual. Saf.* **2012**, *21*, i19–i21. Available online: www.ncbi.nlm.nih.gov/pubmed/23173184 (accessed on 12 October 2015).

4

The Hidden Role of Community Pharmacy Technicians in Ensuring Patient Safety with the Use of E-Prescribing

Olufunmilola K. Odukoya [1,*], Loren J. Schleiden [1] and Michelle A. Chui [2]

[1] Pharmacy and Therapeutics, School of Pharmacy, University of Pittsburgh, 3501 Terrace St, 720 Salk Hall, Pittsburgh, PA 15213, USA; E-Mail: ljs24@pitt.edu

[2] Social & Administrative Sciences, School of Pharmacy, University of Wisconsin-Madison, 777 Highland Avenue, Madison, WI 53705, USA; E-Mail: michelle.chui@wisc.edu

* Author to whom correspondence should be addressed; E-Mail: oodukoya@pitt.edu

Academic Editor: Reem Kayyali

Abstract: Objectives: It has been reported that supportive personnel, such as pharmacy technicians, are key participants in the use of health information technology. The purpose of this study was to describe how pharmacy technicians use e-prescribing and to explore the characteristics of technicians that support pharmacists in ensuring patient safety. Methods: This was a qualitative study that used observations, interviews, and focus groups to understand the role of pharmacy technicians in e-prescribing. Fourteen pharmacy technicians and 13 pharmacists from five community pharmacies participated. Observations lasted about nine hours in each pharmacy. Follow-up interviews and two separate focus groups were later conducted. Observation field notes and audio recordings were transcribed and thematically analyzed. Results: Pharmacy technicians were primarily responsible for all steps leading up to pharmacist review of the e-prescription and dispensing of medications to the patient. Technician characteristics, including experience, certification status, and knowledge of appropriate medication use, were reported as important factors in supporting a pharmacist's role in ensuring patient safety with the use of e-prescribing. Conclusion: Study findings indicate that pharmacy technicians have an important role in supporting pharmacists to prevent medication errors. Certain characteristics of pharmacy technicians were identified with the potential to improve the e-prescription medication dispensing process and decrease patient harm through the identification and resolution of errors.

Keywords: pharmacy technicians; electronic prescribing; e-prescribing; patient safety; community pharmacies

1. Introduction

Medication errors are a significant problem in healthcare settings [1–3]. Medication errors can lead to suboptimal outcomes in patients, including increased cost [3], longer hospitalization [4], injury [5] and death [6]. One form of health information technology (health IT) that has been promoted to reduce medication errors in various healthcare settings is electronic prescribing (e-prescribing) [7–9]. E-prescribing systems allow physicians to electronically generate and transmit prescriptions to community pharmacies. In the United States, e-prescriptions are entered by the prescriber and transmitted to a transaction hub, which links the prescriber, preferred pharmacy system, and pharmacy benefits manager. E-prescribing presents an alternative to more traditional methods of transmitting prescriptions via phone, fax, or paper. E-prescribing system use has seen tremendous growth over the past decade, from 29 million e-prescriptions generated in 2007 to 1.20 billion in 2014 [10]. In community pharmacies that are primarily responsible for processing prescriptions, it is estimated that prescription error rates are as low as 0.23% and as high as 11% [11–18]. Despite the emergence of e-prescribing as a major method of sending prescriptions from the prescriber offices directly to community pharmacies, there is evidence that e-prescribing does not reduce prescription error rates [19].

E-prescriptions sent to community pharmacies are often first received and processed by pharmacy technicians [20]. However, little is known about the role of pharmacy technicians in using e-prescribing and their contributions to preventing medication errors in community pharmacies. Pharmacy technicians are supportive staff who can work in a variety of pharmacy settings, such as community, hospital, and assisted living facility pharmacies. Pharmacy technicians at community pharmacies are typically responsible for all of the steps in preparing a medication to be reviewed by a pharmacist and subsequent dispensation to the patient [21].

There is compelling evidence of the impact of similar types of medical supportive staff, such as nurses, physician assistants, and medical assistants, in making important contributions to improving patient safety in healthcare settings [22–30]. Studies of the characteristics of supportive staff have given insight into their significance in improving patient safety, including reduction of healthcare-associated infections through implementation of a unit-based quality nurse [30], association of reduced failure to rescue with an increased nurse to patient ratio [22], association of hospital nurse educational level and surgical patient mortality [23] and the decrease of the length of stay and patients who leave without being seen at emergency departments through the addition of a physician assistant as a triage liaison provider [24].

While there is convincing evidence of the significance of other types of medical supportive staff in improving patient safety [25–29], there has been little attention given to the role of pharmacy technicians in using health IT, such as e-prescribing to improve medication safety. It has been reported that about 11% of e-prescriptions sent to community pharmacies from prescriber offices have medication errors [19]. Since pharmacy technicians are the first personnel in community pharmacies to handle processing of prescriptions and the high rate of e-prescription errors encountered, it is important to explore how the characteristics of pharmacy technicians influence patient safety. Previous research on e-prescriptions in England has investigated types of errors encountered in community pharmacies along with implications for increasing efficiency in the process, such as keeping databases used by dispensing systems updated [31,32]. Examining the processes involved in preventing, identifying and resolving e-prescription errors in the United States could inform efforts at community pharmacies to prevent e-prescription errors from happening, identify e-prescription errors when they do happen, and fix e-prescription errors in an efficient and effective manner.

2. Objective

The purpose of this study was to describe how supportive personnel in community pharmacies, specifically pharmacy technicians, use e-prescribing and the characteristics of technicians that ensure medication safety.

3. Methods

Pharmacist technicians and pharmacists at five Southwest Wisconsin community pharmacy sites (two chain pharmacies, three independent pharmacies) with previous collaborative relationships were invited to participate in this study from October 2012 to April 2013. Participants gave informed consent and were remunerated $50 each for their participation. Approval for this research was granted by the University of Wisconsin-Madison Institutional Review Board. This research was part of a larger study that explored e-prescription error recovery in community pharmacies, and additional details of the methods can be found in previous publications [20,33]. Data were collected using three different methods: observation, interviews and focus groups. These methods were used to understand how technicians handled e-prescriptions and prevented associated medication errors.

4. Direct Observations

Direct observations were used to understand how pharmacy technicians processed e-prescriptions and dealt with any medication errors as they were encountered. Pharmacy technicians were observed in four-hour intervals on two separate days, and these intervals typically took place on weekdays during the hours of 8 a.m. and 8 p.m. Observations on the first day took place during the early hours of operation, and observation on the second day took place during the later hours of operation. Two researchers with prior patient safety research experience (one pharmacist and one human factors engineer) observed participants as they processed e-prescriptions. Participants were instructed to perform their regular duties as usual and to notify the observing researcher when they encountered a medication error. Researchers took extensive field notes on how e-prescriptions were processed by pharmacy staff, which were transcribed within 24 hours of the observation period. A total of 26 pharmacy personnel participated in direct observations, including 15 technicians and 11 pharmacists. All direct observations were conducted before any participants were interviewed. Data gathered from direct observations were used to inform interviews with participants.

5. Interviews

Semi-structured interviews were administered in order to collect additional information on how e-prescriptions were processed by pharmacy technicians, including the process of dealing with medication errors when they were encountered. An interview guide was developed to provide predetermined questions, prompts, and probes to help elicit additional information about how e-prescriptions were processed and how medication errors were dealt with. Questions in the interview guide were designed to be neutral and open in order to keep from educing socially desirable responses [34]. Questions were also examined for content validity by five experts, including four pharmacists and one human factors engineer.

Two researchers conducted the interviews, which lasted approximately one hour each, with one researcher facilitating the interview while the second researcher took notes and provided support in asking questions and prompting for more information from participants. Nine pharmacy technicians and eleven pharmacists were interviewed. Of the 20 interview participants, 17 had also participated in the direct observations. Each interview was audio-taped, and all audio recordings were professionally transcribed. Interview transcripts were verified for accuracy by listening to eight audio-recordings of interviews (40%). The interview transcripts and data analysis plan were discussed by three researchers. Data obtained from direct observations and interviews were used to inform the focus groups with participants.

6. Focus Groups

Two separate focus groups were conducted: a technician focus group and a pharmacist focus group. Both focus groups took place after all interviews were completed, and both were facilitated by the first author. A focus group guide was created by triangulating and summarizing direct observation and interview data from all pharmacies and was used to help direct focus group discussions. This guide gave participants the chance to: (1) provide additional information not captured during observations and interviews; (2) learn about data gathered from other pharmacies; and (3) verify the interpretations of and to give the data collected. The guide also sought to examine in more depth the role of technicians in processing e-prescriptions and handling medication errors. Questions and summary data documents were reviewed by three researchers and presented to participants in the form of summaries of strategies used to process e-prescriptions and handle medication errors from all pharmacies. Focus group participants were emailed the focus group questions and documents one week prior to the focus group session.

Four technicians participated in the technician focus group held eight weeks after the last interview (March 2013). Eight pharmacists participated in the pharmacist focus group held in early April 2013, with one pharmacist joining the focus group via telephone. All focus group participants had previously participated in the individual interviews. Each focus group lasted approximately 90 minutes. Researchers held a debriefing session immediately after completion of the first focus group (technician focus group) to review the focus group questions and discuss changes needed for participants in the second focus group (pharmacist focus group). Both focus groups were tape-recorded and transcribed by a professional transcriptionist. The first author verified the accuracy of the transcription process by listening to both focus groups. A comprehensive summary, including transcripts of audiotapes, anecdotal notes and field notes, was generated following the completion of both focus groups.

7. Data Analysis

Observation field notes, interview transcripts and focus group questions were imported into the qualitative analysis software NVivo 10 and subjected to content analysis [35]. Two researchers reviewed field notes and transcripts line by line to identify sections of the text that were assigned codes. Codes were further reviewed to identify patterns and themes that were summarized into higher-level themes. The third author reviewed these themes, and the research team met to address disparities and inconsistencies within the data and to create final descriptions of the study findings.

8. Results

8.1. Characteristics of Technicians and Pharmacies

On average, participating pharmacies processed about 120 to 400 e-prescriptions daily. Each pharmacy generally had about two to five technicians on staff daily. The age range of technicians was 22 to 59 years old, and their experience in pharmacy practice ranged from 3 to 30 years. A few of the technicians had received formal technician training and were certified technicians.

8.2. E-Prescription Processing: Pharmacy Technician's Role in Ensuring Safety

Technicians were primarily responsible for processing e-prescriptions in community pharmacies. The general process for processing e-prescriptions in community pharmacies is shown in Figure 1. In the initial step of e-prescriptions processing, a notification was received that an e-prescription had been sent from the prescriber's office directly into the e-prescribing queue in the pharmacy's computer system. In some of the study pharmacies, the e-prescription was then printed by the technician and the information either manually re-inputted or electronically auto-populated into the patient's profile in the pharmacy system (the inputting phase). For pharmacies in which e-prescriptions were first printed, technicians gave three main reasons for printing e-prescriptions: (1) to prevent errors during inputting of information; (2) for easy verification of information; and (3) for record keeping purposes. The e-prescription information, such as a patient's or physician's information (name, date of birth, address, telephone number) and drug information (name, strength, dosing directions, quantity), did not always enter the pharmacy system directly. Such information was sometimes manually typed into the patient's prescription profile in the pharmacy system.

> Pharmacist: "The primary responsibility for processing prescription is the technicians. So generally they will receive the notification that there is an e-prescription in the queue, and then they will process it in the computer. And after they processed it, a paper version of the e-prescription will print out to be used as a check during the checking process and filling process of the prescription. And then as the pharmacist, we'll receive the paper version that's been printed off and use that to check the accuracy of the filled prescription."

> Technician: "We just don't fill them from the e-prescription…The directions, if you do fill it off of [the computer], without printing it out, all those directions will be on there. So if you, let's say, don't catch the two different directions on there, both directions are going to be on that prescription for that patient unless you would delete it or change it. So nothing is,

you know, there isn't one thing that would probably ever be right if you were to fill it off of an e-prescription."

Technician: "And so I print out the hard copy, and then I go through and, I'll actually use the computer, I'll take the hard copy and then just use that to compare against what comes up on the screen for the patient and everything… Then you look at the physical prescription there. And then you look down at the doctor's name, make sure that that matches up. And then I usually give the prescription one more look-over. I'll circle the date on the front of the prescription."

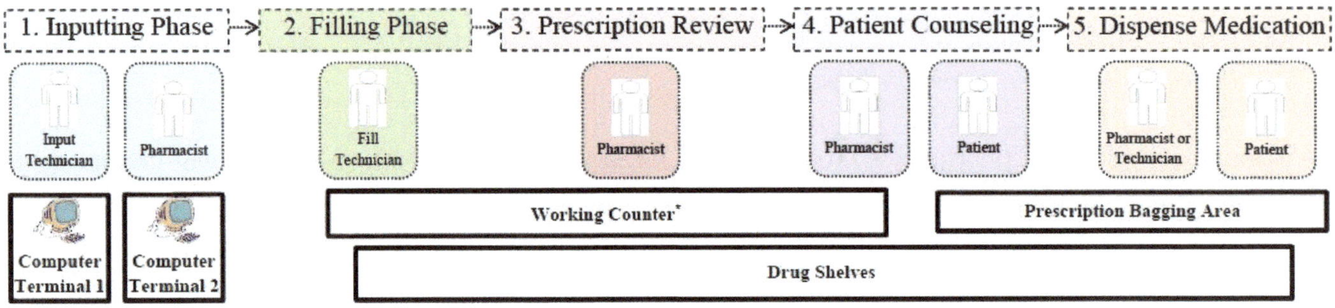

Figure 1. E-prescription processing and layout of community pharmacies. Notes: * Working Counter is used for inputting, filing, checking, and dispensing medications. Holds tools used for prescription processing, such as prescription dispensing bins, calculators, labels and computers.

Technicians also played a significant role in detecting e-prescription errors during inputting and filling through verification of prescription information. The input technician typically initiated the inputting of the e-prescription into the pharmacy system; however, in one pharmacy, the pharmacist was responsible for inputting e-prescriptions into the pharmacy system. One participant reported that input of an e-prescription was done very fast and took about 30 seconds, and this was also witnessed by researchers during the observation periods.

Technician: "Most of the time, they enter so fast, which is a nice thing. I mean, it takes you like 30 seconds to enter an e-prescription. So you can do them fast."

During the inputting phase, the input technician or pharmacist verified the e-prescription information as it was being entered into the patient's profile and then printed the appropriate labels. During inputting, the patient's medication profile was sometimes reviewed to determine if the prescription was appropriate for the patient. For example, the inputting technician verified patient allergies, how often the patient was receiving the prescriptions and compared past dosing regimen with the e-prescription being inputted.

Technicians: "The e-prescriptions are seen by the technician first."

The filling phase (second check) was the next step; this was done mainly by the designated filling technicians. The input technician placed the printed e-prescription and medication label in a dispensing bin that was then passed down to the fill technician. The fill technician was responsible for picking medications from the shelves or dispensing robot, counting medications, and placing them in dispensing bottles, attaching appropriate labels, and ensuring that the number of counted pills filled matched the printed e-prescription label. Once the prescriptions were filled and labeled, they were put into specific colored dispensing bins and passed down the workflow for final check and review by the pharmacist. Different colors of dispensing bins were used to notify the pharmacist of the type of prescription or if the patient was waiting to pick up their medications. However, all five pharmacies used different colors to designate prescription information. For example one pharmacy used the pink dispensing bins to indicate that patients were waiting in the pharmacy to pick up the prescriptions and used green colored dispensing bins to indicate that an e-prescription had an error or an unresolved problem. Another pharmacy used white bins to indicate that the e-prescription was a refill medication, and a red bin meant the patient was waiting to pick up the medication.

> Technician: "What we do also is when we fill the prescription, then when we go, well, we fill it in the computer, and then we actually count out the pills ourselves and then pass it down to the pharmacist. But what we do when we're filling too, after we're done, we'll take the bottle, look at the NDC underline the NDC number, make sure we got the right bottle off the shelf to match your label, and then we circle the quantity and make sure we had counted out the right quantity, so it eliminates the error there."
>
> (NDC: National Drug Code, a unique number used to identify medications in the United States)

The next phase was the pharmacist overall review of the e-prescription and filled medication (third and final check). Pharmacists were primarily responsible for checking the accuracy of the e-prescription filled and inputted by the technicians; this was commonly described by participants as performing "DUR" (drug utilization review). The pharmacist's review of the e-prescription consisted of verification of the following: (1) information entered by the input technician; (2) the corresponding medication filled by the fill technician; (3) drug-drug interactions; (4) dosage changes; and (5) overall medication profile history of the patient. Finally, pharmacists bagged the prescription and proceeded to counsel the patient before dispensing the medication to the patient (patient counseling and dispensing of medication).

8.3. What Pharmacy Technicians Do to Support Pharmacists' Role in E-Prescribing

Technicians performed a variety of tasks when processing e-prescriptions to enable the pharmacist to be more efficient in making sure medications were accurately dispensed. For instance, technicians memorized pharmacist preferences, assisted the pharmacist to look up drug information using online tools, and performed a second check to drug or patient information inputted by the pharmacist into the pharmacy's e-prescribing system.

Of particular importance for technicians was having a general awareness of what was going in the pharmacy. For instance, technicians were usually the first set of eyes to review e-prescriptions and to detect errors. A primary role of technicians in e-prescription processing was ensuring patient safety by detecting medication errors, because most were caught during the inputting of the e-prescription information. One technician expressed that technicians were the first individuals in the pharmacy to review e-prescription for errors, and it was their job to detect errors.

> Technician: "Well, a lot of the times, you're like the first, well, at least I'm the first person to see it if I'm sitting there and entering whatever. So I think it's just my job if I'm there like

first, or I'm late instead of passing it on and making the second technician and finally the pharmacist finds it, and then the patient is there already. So I think like since I'm the first set of eyes, it's my job to find errors first and to be looking for them."

Technicians made sure to communicate with the pharmacist on shift about e-prescription errors that were detected. Technicians were also proactive in using a variety of strategies, such as colored bins or flags to distinguish that an error was suspected, to ensure the pharmacist performed a double check on an e-prescription that they suspected had an error. Pharmacy technicians also examined the patient's medication profile prior to the pharmacist's review of the e-prescription so as to be proactive in alerting the pharmacist of a medication error. Technicians also served as second check or a "second set of eyes" to look over e-prescriptions that had been previously reviewed by a pharmacist for things like inputting or spelling errors.

Technician: "I do three checks along the way. Like I check the NDC when I'm grabbing it off the shelf. I check the NDC when I'm pouring the excess back into the bottle. And when I set it down, I check NDC and quantity that I've just counted, and I figure I'm doing it three times along the way. Even If I miss one of those, I'm still doing it twice, so just, you know, having a very good system and like trying to stick to it is really good for reducing errors."

Technician: "I mean, and that may just be an entering error rather than a prescription error, but I'm the spell check for the pharmacy too, so I just make sure that there's nothing weird in there. And, I mean, we have short codes for entering stuff in, because the way our software works, you only get so many characters. Like the characters that can be on the label are greater. The characters will let you type in the field, so they have short codes that are separated by semicolons. If they like don't hit the semicolon or something, then you just end up with the short code in it rather than the actual words. So I keep an eye out for that and make sure that everything is actually, you know, real words and not abbreviations."

The goal of reviewing prescription was to make sure the medication order was accurately inputted into the pharmacy system and that patient or drug information matched up correctly with the intention of the prescriber. Technicians' knowledge of appropriate medication use was useful to the pharmacist because the technician could be proactive about calling the prescriber to address errors on the e-prescriptions, especially when the pharmacist was busy. Some pharmacists gave technicians autonomy to contact prescribers directly without asking the pharmacists, particularly when they perceived that the e-prescription error was minor and would not be complicated to resolve. In these cases, the technician was able to reduce the pharmacist's workload and prevent the task from interrupting the pharmacist.

Technicians also tried to keep abreast of patient information, such as drug allergies, to easily detect errors. Overall, a high attention to detail was important for technicians to contribute to enhancing patient safety.

Technician: "We have one patient that has a yellow dye allergy, so whenever they get a new medication, I, like just on my own, like I just go grab the thing, grab the insert, take a look at all the ingredients and make sure there's not yellow dye in that."

During the focus groups, technicians stated that it was helpful to learn about strategies used by technicians in other pharmacies to ensure e-prescribing safety. The focus group served as a learning session to compare the role of technicians in other pharmacies and how useful strategies could be incorporated into their respective pharmacy settings.

> Technician: "...if they have other strategies for what they do, it might work for us, just as our strategies might help them."

> Technician: "...it was interesting to learn that the same problems that we deal with..., everyone else, you guys deal with."

8.4. How Do the Characteristics of Pharmacy Technicians Impact Medication Safety with E-Prescribing?

During the pharmacist focus group, pharmacists discussed various characteristics of pharmacy technicians that would have an impact on their ability to detect errors. These included having more pharmacy practice experience, certification as a pharmacy technician, a high level of commitment, critical thinking skills, close attention to detail, and a proactive personality.

> Pharmacist: "It's level of experience, for one. The longer they've been in this field or in its employ, that is tremendous. Those who are, those who have been, are certified technicians, have also indicated, you know, a higher level of commitment. I look at that as someone has a higher level of commitment, you know, in wanting to make this and everything more of a career for them. So I think that helps tremendously."

Pharmacists indicated that having a full-time pharmacy technician on their shift makes their jobs easier, as full-time technicians who deal with working in a pharmacy on a daily basis may have more familiarity with common e-prescribing issues.

> Pharmacist: "One thing that makes it a little bit easier is that we typically have a full-time technician on every shift. So there's somebody that has a lot of experience dealing with e-prescriptions, so they're familiar with a lot of the common issues. And they're, they tend to be more experienced technicians as well, so they, they're helpful at identifying issues or supporting me when I need to address an issue and contact a physician."

Pharmacists reported that a pharmacy technician being overconfident, rushing or not being well trained could lead to medication errors getting through to the pharmacist or patient.

> Pharmacist: "...while our technicians help us, they can also make a barrier, whether they're not as well trained, or they are overconfident, or they go too fast, or whatever it is, where they're not checking their work, and that could be a barrier."

> Pharmacist: "I think one thing that hurts is that you don't really get a whole lot of training on e-prescriptions. It's just sort of a, you get used to doing them over time, just practice. So I don't know that, I don't know that it's a whole lot different from other prescription filling that we do though, so. It could just make it a little bit more confusing when you're working with a newer technician, because they may not be as familiar with the ins and outs of the e-prescribing processing."

8.5. What Can Pharmacists Do to Encourage Valuable Contribution From Pharmacy Technicians?

The quality of interaction between pharmacists and pharmacy technicians was reported as a factor that could enhance pharmacy technicians' ability to properly handle medication errors. Pharmacists in the focus group reported that trusting technicians to process e-prescriptions and handle any medication errors that might be encountered, empowering technicians to call physician offices to fix medication errors, and reassuring and providing positive reinforcement to technicians could result in further valuable contributions from technicians in processing e-prescriptions. For technicians with different experiences and employment histories, not all technicians will have the same concept of what they can and cannot do within their roles. By providing consistent trust, encouragement, and positive reinforcement, pharmacists stated that technicians may be more confident and knowledgeable in their roles and, thus, more likely to contribute in appropriate situations.

> Pharmacist: "...empower the technician to go ahead and do so. In other words, if you let them know that you have the trust, okay, because, you know what, because they earned it, I think that really kind of goes a long way too."

> Pharmacist: "Or maybe it takes a couple times of you giving them the reassurance. Like it's fine if you want to just go ahead and call on that, or you, yeah, that's good, that's a good catch. You know, why don't you check on it. And then after a few times, then they realize..."

9. Discussion

Community pharmacies are healthcare settings where prescribed medications are frequently dispensed to patients. Pharmacists practicing in these settings act as middle men between prescribers and patients to ensure that patients receive the right medications, thus playing a key role in intercepting prescribing errors and ensuring medication safety. Due to increasing workload and prescriptions volume (an estimated 3.3 billion annually) in community pharmacies [36–39], pharmacy technicians are increasingly playing important roles in the dispensing of medications. Within these settings, pharmacy technicians perform a variety of tasks related to the processing of these prescriptions under the guidance of a community pharmacist [40]. E-prescribing is now the primary way community pharmacies receive prescriptions from physician offices [10]. As e-prescribing becomes more widely used, it is important to examine the role of technicians in ensuring medication safety with this health information technology. Ensuring the safety of e-prescriptions has become paramount, because 11% of e-prescriptions received in community pharmacies have medication errors [19]. Findings from this study highlight the role of pharmacy technicians in processing e-prescriptions in community pharmacies and efforts they make to prevent medication errors from reaching patients.

The findings from this study indicate that all of the steps in the inputting and filling phases of processing an e-prescription were typically conducted by pharmacy technicians prior to verification by a pharmacist. Pharmacy technicians can receive traditional and electronic prescriptions, review for accuracy, prepare orders, package and label medicine, assist patients and maintain patient records. Pharmacy technicians in this study reported that they used a variety of strategies to review prescriptions and to ensure that any medication errors were identified and either: (1) resolved if the error was not complicated; or (2) communicated with the pharmacist if the error was beyond the expertise of the pharmacy technician.

Despite their integral role in processing a prescription, there is still no uniform national requirement for pharmacy technician training. While some pharmacy technicians have completed an educational program to achieve an associate's degree, diploma, certificate or license, others have been trained on the job [41]. Consistent training of pharmacy technicians through continuing education or taking advantage of on the job learning opportunities could improve their job performance. However, continuing education is not required among all pharmacy technicians, and on the job training may be inconsistent and depend on the availability and ambition of the pharmacy technician. In a recent study, only 16.8% of pharmacy technician respondents reported that, in their most recent medication preparation error, pharmacists provided instruction on how to reduce the chance of a similar error in the future [42]. Findings from our study indicate that pharmacist-technician working relationships can be improved by pharmacists trusting, empowering, reassuring and providing positive reinforcement to help a pharmacy technician to gain confidence and knowledge in his or her roles. Targeting pertinent continuing education topics, taking advantage of possible on the job learning opportunities and promoting confidence and knowledge in their roles could lead to enhanced effectiveness in pharmacy technicians being able to identify and correct medication errors before they reach the pharmacist or patient.

Previous studies have reported that education level, continuing education, training, and related characteristics of other similar types of supportive personnel have been associated with impacting patient safety outcomes [22–30]. Considering the important role pharmacy technicians have in processing e-prescriptions, it is reasonable to surmise similar impacts of the characteristics of pharmacy technicians on patient safety outcomes related to medication errors. Pharmacists in this study reported that person-specific characteristics, such as experience, certification, commitment, critical thinking skills, close attention to detail, a proactive personality, and full- *versus* part-time status, impacted how well a technician could perform his or her patient care responsibilities. These associations could have implications on clinical outcomes, such as performance or accuracy in processing e-prescriptions, identification of medication errors, and efficiency in resolving errors when they do occur. The positive implications of optimizing these outcomes include less prescriber, pharmacist and technician time and resources taken to resolve medication errors and fewer medication errors possibly reaching patients and causing harm.

10. Study Limitations

The nature of this study was exploratory and only involved five community pharmacy sites in Southwest Wisconsin, the United States. As such, these results may not be generalizable to all community pharmacy sites across the nation and other types of pharmacy settings.

11. Conclusions

Pharmacy technicians have been shown to play an important role in the e-prescription process and medication dispensing community pharmacies. Many specific characteristics of pharmacy technicians were reported to be associated with better support of pharmacists in fulfilling their patient care responsibilities and more efficient identification and resolution of medication errors. The true magnitude of these associations with key outcomes, such as productivity and patient safety, are currently unknown. Future research could be done to determine these associations; interventions could be better informed to target potential areas of improvement in an effort to optimize the e-prescription process and robustness of pharmacy technician training to improve medication safety.

Acknowledgements

This study was funded by the Community Pharmacy Foundation. Michelle Chui was supported by the Clinical and Translational Science Award (CTSA) program, through the NIH National Center for Advancing Translational Sciences (NCATS), grant UL1TR000427. The content is solely the responsibility of the authors and does not necessarily represent the official views of the NIH.

Author Contributions

Olufunmilola K. Odukoya was responsible for study conceptualization, data collection, analysis, and writing this final report. Loren J. Schleiden contributed to preparing this manuscript for publication, data analysis, and interpretation of results. Michelle A. Chui was involved in study design, data interpretation, and drafting the final manuscript. All authors have reviewed the paper and agree to its publication.

Conflicts of Interest

The authors declare no conflict of interest.

References

1. Bates, D.W.; Boyle, D.L.; Vander Vliet, M.B.; Schneider, J.; Leape, L. Relationship between medication errors and adverse drug events. *J. Gen. Intern. Med.* **1995**, *10*, 199–205.
2. Meredith, S.; Feldman, P.H.; Frey, D.; Hall, K.; Arnold, K.; Brown, N.J.; Ray, W.A. Possible medication errors in home healthcare patients. *J. Am. Geriatr. Soc.* **2001**, *49*, 719–724.
3. Samp, J.C.; Touchette, D.R.; Marinac, J.S.; Kuo, G.M. Economic evaluation of the impact of medication errors reported by U.S. clinical pharmacists. *Pharmacotherapy* **2014**, *34*, 350–357.
4. Roughead, E.E.; Semple, S.J. Medication safety in acute care in Australia: Where are we now? Part 1: a review of the extent and causes of medication problems 2002–2008. *Aust. New Zealand Health Policy* **2009**, *6*, 18. doi:10.1186/1743-8462-6-18.
5. Ferner, R.E.; Aronson, J.K. Medication errors, worse than a crime. *Lancet* **2000**, *355*, 947–948.
6. Phillips, D.P.; Christenfeld, N.; Glynn, L.M. Increase in US medication-error deaths between 1983 and 1993. *Lancet* **1998**, *351*, 643–644.
7. Lapane, K.L.; Waring, M.E.; Schneider, K.L.; Dubé, C.; Quilliam, B.J. A mixed method study of the merits of e-prescribing drug alerts in primary care. *J. Gen. Intern. Med.* **2008**, *23*, 442–446.
8. Bell, D.S.; Friedman, M.A. E-prescribing and the medicare modernization act of 2003. *Health Aff. (Millwood)*. **2005**, *24*, 1159–1169.
9. Moniz, T.T.; Seger, A.C.; Keohane, C.A.; Seger, D.L.; Bates, D.W.; Rothschild, J.M. Addition of electronic prescription transmission to computerized prescriber order entry: Effect on dispensing errors in community pharmacies. *Am. J. Health Syst. Pharm.* **2011**, *68*, 158–163.
10. Surescripts. 2014 National Progress Report and Safe-Rx Rankings 2015. Available online: http://surescripts.com/news-center/national-progress-report-2014 (accessed on 19 October 2015).

11. Knudsen, P.; Herborg, H.; Mortensen, A.R.; Knudsen, M.; Hellebek, A. Preventing medication errors in community pharmacy: frequency and seriousness of medication errors. *Qual. Saf. Health Care* **2007**, *16*, 291–296.
12. Buurma, H.; de Smet, P.A.; van den Hoff, O.P.; Egberts, A.C. Nature, frequency and determinants of prescription modifications in Dutch community pharmacies. *Br. J. Clin. Pharmacol.* **2001**, *52*, 85–91.
13. Chen, Y.F.; Neil, K.E.; Avery, A.J.; Dewey, M.E.; Johnson, C. Prescribing errors and other problems reported by community pharmacists. *Ther. Clin. Risk Manag.* **2005**, *1*, 333–342.
14. Hawksworth, G.M.; Corlett, A.J.; Wright, D.J.; Chrystyn, H. Clinical pharmacy interventions by community pharmacists during the dispensing process. *Br. J. Clin. Pharmacol.* **1999**, *47*, 695–700.
15. Leemans, L.; Veroeveren, L.; Bulens, J.; Hendrickx, C.; Keyenberg, W.; Niesten, F.; Vandeberg, J.; Van Hoof, J.; Laekeman, G. Frequency and trends of interventions of prescriptions in Flemish community pharmacies. *Pharm. World Sci.* **2003**, *25*, 65–69.
16. Westein, M.P.; Herings, R.M.; Leufkens, H.G. Determinants of pharmacists' interventions linked to prescription processing. *Pharm. World Sci.* **2001**, *23*, 98–101.
17. Rupp, M.T.; Schondelmeyer, S.W.; Wilson, G.T.; Krause, J.E. Documenting prescribing errors and pharmacist interventions in community pharmacy practice. *Am. Pharm.* **1988**, *NS28*, 30–37.
18. Rupp, M.T.; DeYoung, M.; Schondelmeyer, S.W. Prescribing problems and pharmacist interventions in community practice. *Med. Care* **1992**, *30*, 926–940.
19. Gilligan, A.M.; Miller, K.; Mohney, A.; Montenegro, C.; Schwarz, J.; Warholak, T.L. Analysis of pharmacists' interventions on electronic versus traditional prescriptions in 2 community pharmacies. *Res. Social Adm. Pharm.* **2012**, *8*, 523–532.
20. Odukoya, O.K.; Stone, J.A.; Chui, M.A. How do community pharmacies recover from e-prescription errors? *Res. Social Adm. Pharm.* **2014**, *10*, 837–852.
21. Witte, D.; Dundes, L. Prescription for error: Process defects in a community retail pharmacy. *J. Patient Saf.* **2007**, *3*, 190–194.
22. Ghaferi, A.A.; Osborne, N.H.; Birkmeyer, J.D.; Dimick, J.B. Hospital characteristics associated with failure to rescue from complications after pancreatectomy. *J. Am. Coll. Surg.* **2010**, *211*, 325–330.
23. Aiken, L.H.; Clarke, S.P.; Cheung, R.B.; Sloane D.M.; Silber, J.H. Educational levels of hospital nurses and surgical patient mortality. *JAMA*. **2003**, *290*, 1617–1623.
24. Nestler, D.M.; Fratzke, A.R.; Church, C.J.; Scanlan-Hanson, L.; Sadosty, A.T.; Halasy, M.P.; Finley, J.L.; Boggust, A.; Hess, E.P. Effect of a physician assistant as triage liaison provider on patient throughput in an academic emergency department. *Acad. Emerg. Med.* **2012**, *19*, 1235–1241.
25. Hooker, R.S.; Everett, C.M. The contributions of physician assistants in primary care systems. *Health Soc. Care Community* **2012**, *20*, 20–31.
26. Budzi, D.; Lurie, S.; Singh, K.; Hooker, R. Veterans' perceptions of care by nurse practitioners, physician assistants, and physicians: A comparison from satisfaction surveys. *J. Am. Acad. Nurse Pract.* **2010**, *22*, 170–176.
27. Rogers, A.E.; Dean, G.E.; Hwang, W.T.; Scott, L.D. Role of registered nurses in error prevention, discovery and correction. *Qual. Saf. Health Care* **2008**, *17*, 117–121.
28. Rogers, A.E.; Hwang, W.T.; Scott, L.D.; Aiken, L.H.; Dinges, D.F. The working hours of hospital staff nurses and patient safety. *Health Aff. (Millwood)* **2004**, *23*, 202–212.

29. Aiken, L.H.; Cimiotti, J.P.; Sloane, D.M.; Smith, H.L.; Flynn, L.; Neff, D.F. Effects of nurse staffing and nurse education on patient deaths in hospitals with different nurse work environments. *Med. Care* **2011**, *49*, 1047–1053.
30. Thom, K.A.; Li, S.; Custer, M.; Preas, M.A.; Rew, C.D.; Cafeo, C.; Leekha, S.; Caffo, B.S.; Scalea, T.M.; Lissauer, M.E. Successful implementation of a unit-based quality nurse to reduce central line-associated bloodstream infections. *Am. J. Infect. Control.* **2014**, *42*, 139–143.
31. Franklin, B.D.; Reynolds, M.; Sadler, S.; Hibberd R.; Avery A.J.; Armstrong, S.J.; Mehta, R.; Boyd, M.J.; Barber, N. The effect of the electronic transmission of prescriptions on dispensing errors and prescription enhancements made in English community pharmacies: A naturalistic stepped wedge study. *BMJ Qual. Saf.* **2014**, *23*, 629–638.
32. Franklin, B.; Reynolds, M.; Hibberd, R.; Sadler, S.; Barber, N. Community pharmacists' interventions with electronic prescriptions in England: An exploratory study. *Int. J. Clin. Pharm.* **2013**, *35*, 1030–1035.
33. Odukoya, O.K.; Stone, J.A.; Chui, M.A. Barriers and facilitators to recovering from e-prescribing errors in community pharmacies. *J. Am. Pharm. Assoc.* **2015**, *55*, 52–58.
34. Roulston, K. Interviews in Qualitative Research. In *The Encyclopedia of Applied Linguistics*; Blackwell Publishing Ltd.: Hoboken, NJ, USA, 2012.
35. Graneheim, U.H.; Lundman, B. Qualitative content analysis in nursing research: Concepts, procedures and measures to achieve trustworthiness. *Nurse Educ. Today* **2004**, *24*, 105–112.
36. Flynn, E.A.; Barker, K.N.; Carnahan, B.J. National observational study of prescription dispensing accuracy and safety in 50 pharmacies. *J. Am. Pharm. Assoc.* **2003**, *43*, 191–200.
37. Mott, D.A.; Doucette, W.R.; Gaither, C.A.; Pedersen, C.A.; Schommer, J.C. Pharmacists' attitudes toward worklife: Results from a national survey of pharmacists. *J. Am. Pharm. Assoc.* **2004**, *44*, 326–336.
38. Skrepnek, G.H.; Armstrong, E.P.; Malone, D.C.; Abarca, J.; Murphy, J.E.; Grizzle, A.J.; Rehfeld, R.A.; Woosley, R.L. Workload and availability of technology in metropolitan community pharmacies. *J. Am. Pharm. Assoc.* **2006**, *46*, 154–160.
39. Westrick, S.C. Forward and backward transitions in pharmacy-based immunization services. *Res. Social Adm. Pharm.* **2010**, *6*, 18–31.
40. World Health Organization. Classifying health workers Geneva. Available online: http://www.who.int/hrh/statistics/Health_workers_classification.pdf (accessed on 5 February 2014).
41. Alkhateeb, F.M.; Shields, K.M.; Broedel-Zaugg, K.; Bryan, A.; Snell, J. Credentialing of pharmacy technicians in the USA. *Int. J. Pharm. Pract.* **2011**, *19*, 219–227.
42. Desselle, S.P. Certified pharmacy technicians' views on their medication preparation errors and educational needs. *Am. J. Health Syst. Pharm.* **2005**, *62*, 1992–1997.

5

Do not Lose Your Students in Large Lectures: A Five-Step Paper-Based Model to Foster Students' Participation

Mona Hassan Aburahma

Department of Pharmaceutics and Industrial Pharmacy, Faculty of Pharmacy, Cairo University, Kasr El-Aini Street, Cairo 11562, Egypt; E-Mail: mona_aburahma@hotmail.com

Academic Editor: Maree Donna Simpson

Abstract: Like most of the pharmacy colleges in developing countries with high population growth, public pharmacy colleges in Egypt are experiencing a significant increase in students' enrollment annually due to the large youth population, accompanied with the keenness of students to join pharmacy colleges as a step to a better future career. In this context, large lectures represent a popular approach for teaching the students as economic and logistic constraints prevent splitting them into smaller groups. Nevertheless, the impact of large lectures in relation to student learning has been widely questioned due to their educational limitations, which are related to the passive role the students maintain in lectures. Despite the reported feebleness underlying large lectures and lecturing in general, large lectures will likely continue to be taught in the same format in these countries. Accordingly, to soften the negative impacts of large lectures, this article describes a simple and feasible 5-step paper-based model to transform lectures from a passive information delivery space into an active learning environment. This model mainly suits educational establishments with financial constraints, nevertheless, it can be applied in lectures presented in any educational environment to improve active participation of students. The components and the expected advantages of employing the 5-step paper-based model in large lectures as well as its limitations and ways to overcome them are presented briefly. The impact of applying this model on students' engagement and learning is currently being investigated.

Keywords: large lectures; paper-based approach: economic constrains; active learning; feedback; writing

---

1. Introduction

In the Middle East, Egypt pioneered in introducing pharmacy education, which started at Cairo University in 1824. Although Egypt has the largest number of pharmacy colleges in the Middle East, either public or private, that results in more than 13,000 pharmacist graduates annually [1], pharmacy colleges are still experiencing significant growth in students' enrollments annually. Accordingly, lecturers in the pharmacy colleges are forced to rely on traditional lectures that span typically for 1 h for one-way transmission of factual information to passive students. The wide spread of large lectures in the Egyptian public universities represents an economic necessity born due to resource restrictions associated with the large number of students.

In educational literature, there is great discrepancy in defining the term "large lectures" [2], nevertheless, in this article, the large lecture is a representation of any lecture that contains more than 100 students.

Generally speaking, lectures are ideal for presenting information or delivering educational content to a large number of students in a cost-effective way [3]. In addition, lectures permit maximum teacher control regarding the pacing and range of material presented. In relation to students, lectures present the least threat to students, since they are not obliged to participate in comparison to workshops or tutorials [3]. In addition, lectures represent a consistent learning experience for all students [4].

On the other hand, large lectures suffer from significant shortcomings due to the impersonal nature between students and the lecturer that sometimes leads to students frustration or disconnection from the educational environment [3,4]. In addition, traditional didactic lectures have serious educational limitations as they mainly improve the students' ability to recall knowledge and do not suit higher levels of learning that require active participation and engagement of students within the educational environment [5,6]. Further, didactic lectures might not be the optimum mean to teach students who differ greatly in their cognitive skills and background knowledge. Nevertheless, as the lecture proceeds, the students' attention, which has been reported to be around 15–20 min [7,8], wanes rapidly when the lecturer relies on just reading or explaining the information present on the PowerPoint slides projected onto a screen [9]. More recently, it was reported that the current generation learners have even shorter attention span that lasts 7 min [10] or less [11]. Another drawback of large lectures is the lack of instant feedback on students' understanding or progress during information delivery [3].

Opposing didactic lectures where students just passively listening to the lecturer, active learning strategies address the educational contents in an interactive manner. As learning basically relies on what the learner does not the lecturer [3]. In active learning, the students perform instructional activities and think about what they are doing through reading, writing, discussing, or being engaged in solving problems [3]. This allows the students to reflect back upon what they have learnt and eventually produce significant improvement in terms of the learning outcomes. Ideal active learning environments are rich in instructional activities that engage students in higher-order thinking activities such as analysis, evaluation and synthesis to improve conceptual understanding, problem-solving and critical thinking in students [12–14].

2. Reported Techniques to Initiate Active Participation in Lectures

To mend the weaknesses of large lectures for more pedagogically fruitful environment, many lecturers have proposed different ways to promote active participation of students and reduce the complete dependence on traditional lecturing [15,16]. Typical techniques encompassed engaging the students in small group discussions during the lectures. Yet, limitations were reported for these methods, wherein it was tough to manage group discussion in large lectures and ensure active involvement of all students [17]. Henley and Oakley (1998) integrated group debates in lectures to improve student-student interaction. However, this approach might not be suitable for class size that exceeds 100 students and lasts for 1 h [18]. In other cases, the large lectures based courses were split into smaller-group courses encompassing discussion to foster active participation [19]. Yet, this approach often requires a complete curriculum review that is somehow beneficial, however, many lecturers are not in a position to do this and they do not have choice in the lecture size that they teach.

Recently, different studies have included technology-based approaches like personal response systems or clickers to engage and motivate students within the lectures [20,21]. Yet, financial barriers limit the adoption of these engaging pedagogies due to the unavailability of laptops or tablets for all students in public pharmacy colleges . It is worth noting that colorcolored cards can be used as a low cost and low tech replacement for clickers. Another published way to amend the dynamics of large lectures and widen students' participation was by allowing them to tweet their questions to the lecturer via Twitter. However, the main drawback is that tweeting can divert students' attention away from the lecture and disrupt the learning process [22–24]. Not to mention that this method discourages the face-to-face (student/teacher and student/student) interaction and communication.

3. Description of the 5-Step Paper-Based Model

Under all conditions and regardless of the number of students in the lecture, any learning environment should provide an opportunity for deep understanding of the material for all students. Accordingly, lecturers are obliged to identify and implement viable methods of instruction for large lectures to optimize students' involvement using the available resources either low-cost or expensive.

In the current article, a simple 5-step paper based-model comprising various student centered activities is presented to initiate students' engagement in large lectures. The main components of the 5-step paper-based approach are presented in Figure 1.

The key advantage to implementing this model is that it does notdoes not require any additional resources except photocopying the 5-step paper.

A brief outline for the 5-step paper-based model using a "Rheology and Viscosity" lecture delivered for pharmacy students as an example is presented in Figure 2.

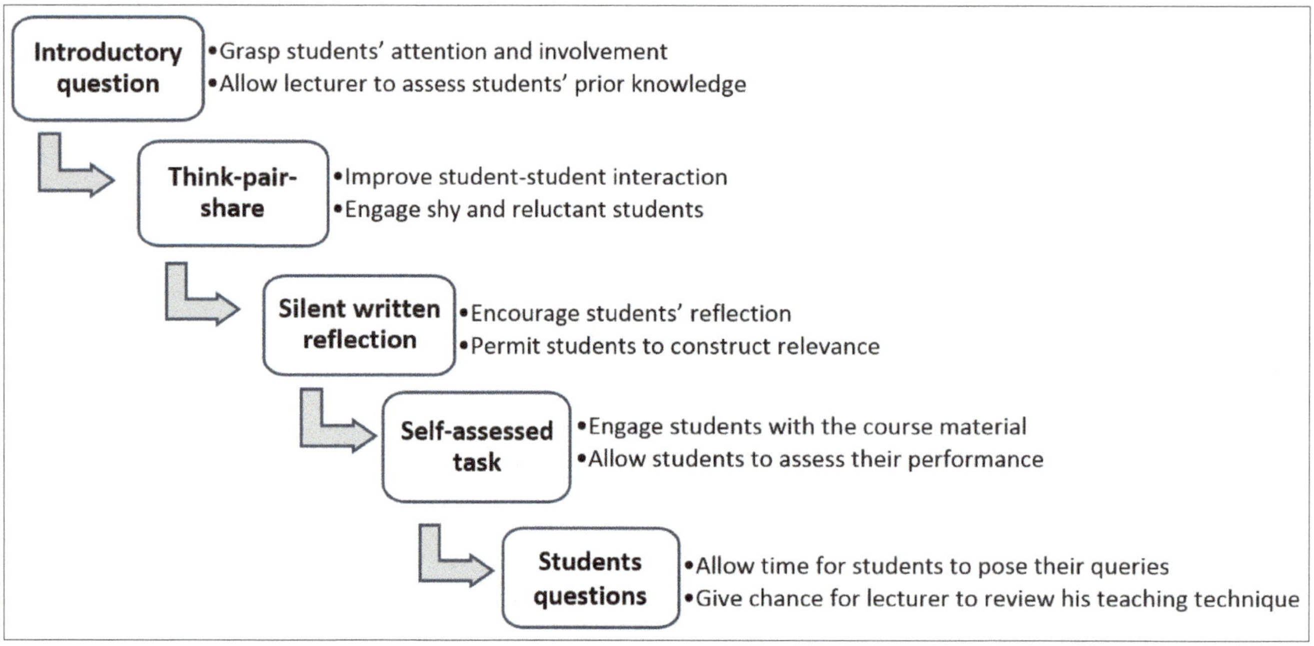

Figure 1. The main components of the 5-step paper-based approach.

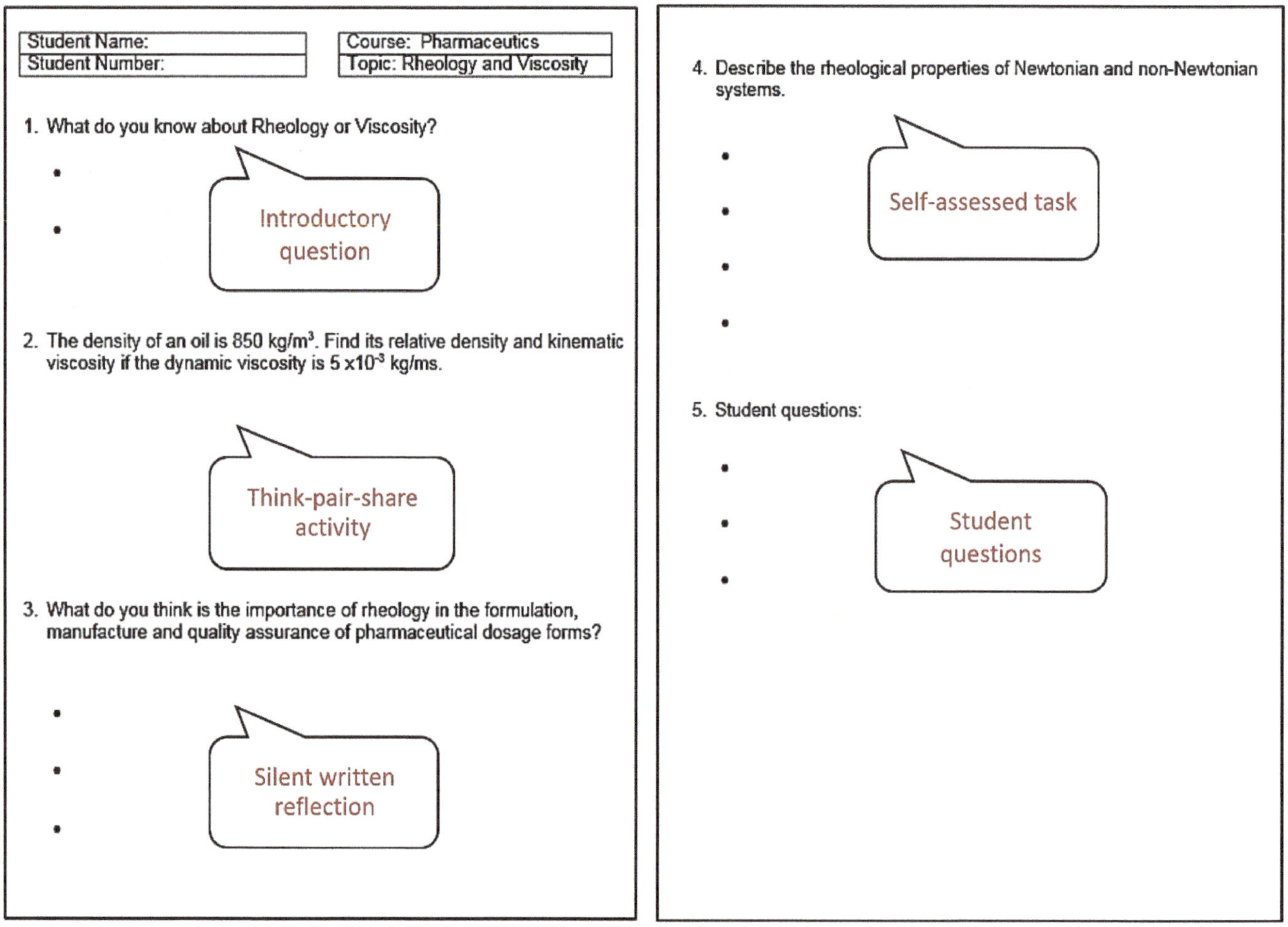

Figure 2. Sample outline for the 5-step paper-based model using a "Rheology and Viscosity" lecture delivered to pharmacy students.

To create time for active learning in the lecture, the students were instructed to read and prepare the lecture before class to gain background information. At the beginning of the lecture, the 5-step papers are placed at the entry of the lecture hall so that students would take their papers while entering. To encourage them to take the process seriously and provide them with a sense of ownership, the students are required to write their names and respond to all the tasks on the 5-step paper at the set time. For each task, the students are committed to condense and present their ideas/responses in short written statements in the provided space. Writing is an integral component in this model to active engage students and keep them involved in tasks [25]. At the end of the lecture, the 5-step papers will ultimately be collected from the students although they are unassessed and do not count for points or grades in the course.

Based on the proposed model, the lecture is divided into approximately 3 or 4 lecture chunks/main points dispersed with preset writing tasks involving students discussion, reflection, and self-assessment to balance lecturing-style instructions with students-centered activities. The students' tasks are integrated at certain timings during the 1-hour lecture as presented in Figure 3.

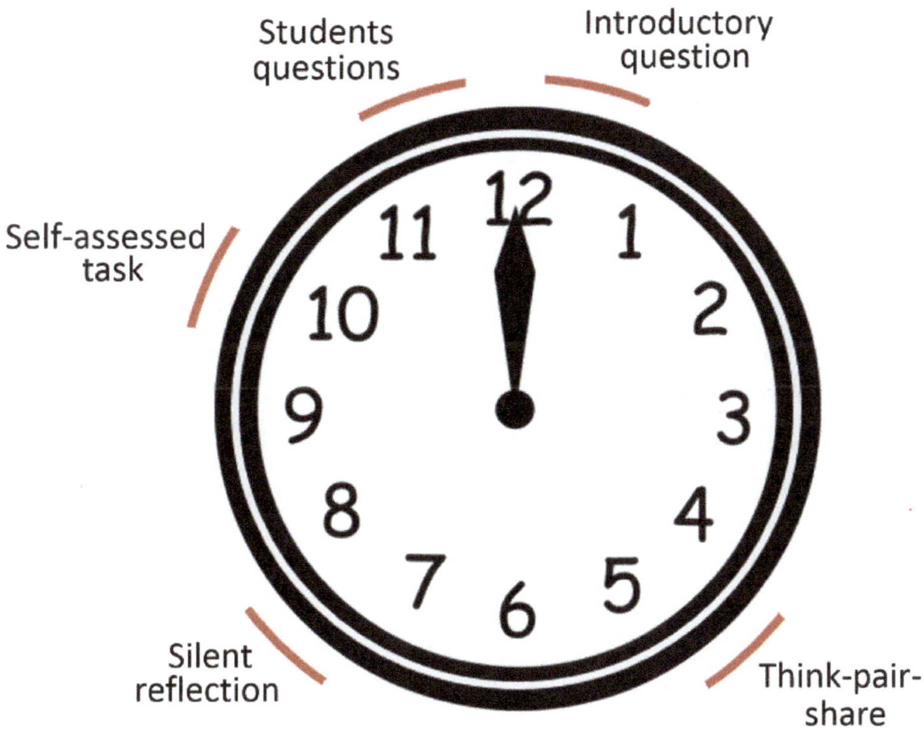

Figure 3. 5-step paper-based model components dispersed during 1-hour lecture.

Such pacing by breaking down the 1 h lecture into short segments is essential to maintain students' attention during the whole lecture by restarting their attention clock. After each task, lecturer feedback is given to students regarding their progress. A clear explanation of the components/tasks of the 5-step paper-based approach is presented hereafter:

3.1. Introductory Question

Incorporating an effective question at the beginning of the lecture is essential to reinforce students' attention early on by challenging them to think and encouraging immediate participation [26,27]. The lecturer can also use this introductory question to determine the level of students' prior knowledge for key concepts related to the lecture topic to build upon his new information [28]. Using this initially engaging approach, the lecturer brings the students "on lecture stage" with him/her instead of leaving them to passively hear the lecture. All the students are encouraged to write their responses on the submitted paper and few students are randomly selected to state their responses. It is worth mentioning that the lecturer ought to deal tactfully with all students' contributions irrespective of the accuracy of the received responses.

3.2. Think-Pair-Share

In this section, the students are given a question, preferably a challenging one, to elicit higher level thinking. All the students are allowed to think then construct their responses individually, then, pair with the neighboring student to share their ideas followed by writing their response. Randomly selected pairs of students are given the opportunity to share their response in the lecture followed by lecturer feedback. The verbal articulation between the students in this activity offers the students, especially the shy or reluctant ones who find responding in large lectures intimidating, an opportunity to discuss and confirm their responses with peers resulting in more confidence and openness to share ideas. Educational researches indicated that peer discussions lead not only to improvements in students' conceptual understanding and performance but also nurture greater involvement and self-confidence [29,30].

3.3. Silent Written Reflection

In this section, the students are given time to silently reflect on the key ideas presented in the lecture then seek their relevance or application in real life. The students are allowed to write their responses then randomly selected students share their ideas with the whole class followed by feedback from the lecturer. This activity helps the students to appreciate the relevance of the taught content to their future career which arise their interest and motivation in the subject content [31].

3.4. Self-Assessed Task

In this section, the students are given time to either summarize the main ideas delivered during the whole lecture or answer a comprehensive question in a pre-set time interval. After that, the lecturer presents the expected model answer and allow students to self-assess their written responses. Getting students to present their ideas in writing is a good approach for them to identify their misconceptions. This approach also assists the students in monitoring and evaluating the quality of their thinking and allow them to easily identify discrepancies between their current performance and the desired performance [3,32].

3.5. Student Questions

Finally, before the end of the lecture, the students are allowed to think, formulate and write down any questions they have. It is reported that students need time to actually reflect on previous instructions and articulate questions [33]. This simple practice of providing students adequate time to frame a question normally increase students' contribution. Subsequently, that lecturer responds to the students questions.

At the end, the 5-step papers are collected from the students so that the lecturer would have the chance to gauge their participation and performance and address the unanswered questions, if present, in the coming lectures.

4. Advantages and Limitations of the 5-Step Paper-Based Model

This article describes a basic 5-step paper-based model that is based on a mixed-format to improve the pedagogy of large lectures in educational environment with limited resources.

The components of the 5-step paper based model are considered to emotionally and intellectually enhance interactions among students, the lecturer, and the lecture content using several tasks completed by students in writing.

In this model, the immediate feedback, whether to or from students, represents an essential element that caters for a two-way learning experience. Lecturer's feedback helps the students in validating their understanding of concepts and apprehending their progress. In addition, students' feedback give the lecturer an opportunity to evaluate students' understanding and ascertain difficulty areas and adapts his teaching pace and methodology to meet their learning needs [34].

According to Biggs [35], four key components are essential in a learning process for students to achieve deeper learning: (a) Motivational context: where students are required to realize that the learning goals and processes are relevant to them, (b) Learner activity: where students are required to be active as deep learning is connected with doing rather than receiving passively, (c) Interaction with others: as discussions with peers promote students' learning, and (d) Well-structured knowledge base: as new learning needs to be built on students' prior knowledge and experience. Mapping of the presented 5-step paper-based model to Biggs four key features to achieve deeper learning is presented in Figure 4.

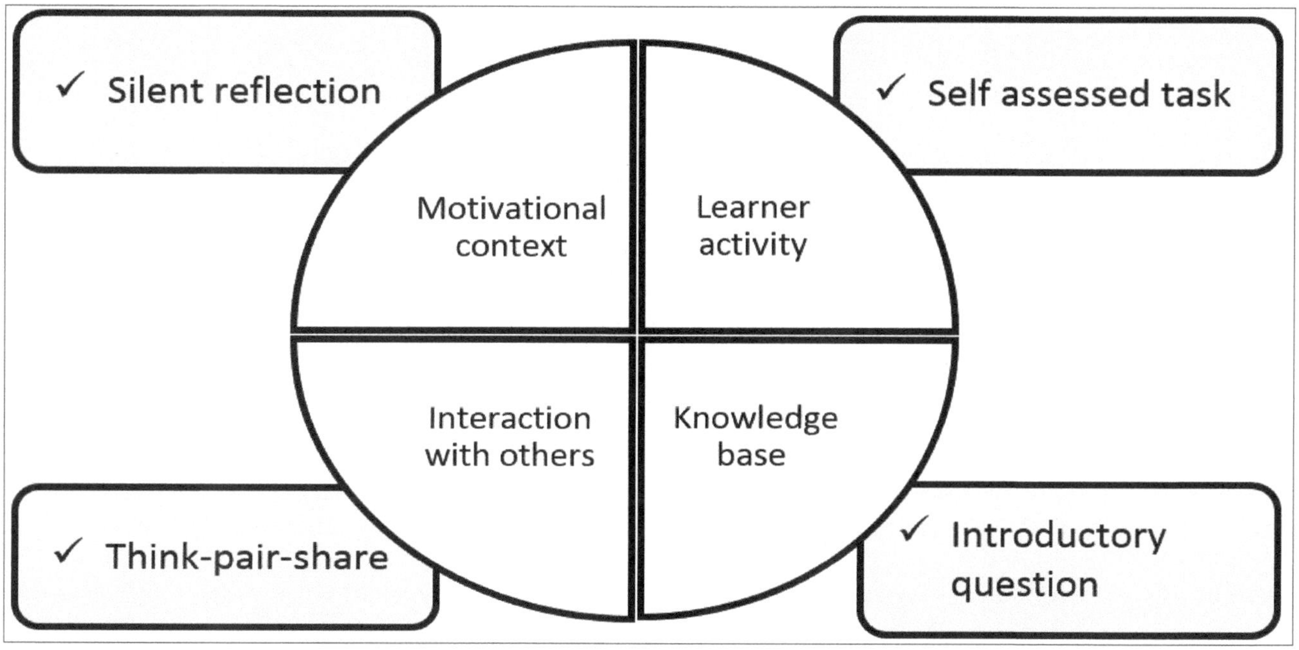

Figure 4. Mapping of 5-step paper-based model to Biggs four key features for deeper learning.

Table 1 summarizes the anticipated limitations that might be encountered when applying the 5-step paper-based model and types of solutions that may be employed.

Table 1. Issues that might arise during implementing the 5-Step paper based approach.

Problem	Potential Solution
Some students might find it hard to speak up in front of the whole class	Giving the student time to think about the question and then write their answer may be helpful. Think-pair-share activity allow shy students to present ideas to their partner giving them more confidence in their responses.
Some students are reluctant to participate in the activities	Allowing students to write their responses may motivate them to participate. Collecting the papers at the end of the lecture may facilitate tracking of non-participating students.
Off topic discussions between students during the think-pair-share activity	Short time limit- given for the think-pair-share activity decreases the chance for off-topic discussion.
High load for the lecturer to track students participation and questions posed from the collected papers	A quick scan of the papers can give an overview of the whole class participation in activities. Involving teaching assistants to compile the unanswered students' questions. This might be a good learning excersise for them as it aquaints them with their future roles.
More time is consumed during the lecture than what was already anticipated for each task	Putting a tight time limit for each activity and limiting the writing space for each activity so that the students are concise in their replies.
Distribution and collection of papers at the beginning of the lecture and at the end is tedious and time consuming	Placing the papers at the entry of the lecture hall so that the studunts can collect them when they enter the lecture. Assigning students to collect the papers at the end of the lecture. The collected papers can be a good representation of students' attendance in large lectures where their attendance is not usually tracked.
Not covering all the lecture contents as time is consumed in the students tasks	Assigning some topics for students to study on their own to promote their self-study abilities.
Lecturer time is consumed in preparing the 5-step paper based approach, redesign the lectures and realigning the self-study content	Initially, time is needed for lectures modification and designing the 5-step paper. However, once designed, they can be used for future classes with only slight modification if necessary.
Students may be distracted by the activities and attempt to read them before the lecturer permits	The paper may contain uncompleted questions that would be presented in the lecture slides at the preset time.
Photocopying is an additional expense	Providing small space for responding to each task so that the students are concise in their replies and not more than one paper is required for each student in the lecture.
Redundancy of the same presented format in all the lectures might decrease attention due to the loss of novelty.	Include other low cost active learning and collaborative activities that suit large lecture settings.

5. Implications for Implementing the 5-Step Paper-Based Model

In the 5-step paper-model, proper planning for how the content would be taught and ensuring that the students' activities address the learning outcomes of the lecture is a necessity to creatively use the lecture time. The questions/tasks presented must be effectively designed to simulate deeper understanding and enhance pedagogical goals beyond just content memorizing [36].

The included students' tasks should be specific to prevent students' confusion. In addition, the lecturer should be strict with timekeeping of each task to efficaciously present and conclude the lecture content and discuss troublesome concepts within the allotted time. Collectively, the tasks of the 5-step paper-based model should not take more than 20 min of a 1 h lecture.

Although the lecturers are mainly held responsible for students' learning, the recruitment of one or two teaching assistants in large lectures may be required to assist in reviewing the students' questions section in the 5-step paper-based model, and to address the unanswered questions during the subsequent lectures or laboratory sessions to complete the feedback loop. It is of paramount importance to make sure that all the students' questions are being recognized to motivate them to pose their queries in the coming lectures.

It is of no doubt that implementing active learning techniques takes time away from lectures, allowing insufficient time to complete the lecture content. In this context, different researches suggested that it is not essential to cover all the topics in the lectures. Some topics could be independently learned by the students to prepare them for their role as self-directed and lifelong learners [30].

For successful implementation of such approach in large lectures, it is advisable to delegate activities to different students in each lecture, like collecting and distributing the papers. In general, involving the students in the educational process might be helpful to develop their sense of responsibility and allow more intimate interaction with their lecturers.

6. Conclusions

Based on the anticipated increase in students' enrollment in the public pharmacy colleges in Egypt, large lectures will continue to be the main method of teaching at least during the coming 10–15 years. Therefore, researches that investigate active and collaborative teaching methods that suit large lectures are paramount.

This article presents a simple 5-step paper-based model as an inclusive and engaging mean to increase students' participation in large lectures in colleges with economic barriers. All that is required is the distribution of the 5-step paper to the students at the beginning of the lecture to engage them within the educational process using different writing tasks that involve students' interaction, reflection and self-assessment, then collecting the papers at the end of the lecture. The presented model can be adapted or modified to suit individual lecture contents, course outcomes and teaching style. Although it is presented and discussed in terms of pharmacy discipline in this article, the 5-step paper-based model is relevant to teaching and learning in all disciplines. This model might also provide a valuable direction for lecturers to re-evaluate their routine in large lectures and serve as a basic tool to help them in adapting and ideally improving their lecturing technique.

7. Implications for the Future

This article presents a simple attempt to improve the teaching experience in large lectures instead of accepting its weaknesses. Moreover, the presented model might encourage lecturers who are wedged with large lectures to advance their lecturing practices and strive for excellence using available resources.

This paper-based model will be implemented in lectures for different courses in the pharmacy college to demonstrate its applicability. Both, unbiased lecturers' perspectives along with students' perspectives using different survey instruments that include questionnaires and open-ended questions in addition to pre- and post-intervention students test scores would be analyzed to assess the effectiveness of this model and give more realistic insight into its value and limitations.

8. Declaration

The views expressed in this paper are of the author and not an official position of the affiliated institute.

Conflicts of Interest

The author reports no conflict of interest.

References

1. Kheir, N.; Zaidan, M.; Younes, H.; Hajj, M.E.; Wilbur, K.; Jewesson, P.J. Pharmacy education and practice in 13 Middle Eastern countries. *Am. J. Pharm. Educ.* **2008**, *72*, Article 133.
2. Christopher, D.A. Interactive large classes: The dynamics of teacher/student interaction. *J. Bus. Econ. Res.* **2003**, *1*, 81–98.
3. Bonwell, C.; Eison, J. *Active Learning: Creating Excitement in the Classroom* (*ASHE-ERIC Higher Education Reports*); George Washington University: Washington, DC, USA, 1991. Available online: http://files.eric.ed.gov/fulltext/ED336049.pdf (accessed on 1 April 2015).
4. Carpenter, J.M. Effective teaching methods for large classes. *J. Fam. Con. Sci. Educ.* **2006**, *24*, 13–23.
5. De Caprariis, P.; Barman, C.; Magee, P. Monitoring the benefits of active learning exercises in introductory survey courses in science: An attempt to improve the education of prospective public school teachers. *J. Scholarsh. Teach. Learn.* **2001**, *1*, 1–11.
6. Powell, K. Science education: Spare me the lecture. *Nature* **2003**, *425*, 234–236.
7. Stuart, J.; Rutherford, R. Medical student concentration during lectures. *Lancet* **1978**, *312*, 514–516.
8. Frederick, P.J. The lively lecture-8 variations. *College Teach.* **1986**, *34*, 43–50.
9. Schwerdt, G.; Wuppermann, A.C. Is traditional teaching really all that bad? A within-student between-subject approach. *Econ. Educ. Rev.* **2011**, *30*, 365–379.
10. Baker, R.; Matulich, E.; Papp, R. Teach me in the way I learn: Education and the internet generation. *J. College Teach. Learn.* **2007**, *4*, 27–32.
11. Bunce, D.M.; Flens, E.A.; Neiles, K.Y. How long can students pay attention in class? A study of student attention decline using clickers. *J. Chem. Educ.* **2010**, *87*, 1438–1443.

12. Eison, J. *Using Active Learning Instructional Strategies to Create Excitement and Enhance Learning*; 2010. Available online: http://www.cte.cornell.edu/documents/presentations/Eisen-Handout.pdf (accessed on 1 April 2015).
13. Allen, D.; Tanner, K. Infusing active learning into the large-enrollment biology class: Seven strategies, from the simple to complex. *Cell Biol. Educ.* **2005**, *4*, 262–268.
14. Armbruster, P.; Patel, M.; Johnson, E.; Weiss, M. Active learning and student-centered pedagogy improve student attitudes and performance in introductory biology. *CBE Life Sci. Educ.* **2009**, *8*, 203–213.
15. Macgregor, J.; Cooper, J.L.; Smith, K.A.; Robinson, P. (Eds). Strategies for Energizing Large Classes: From small groups to learning communities. In *New Directions for Teaching and Learning*; Jossey-Bass Inc.: San Francisco, CA, USA, 2000; Volume 81.
16. Bligh, D.A. *What's the Use of Lectures*? Jossey-Bass Publishers: San Francisco, CA, USA, 2000.
17. Nicol, D.J.; Boyle, J.T. Peer instruction *versus* class-wide discussion in large classes: A comparison of two interaction methods in the wired classroom. *Stud. High. Educ.* **2003**, *28*, 457–473.
18. Hensley, T.; Oakley, M. The challenge of the large lecture class: Making it more like a small seminar. *Polit. Sci. Polit.* **1998**, *31*, 47–51.
19. Persky, A.M.; Pollack, G.M. Transforming a large-class lecture course to a smaller-group interactive course. *Am. J. Pharm. Educ.* **2010**, *74*, Article 170.
20. Liu, F.C.; Gettig, J.P.; Fjortoft, N. Impact of a student response system on short- and long-term learning in a drug literature evaluation course. *Am. J. Pharm. Educ.* **2010**, *74*, Article 6.
21. Titman, A.C.; Lancaster, G.A. Personal response systems for teaching postgraduate statistics to small groups. *J. Stat. Educ.* **2011**, *19*, 1–20.
22. Bussieres, J.F.; Metras, M.E.; Leclerc, G. Use of Moodle, ExamSoft and Twitter in first-year pharmacy course. *Am. J. Pharm. Educ.* **2012**, *76*, Article 94.
23. Mistry, V. Critical care training: Using Twitter as a teaching tool. *Br. J. Nurs.* **2011**, *20*, 1292–1296.
24. Fox, B.I.; Varadarajan, V. Use of Twitter to encourage interaction in a multi-campus pharmacy management course. *Am. J. Pharm. Educ.* **2011**, *75*, Article 88.
25. Bridgeman, A.J. Using very short writing tasks to promote understanding in chemistry. In Proceedings of the Australian Conference on Science and Mathematics Education, University of Sydney, Sydney, Australia, 26 September 2012; pp. 110–117.
26. Dewinstanley, P.; Bjork, R. Successful lecturing: Presenting information in ways that engage effective processing. *New Dir. Teach. Learn.* **2002**, *89*, 19–31.
27. Frederick, P. Engaging students actively in large lecture settings. In *Engaging Large Classes: Strategies and Techniques for College Faculty*; Stanley, C., Porter, M., Eds.; Anker Publishing Company: Bolton, MA, USA, 2002; pp. 58–66.
28. Ashwin, P.; Trigwell, K. Evoked prior experiences in first-year university student learning. *High. Educ. Res. Dev.* **2012**, *31*, 449–463.
29. Perkins, D.; Saris, N. A jigsaw classroom technique for undergraduate statistics courses. *Teach. Psychol.* **2001**, *28*, 111–113.
30. Yoder, J.; Hochevar, C. Encouraging active learning can improve students' performance on examinations. *Teach. Psychol.* **2005**, *32*, 91–95.

31. Frymier, A.B.; Schulman, G.M. "What's in it for me?" Increasing content relevance to enhance students' motivation. *Commun. Educ.* **1995**, *44*, 40–50.
32. McDonald, B.; Boud, D. The impact of self-assessment on achievement: The effects of self-assessment training on performance in external examinations. *Assess. Educ.* **2003**, *10*, 209–220.
33. Rowe, M.B. Wait time: Slowing down may be a way of speeding up. *J. Teach. Educ.* **1986**, *37*, 43–50.
34. Nicol, D.J.; Macfarlane-Dick, D. Formative assessment and self-regulated learning: A model and seven principles of good feedback practice. *Stud. High. Educ.* **2006**, *31*, 199–218.
35. Biggs, J.B. Approaches to the enhancement of tertiary teaching. *High. Educ. Res. Dev.* **1989**, *8*, 7–25.
36. Newble, D.; Cannon, R. A handbook for teachers in universities and colleges. In *A Guide to Improving Teaching Methods*, 4th ed.; Kogan Page: London, UK, 2000.

6

A European Competence Framework for Industrial Pharmacy Practice in Biotechnology

Jeffrey Atkinson [1,*], Pat Crowley [2], Kristien De Paepe [3], Brian Gennery [4], Andries Koster [5], Luigi Martini [4], Vivien Moffat [6], Jane Nicholson [7], Gunther Pauwels [8], Giuseppe Ronsisvalle [9], Vitor Sousa [10], Chris van Schravendijk [11] and Keith Wilson [12]

[1] Pharmacolor Consultants Nancy (pcn-consultants), 12 rue de Versigny, 54600 Villers, France

[2] Callum Consultancy, 571 Berwyn Baptist Road, Devon, PA 19333, USA; E-Mail: ktcrowley@msn.com

[3] Vrije Universiteit Brussel (VUB), Laarbeeklaan 103, 1090 Brussels, Belgium; E-Mail: kdepaepe@vub.ac.be

[4] Department of Pharmacy, Waterloo Campus, King's College London, 150 Stamford Street SE1, 9NH, London, UK; E-Mail: brian.gennery@kcl.ac.uk (B.G.); luigi.martini@kcl.ac.uk (L.M.)

[5] European Association of Faculties of Pharmacy (EAFP), Department Pharmaceutical Sciences, Utrecht University, PO Box 80082, 3508 TB Utrecht, The Netherlands; E-Mail: A.S.Koster@uu.nl

[6] European Federation of Pharmaceutical Industries and Associations (EFPIA), Rue du Trône, 108, 1050 Brussels, Belgium; E-Mail: vivien.moffat@amgen.com

[7] European Industrial Pharmacists' Group (EIPG), 4 avenue Ruysdael, Paris, France; E-Mail: jane@nicholj.plus.com

[8] Genzyme Flanders, Cipalstraat 8, 2440 Geel, Belgium; E-Mail: gunther.pauwels@Genzyme.com

[9] Pharmacy Department, Universitá di Catania, Viale Andrea Doria 6, 95125, Catania, Italy; E-Mail: giuseppe.ronsisvalle@unict.it

[10] Areta International, via Roberto LePetit, 21040 Gerenzano, Italy; E-Mail: vsousa@aretaint.com

[11] Vrije Universiteit Brussel (VUB), Laarbeeklaan 103, 1090 Brussels, Belgium; E-Mail: chrisvs@vub.ac.be

[12] Life and Health Sciences, Aston University, Aston Triangle, B75 6D9 Birmingham, UK; E-Mail: K.a.wilson@aston.ac.uk

* Author to whom correspondence should be addressed; E-Mail: Jeffrey.atkinson@univ-lorraine.fr

Academic Editor: Maree Donna Simpson

Abstract: The PHAR-IN ("*Competences for industrial pharmacy practice in biotechnology*") looked at whether there is a difference in how industrial employees and academics rank competences for practice in the biotechnological industry. A small expert panel consisting of the authors of this paper produced a biotechnology competence framework by drawing up an initial list of competences then ranking them in importance using a three-stage Delphi process. The framework was next evaluated and validated by a large expert panel of academics (n = 37) and industrial employees (n = 154). Results show that priorities for industrial employees and academics were similar. The competences for biotechnology practice that received the highest scores were mainly in:

- "Research and Development",
- ""Upstream" and "Downstream" Processing',
- "Product development and formulation",
- "Aseptic processing",
- "Analytical methodology",
- "Product stability", and
- "Regulation".

The main area of disagreement was in the category "Ethics and drug safety" where academics ranked competences higher than did industrial employees.

Keywords: education; pharmacy; industry; Europe; biotechnology

1. Introduction

The PHAR-IN ("*Competences for industrial pharmacy practice in biotechnology*") [1] consortium consists of professional organisations representing industrial employees, *viz*, the European Industrial Pharmacists' Group (EIPG) [2], and the European Federation of Pharmaceutical Industries and Associations, (EFPIA) [3], together with pharmacy academics from the European Association of Faculties of Pharmacy (EAFP) [4]. Amongst other projects, the PHAR-IN consortium looked at whether there is a difference in how industrial employees and academics rank competences for practice in the biotechnological industry. A small expert panel consisting of the authors of this paper produced a biotechnology competence framework by drawing up an initial list of competences then ranking them in importance using a three-stage Delphi process. The framework was next evaluated and validated by a large expert panel of academics drawn from EAFP (n = 37), and by industrial employees that were members of EIPG, EFPIA and European Federation for Pharmaceutical Sciences (EUFEPS [5]) (n = 154).

The PHARMINE study (*Pharmacy Education in Europe*) found that a substantial number (37,308) of European pharmacists (6% of the total workforce) work in industry [6], this is similar to the world-wide figure of 10% given by the International Pharmaceutical Federation [7]. Recent publications have outlined the many profound changes in the drug industry, one of the most notable of which is a switch towards biotechnology [8,9]. The question arises, therefore, as to how to adapt pharmacy education to this switch towards biotechnology; this is under discussion in Europe [10], Australia [11] and the USA [12]. The PHARMINE study cited above found that in addition to the traditional courses in pharmaceutical technology (representing an average of 12% of contact hours of the five-year European pharmacy course), some pharmacy departments (10/31 studied) do give elective pre-graduate courses in industrial pharmacy but these are mainly concerned with chemical production of drugs and other matters such as regulatory affairs. The PHARMINE study also found that 11/31 departments give post-graduate courses in industrial pharmacy.

A potential mismatch may exist between the competences of recently graduated pharmacists and the professional requirements in industry if sufficient input from industrial stake-holders is not obtained. Furthermore, although many academics are actively involved in research, fewer are involved in the drug industry. The above situation requires that the educational system be capable of offering the right courses to produce the right person with the right competences at the right time. This paper presents a European competence framework for biotechnological practice in industry, the methodology by which this framework was produced, and the rankings of competences by industrial employees and academics.

2. Methodology

The competence framework was produced by the Delphi technique [13]. Delphi methodology has been used to produce consensus competence frameworks for healthcare professionals such as nurses [14] and medical doctors [15]; it has also been used to produce competence frameworks for secondary level teachers in biotechnology [16,17]. To our knowledge, Delphi has not been used to produce a competence framework for professionals working in biotechnology.

A small expert panel consisting of the 13 authors of this paper (six with an academic background, seven with an industrial background) produced a proposal for a competence framework, starting with an initial framework produced by two industrial consultants (BG and PC) and based on their expert knowledge and on recent literature in biotechnology. This version was then subjected to three Delphi rounds within the small expert panel producing a version that contained 46 proposals for competences in 13 categories. This competence framework was then evaluated and validated by a large expert panel consisting of (1) academics (members of EAFP), and (2) industrial employees (members of EIPG, EFPIA, EUFEPS and the Innovative Medicines Initiative (IMI) [18]) (using *surveymonkey* [19], see Appendix).

The large expert panel was invited to rank the 46 proposed competences using a uni-dimensional Likert ranking method [20] with a scale of 1 to 4. This scale with an even number of choices contrasts with scales with an odd number of choices that allow for a "neutral" option. The expert panel also had the possibility to check a "I am unable to rank this premise" box There was also the possibility of skipping a competence by not replying at all (blank).

The panel could also comment on the various competences.

3. Statistical Analysis

Response rates were calculated as the sum of the responses in ranks 1 through 4 divided by the total number of responses possible (=46 competences × 153 industrial respondents or × 35 academic respondents). Blanks and "I am unable to rank this premise" were pooled.

Ranking scores are expressed as means; this is for descriptive purposes only. Statistical significance was based on the Wilcoxon signed rank test for differences from the global median of the population (industrial employees or academics). The overall median was calculated from all answers given in order to make it possible to identify answers which score higher (or lower) than this overall median. Chi-square was used to compare results of academics with those of industrial employees.

Ordinal consensus was calculated using the Leik technique [21].

The statistical tests used are described on the GraphPad website [22].

4. Results

The distribution of academic and industrial respondents over the different European countries was not equal (chi-square = 72, d.f. = 1 and 19, $p < 0.0001$) (Table 1, top). There was no significant difference for age distribution; the main age groups represented were in the 41–60 years range (Table 2, bottom).

Table 1. Survey population characteristics.

Country of residence.

	Industrial Employees		**Academics**	
	Number	**%**	**Number**	**%**
Country of residence				
Austria	1	0.6		
Belgium	12	7.8	5	13.5
Bulgaria	2	1.3	4	10.8
Czech Republic	1	0.6		
Denmark	5	3.2		
Finland	18	11.7		
France	15	9.7	1	2.7
Germany	8	5.2		
Greece		0.0	2	5.4
Hungary	1	0.6		
Ireland	8	5.2		
Italy	6	3.9	17	45.9
Malta			1	2.7
Portugal	14	9.1	1	2.7
Serbia	1	0.6		
Spain	1	0.6		
Sweden	3	1.9		
Switzerland	20	13.0		
The Netherlands	15	9.7	1	2.7
UK	23	14.9	5	13.5
Total	154 (1 did not reply)	100	37 (2 did not reply)	100

Chi-square = 72, d.f. 19, p value < 0.0001.

Age group.

	Industrial Employees		Academics	
	Number	%	Number	%
Age group (years)				
18–30	13	8.4	3	7.7
31–40	29	18.7	9	23.1
41–50	46	29.7	13	33.3
51–60	54	34.8	9	23.1
61–70	11	7.1	4	10.3
>70	2	1.3	1	2.6
Total	155	100	39	100

Chi-square = 3.9, d.f. 5, p value 0.5617.

Overall ranking profiles (ranks 1 through 4) and response rates were not different between industrial employees and academics (Table 2).

Table 2. Frequencies of rankings (as % total possible) by industrial employees and academics of 46 competences for biotechnological professionals.

Rank	Industrial Employees (n = 153)	Academics (n = 35)
1	5.0	3.0
2	15.0	13.0
3	22.3	32.5
4	27.5	32.6
Blanks + "I am unable to rank this premise"	30.2	18.9
Total	100	100

Chi-squares on differences between industrial employees and academics regarding frequencies of ranks 1–4 = 2.12, d.f. 6, p value 0.9085.

Leik ordinal consensus based on the frequencies of ranking given in Table 2 was for industrial employees 0.50 and for academics 0.58.

Both academics and industrial employees ranked scores significantly above the global median for categories "Research and Development", '"Upstream" and "Downstream" Processing', "Product development and formulation", "Aseptic processing", "Analytical methodology", "Product stability", and "Regulation". (Appendix Table A1). Only for competences "Describe the range of products available with recombinant DNA technology", "Employ pharmaco-epidemiology skills, including the statistical methodologies to strategically evaluate a drug product and produce a risk management plan", "Interpret clinical trial designs that address specific ethical issues e.g., in special patient populations" and "Design a consent process that ensures that subjects are not coerced into participating in clinical trials" was there a significant difference (chi-square) between academics and industrial employees—academics scoring higher than industrial employees.

There were 59 comments on the following:

- The clarity of the survey
- The context within which answers should be given
- The specificity to biotechnology and not to industrial pharmacy practice in general

- The educational level (foundation or specialist) at which the competence would be acquired
- The balance between the relative importance of different competences

5. Discussion

5.1. Delphi Methodology and Statistics

The Delphi methodology implies that surveying be anonymous and so individuals were not targeted. This contrasts to the survey of pre-selected experts in which the answers obtained depends on the prior selection of the experts. Here, no limitations were fixed on the possibility to participate. Anonymity is a minor issue in this study as the Delphi method requires complete anonymity. In the PHAR-IN study, the identities of the participants were known to the authors but not to each other.

The Delphi technique was also double in that there was first a small expert panel three-round Delphi process and this was followed by a larger panel evaluation and validation. This contrasts to many studies that use the first step (e.g., Stupans, *et al.*,) without the second. It is similar to the methodology used by the MEDINE consortium. It has the advantage that Delphi results are validated by a large group of the professionals actually involved in practice (doctors in MEDINE, biotechnology employees in this PHAR-IN study) and by academics teaching biotechnology.

Regarding statistical analysis, there is an ongoing discussion on the use of parametric or non-parametric statistics when dealing with ordinal data such as Likert scales. Some studies use means and standard variations [23] others use medians (MEDINE). This paper proposes the use of means for descriptive statistics and medians (Wilcoxon) or frequencies (Chi-square) for analysis.

A final issue concerns consensus, which is at the centre of the Delphi process [24]. Leik ordinal consensus values were 0.50 (industrial employees) and 0.58 (academics). Using the scale given by MEDINE [25] this would be qualified as "moderate" consensus.

5.2. Profiles of Respondents

Response rates were high—around 70% for both categories—implying that those participating (both industrial employees and academics) were experienced and knowledgeable enough to reply. There was a significant difference in the distribution of participants across European countries with academics stemming mainly from Bulgaria and Italy and industrial employees from Finland and Switzerland. This discrepancy does not appear to be linked to concentration of pharmacy departments or the pharmaceutical industry in a particular country. Its effect on results is unknown. The UK had approximately equal percentages of academics and of industrial employees. There was no significant difference in age distribution. The main age groups represented were in the 41–60 years range suggesting that replies came from active and experienced participants.

5.3. Ranking Profiles

Categories linked to practical aspects concerned with production: "Research and Development", "Upstream" and "Downstream" Processing", "Product development and formulation", "Aseptic processing", "Analytical methodology", "Product stability", and "Regulation" received high ranking.

Preclinical and clinical categories scored lower with only two out of 19 competences receiving a score higher than the global median. Comments on these areas suggested that some of those replying considered such aspects as "general" competences not specifically linked to biotechnology practice.

Competences in the category "Ethics and drug safety" also received low scores especially on the part of industrial employees. Comments in this area suggested that this matter was self-evident *i.e.*, modern-day pharmaceutical clinical research standards prevent subjects from being coerced into participating in trials.

Finally, in only four out of 46 competences was there a significant difference between rankings of academics and industrial employees. This was mainly in the category "Ethics and drug safety" in which three out of five competences were ranked higher by academics.

6. Conclusions

Several competence frameworks have been proposed, for example, in the UK [26] and at the level of the international pharmaceutical federation [27]. This present study is different in that competences were ranked and validated by a wide European panel—of both industrial practitioners and academics—and were not only the fruit of the expert knowledge of a few. The results show that academics and industrial employees have very similar ideas on the relative importance of different competences for practice in the biotechnological industry. The competences rated as being of highest importance are those concerned with formulation, manufacture and quality control. Thus, academics appear to be in tune with industrial requirements.

7. Perspectives

The consensus framework presented here can be used by academics to examine whether the highly needed competences identified are in fact covered in their existing curricula. If these subjects are not covered in the course, such an examination will open up reflection and discussion on how to cover them. These competences are those of both technicians and research scientists. They may be partially acquired through extra-university and experiential learning on-the-job (APEL) [28]; biotechnological companies have their role to play in APEL—as they do in university master and Ph.D. programmes.

If readers of this paper would like to participate in the PHAR-IN project, they are invited to visit the PHAR-IN webpage [1]

Acknowledgement

This project has been funded with support from the European Commission—538252-LLP-1-2013-BE-ERASMUS-EKA. This communication reflects the views only of the author. The Commission cannot be held responsible for any use which may be made of the information contained therein.

Author Contributions

Jeffrey Atkinson and Kristien De Paepe directed the project. Jeffrey Atkinson ran the survey, analysed the results and wrote the paper. Pat Crowley and Brian Gennery wrote the initial competence framework and gave advice on subsequent versions. Andries Koster interacted with EAFP and critically reviewed early versions of the paper. Luigi Martini and Jane Nicholson distributed the questionnaire to EIPG members; Vivien Moffat distributed the questionnaire to EFPIA members. Gunther Pauwels and Vitor Sousa gave advice based on their knowledge of biotechnology practice; Giuseppe Ronsisvalle and Keith Wilson gave advice based on their knowledge of biotechnology teaching. Chris van Schravendijk provided advice concerning methodology based on his MEDINE experience.

All authors actively participated in the Delphi review by the small expert committee.

Conflicts of Interest

The authors declare no conflicts of interest.

Appendix

The PHAR-IN survey.

The PHAR-IN survey on competences for biotechnology.

Introduction to PHAR-IN.

There is a "knowledge transfer time gap" between industry and education and training.

The time scales in education and industry are substantially different. Education at universities is validated by national agencies on a quadrennial or quinquennial basis and thus tends to change slowly. Industry in order to remain competitive needs to change direction and policy within months. This situation requires that the educational system be capable of adapting within a narrow time frame in order to produce the right person with the right competences at the right time.

The missing link for such a development is a system whereby universities can obtain regular and rapid feedback from industry on what they should be teaching and how, and this in the context of the size of the industry (big pharma, small and medium enterprises…), its activity (R&D, marketing, chemical manufacture, medical devises…), the local/national socioeconomic environment, etc.

The PHARIN consortium (www.phar-qa.eu) will develop a tool for such a feedback process offering a rapid reaction in the quickly evolving field of biotechnology, with the possibility of the creation of cutting edge courses reflecting the progressive nature of this emerging domain. We are especially interested in your ideas on the latest innovations in biotechnology.

We would like you to help us in this endeavor by filling in this questionnaire. Your replies reflect your individual opinions and do not represent the position of an association or institution. Your personal details will not be revealed. You will need 20 minutes to fill in this survey.

Your details.

1. First name?

2. Last name?

3. What is your age?

4. Country of residence.

If you choose other, please specify.

5. email.

6. Profession.

- University staff.
- Industrialist.
- Other (please specify)

The PHAR-IN survey on competences for biotechnology.

7. If you work in industry in which domain do you work?

- ○ R&D
- ○ Regulatory affairs
- ○ Production
- ○ Marketing
- ○ Other (please specify)

8. Do you work in:

- ○ Small and medium enterprise?
- ○ Big pharma?
- ○ Other (please specify)

9. Do you work in a biotechnological environment?

10. In which subject did you obtain your primary degree?

- ○ Pharmacy
- ○ Medicine
- ○ Science

If you checked "Science" please add the domain below:

11. At which stage of your career would like to have had or have the possibility to follow a course in biotechnology?

- ○ In the later stages of the pre-graduate degree course
- ○ As CPD

Research and development.

Please rank the importance of the premises below on a scale from 1 (lowest) to 4 (highest). You also have the possibility of selecting the "unable to rank" box.
Add any comments you may have in the box provided at the end of each premise.

The PHAR-IN survey on competences for biotechnology.

12. Research and development.

	1	2	3	4	I am unable to rank this premise
1. Take an active role in a multidisciplinary team to interpret the key elements of a drug development strategy and use this to design early phase clinical studies	○	○	○	○	○
2. Understand the statistical principles used in preclinical and clinical research	○	○	○	○	○
3. Be able to critically review published studies in preclinical (including safety pharmacology) and clinical research.	○	○	○	○	○

Comments.

Preclinical sciences.

Please rank the importance of the premises below on a scale from 1 (lowest) to 4 (highest). You also have the possibility of selecting the "unable to rank" box.
Add any comments you may have in the box provided at the end of each premise.

The PHAR-IN survey on competences for biotechnology.

13. Preclinical sciences.

	1	2	3	4	I am unable to rank this premise
1. Have an understanding of the choice and predictive value of the nonclinical testing programme as part of the overall drug development plan for chemical and biological compounds.	○	○	○	○	○
2. Be able to describe the general principles of non clinical safety testing.	○	○	○	○	○
3. Know how nonclinical tests are integrated into the overall drug development plan (including scheduling of toxicology tests with respect to clinical trials).	○	○	○	○	○
4. Be able to use animal pharmacokinetics and toxicokinetics to inform the clinical development process.	○	○	○	○	○
5. Describe the importance of the selection of the preclinical animal model in order to have a better and more predictive non-clinical phase.	○	○	○	○	○

Comments.

Biological and advanced therapy.

Please rank the importance of the premises below on a scale from 1 (lowest) to 4 (highest). You also have the possibility of selecting the "unable to rank" box.
Add any comments you may have in the box provided at the end of each premise.

The PHAR-IN survey on competences for biotechnology.

14. Biological and advanced therapy.

	1	2	3	4	I am unable to rank this premise
1. Describe the breadth of advanced therapy medicinal products (ATMPs) that are available and in development, including the scientific principles for the classification in to the categories of gene therapy, somatic cell therapy, tissue engineering and combined ATMPs.	O	O	O	O	O
2. Describe the range of products available with recombinant DNA technology.	O	O	O	O	O
3. Discuss the different needs between the pre-clinical and clinical trial needs of natural proteins and modified proteins	O	O	O	O	O
4. Describe the range of monoclonal antibodies available and those in development and discuss the potential long term safety issues with monoclonal antibodies.	O	O	O	O	O
5. Describe the global need for new and improved vaccines and the barriers to their development.	O	O	O	O	O
6. Define what a therapeutic vaccine is and describe how a therapeutic vaccine could influence therapy in a common disease area.	O	O	O	O	O
7. Describe what is a polysaccharide product and the regulatory and development challenges involved.	O	O	O	O	O

Comments.

The PHAR-IN survey on competences for biotechnology.

Clinical pharmacology.

Please rank the importance of the premises below on a scale from 1 (lowest) to 4 (highest). You also have the possibility of selecting the "unable to rank" box.
Add any comments you may have in the box provided at the end of each premise

15. Clinical pharmacology.

	1	2	3	4	I am unable to rank this premise
1. Take an active role in a multidisciplinary team to design clinical pharmacology studies	O	O	O	O	O
2. Recognise the particular ethical issues of using non patient volunteers in clinical studies	O	O	O	O	O
3. Understand and interpret clinical pharmacodynamic and pharmacokinetic data especially that related to safety issues	O	O	O	O	O
4. Discuss how data from a clinical pharmacology study can inform the future development of a medicine	O	O	O	O	O

Comments.

Clinical development.

Please rank the importance of the premises below on a scale from 1 (lowest) to 4 (highest). You also have the possibility of selecting the "unable to rank" box.
Add any comments you may have in the box provided at the end of each premise.

The PHAR-IN survey on competences for biotechnology.

16. Clinical development.

	1	2	3	4	I am unable to rank this premise
1. Use pre-clinical pharmacology and safety data to prepare a clinical trial plan	○	○	○	○	○
2. Write a protocol for a study including the choice of design, the end points, whether to use a placebo and the inclusion and exclusion criteria	○	○	○	○	○
3. Interpret the elements of GCP that apply to the design and execution of clinical trials	○	○	○	○	○

Comments.

"Upstream" and "Downstream" Processing.

Please rank the importance of the premises below on a scale from 1 (lowest) to 4 (highest). You also have the possibility of selecting the "unable to rank" box.
Add any comments you may have in the box provided at the end of each premise.

The PHAR-IN survey on competences for biotechnology.

17. "Upstream" and "Downstream" Processing.

	1	2	3	4	I am unable to rank this premise
1. Understand "upstream" aspects of biopharmaceutical process development such as cell line development and generation and characterization of Master Cell Banks and Working Cell Banks, cell culture and harvesting	○	○	○	○	○
2. Understand "downstream" aspects of biopharmaceutical process development such as isolation and purification of proteins	○	○	○	○	○
3. Identify Critical Quality Attributes (CQAs), and Critical Process Parameters (CPPs) and define a meaningful set of in-process controls and specifications to ensure quality and consistency of final product.	○	○	○	○	○
4. Have good working knowledge of the principles of "Comparability" as applicable to biopharmaceutical manufacturing changes.	○	○	○	○	○

Comments.

Product development and formulation.

Please rank the importance of the premise below on a scale from 1 (lowest) to 4 (highest). You also have the possibility of selecting the "unable to rank" box.
Add any comments you may have in the box provided at the end of each premise.

The PHAR-IN survey on competences for biotechnology.

18. Product development and formulation.

	1	2	3	4	I am unable to rank this premise
1. Understand the importance of defined quality standards for product and process components used in biopharmaceutical formulation and manufacture, and the potential for interaction with biopharmaceutical macromolecules.	○	○	○	○	○

Comments.

Aseptic Processing.

Please rank the importance of the premises below on a scale from 1 (lowest) to 4 (highest). You also have the possibility of selecting the "unable to rank" box.
Add any comments you may have in the box provided at the end of each premise.

The PHAR-IN survey on competences for biotechnology.

19. Aseptic Processing.

	1	2	3	4	I am unable to rank this premise
1. Understand microbiological principles as they apply to sterility assurance in biopharmaceutical manufacturing.	O	O	O	O	O
2. Understand unit operations in aseptic processing and design of facilities and utilities in sterile manufacturing suite.	O	O	O	O	O
3. Understand concepts of Good Manufacturing Practice (GMP) and Good Distribution Practice (GDP) as applicable to the aseptic production, control, storage and handling of biopharmaceuticals.	O	O	O	O	O

Comments.

Analytical Methodology.

Please rank the importance of the premise below on a scale from 1 (lowest) to 4 (highest). You also have the possibility of selecting the "unable to rank" box.
Add any comments you may have in the box provided at the end of each premise.

The PHAR-IN survey on competences for biotechnology.

20. Analytical Methodology.

	1	2	3	4	I am unable to rank this premise
1. Understand the principles, instrumentation and application of analytical methods (especially bioassay) used to characterize biopharmaceutical raw materials, intermediates and finished products.	O	O	O	O	O

Comments.

Product Stability.

Please rank the importance of the premise below on a scale from 1 (lowest) to 4 (highest). You also have the possibility of selecting the "unable to rank" box.
Add any comments you may have in the box provided at the end of each premise.

21. Product Stability.

	1	2	3	4	I am unable to rank this premise
1. Understand the potential impact of environmental factors (such as temperature, light, oxidation) on biopharmaceutical proteins and consequences for product quality, safety and efficacy.	O	O	O	O	O

Comments.

The PHAR-IN survey on competences for biotechnology.

Regulation.

Please rank the importance of the premises below on a scale from 1 (lowest) to 4 (highest). You also have the possibility of selecting the "unable to rank" box.
Add any comments you may have in the box provided at the end of each premise.

22. Regulation.

	1	2	3	4	I am unable to rank this premise
1. Understand the regulatory framework applicable to the development, manufacture, quality assurance and testing of biopharmaceutical products	O	O	O	O	O
2. Use research skills to find regulatory documents used for the preparation of a Clinical Trial Application.	O	O	O	O	O
3. Use knowledge of specific legislation for biopharmaceuticals to review preclinical and clinical parts of a Marketing Authorisation dossier.	O	O	O	O	O
4. Make decisions based on regulatory and commercial information about what text should be included in a Summary of Product Characteristics and Patient Information for a biopharmaceutical.	O	O	O	O	O
5. Know how National Agencies conduct GXP inspections and how to prepare for them.	O	O	O	O	O
6. Have an appreciation of post-licensing responsibilities for drug safety and how to construct a risk management plan.	O	O	O	O	O
7. Understand the life cycle management of biopharmaceuticals	O	O	O	O	O
8. Understand the current regulatory requirements for biosimilars	O	O	O	O	O

Comments.

The PHAR-IN survey on competences for biotechnology.

Ethics and drug safety.

Please rank the importance of the premises below on a scale from 1 (lowest) to 4 (highest). You also have the possibility of selecting the "unable to rank" box.
Add any comments you may have in the box provided at the end of each premise.

The PHAR-IN survey on competences for biotechnology.

23. Ethics and drug safety.

	1	2	3	4	I am unable to rank this premise
1. Analyse and report adverse event data from clinical trials	O	O	O	O	O
2. Employ pharmacoepidemiology skills, including the statistical methodologies to strategically evaluate a drug product and produce a risk management plan	O	O	O	O	O
3. Interpret clinical trial designs that address specific ethical issues e.g. in special patient populations	O	O	O	O	O
4. Design a consent process that ensures that subjects are not coerced into participating in clinical trials	O	O	O	O	O
5. Utilise their knowledge to ensure that patient safety and patient education are priorities when either an originator biological molecule or a biosimilar molecule is dispensed in practice	O	O	O	O	O

Comments.

Commercialisation.

Please rank the importance of the premise below on a scale from 1 (lowest) to 4 (highest). You also have the possibility of selecting the "unable to rank" box.
Add any comments you may have in the box provided at the end of each premise.

The PHAR-IN survey on competences for biotechnology.

24. Commercialisation..

	1	2	3	4	I am unable to rank this premise
1. Understand of the significance of biomarkers as an integral part of the development process and economic evaluation of biopharmaceuticals	○	○	○	○	○

Comments.

Table A1. Mean rankings by industrial employees (Ind.) and academics (Acad.) of the 46 proposed competences, arranged into 13 categories, for practice in the biotechnological industry (n = number of competence).

Number	Competence	Ranking	
n	1. Research and development.	Ind.	Acad.
1	Take an active role in a multidisciplinary team to interpret the key elements of a drug development strategy and use this to design early phase clinical studies	**3.3**	**3.4**
2	Understand the statistical principles used in preclinical and clinical research	2.9	3.1
3	Be able to critically review published studies in preclinical (including safety pharmacology) and clinical research.	**3.2**	**3.4**
	2. Preclinical sciences.		
4	Have an understanding of the choice and predictive value of the non-clinical testing programme as part of the overall drug development plan for chemical and biological compounds.	3.1	3.2
5	Be able to describe the general principles of non-clinical safety testing.	3.0	2.9
6	Know how non-clinical tests are integrated into the overall drug development plan (including scheduling of toxicology tests with respect to clinical trials).	3.1	3.2
7	Be able to use animal pharmacokinetics and toxicokinetics to inform the clinical development process.	*2.6*	2.8
8	Describe the importance of the selection of the preclinical animal model in order to have a better and more predictive non-clinical phase.	*2.8*	3.2
	3. Biological and advanced therapy.		
9	Describe the breadth of advanced therapy medicinal products (ATMPs) that are available and in development, including the scientific principles for the classification in to the categories of gene therapy, somatic cell therapy, tissue engineering and combined ATMPs.	2.9	3.2
10	Describe the range of products available with recombinant DNA technology.	*2.8*	3.3
11	Discuss the different needs between the pre-clinical and clinical trial needs of natural proteins and modified proteins	*2.8*	3.0
12	Describe the range of monoclonal antibodies available, and those in development, and discuss the potential long term safety issues with monoclonal antibodies.	3.1	3.3
13	Describe the global need for new and improved vaccines and the barriers to their development.	3.0	3.2
14	Define what a therapeutic vaccine is and describe how a therapeutic vaccine could influence therapy in a common disease area.	3.0	**3.4**
15	Describe what is a polysaccharide product and the regulatory and development challenges involved.	2.9	2.7
	4. Clinical pharmacology.		
16	Take an active role in a multidisciplinary team to design clinical pharmacology studies	2.9	3.3
17	Recognise the particular ethical issues of using non patient volunteers in clinical studies	3.0	3.2
18	Understand and interpret clinical pharmacodynamic and pharmacokinetic data especially that related to safety issues	**3.2**	3.3

Table A1. *Cont.*

Number	Competence	Ranking	
19	Discuss how data from a clinical pharmacology study can inform the future development of a medicine	3.3	3.3
	5. Clinical development.		
20	Use pre-clinical pharmacology and safety data to prepare a clinical trial plan	2.9	3.3
21	Write a protocol for a study including the choice of design, the end points, whether to use a placebo and the inclusion and exclusion criteria	2.9	3.3
22	Interpret the elements of GCP that apply to the design and execution of clinical trials	3.2	3.1
	6. "Upstream" and "Downstream" Processing.		
23	Understand ''upstream'' aspects of biopharmaceutical process development such as cell line development and generation and characterization of Master Cell Banks and Working Cell Banks, cell culture and harvesting	3.2	3.1
24	Understand ''downstream'' aspects of biopharmaceutical process development such as isolation and purification of proteins	**3.2**	3.2
25	Identify Critical Quality Attributes (CQAs), and Critical Process Parameters (CPPs) and define a meaningful set of in-process controls and specifications to ensure quality and consistency of final product.	**3.3**	3.2
26	Have good working knowledge of the principles of "Comparability" as applicable to biopharmaceutical manufacturing changes.	**3.3**	3.1
	7. Product development and formulation.		
27	Understand the importance of defined quality standards for product and process components used in biopharmaceutical formulation and manufacture, and the potential for interaction with biopharmaceutical macromolecules.	**3.3**	**3.5**
	8. Aseptic processing.		
28	Understand microbiological principles as they apply to sterility assurance in biopharmaceutical manufacturing.	**3.3**	3.2
29	Understand unit operations in aseptic processing and design of facilities and utilities in sterile manufacturing suite.	3.2	3.1
30	Understand concepts of Good Manufacturing Practice (GMP) and Good Distribution Practice (GDP) as applicable to the aseptic production, control, storage and handling of biopharmaceuticals.	**3.4**	**3.3**
	9. Analytical methodology.		
31	Understand the principles, instrumentation and application of analytical methods (especially bioassay) used to characterize biopharmaceutical raw materials, intermediates and finished products.	3.1	**3.4**
	10. Product stability.		
32	Understand the potential impact of environmental factors (such as temperature, light, oxidation) on biopharmaceutical proteins and consequences for product quality, safety and efficacy.	**3.4**	**3.4**
	11. Regulation.		
33	Understand the regulatory framework applicable to the development, manufacture, quality assurance and testing of biopharmaceutical products	**3.5**	3.3
34	Use research skills to find regulatory documents used for the preparation of a Clinical Trial Application.	*2.8*	2.9

Table A1. *Cont.*

Number	Competence	Ranking	
35	Use knowledge of specific legislation for biopharmaceuticals to review preclinical and clinical parts of a Marketing Authorisation dossier.	2.8	3.0
36	Make decisions based on regulatory and commercial information about what text should be included in a Summary of Product Characteristics and Patient Information for a biopharmaceutical.	3.0	3.0
37	Know how National Agencies conduct GXP inspections and how to prepare for them.	3.0	3.0
38	Have an appreciation of post-licensing responsibilities for drug safety and how to construct a risk management plan.	3.0	3.0
39	Understand the life cycle management of biopharmaceuticals	**3.2**	3.2
40	Understand the current regulatory requirements for biosimilars	3.2	3.1
	12. Ethics and drug safety.		
41	Analyse and report adverse event data from clinical trials	2.9	3.2
42	Employ pharmaco-epidemiology skills, including the statistical methodologies to strategically evaluate a drug product and produce a risk management plan	*2.5*	3.0
43	Interpret clinical trial designs that address specific ethical issues e.g., in special patient populations	*2.6*	3.1
44	Design a consent process that ensures that subjects are not coerced into participating in clinical trials	*2.5*	3.1
45	Utilise their knowledge to ensure that patient safety and patient education are priorities when either an originator biological molecule or a biosimilar molecule is dispensed in practice	2.9	3.2
	13. Commercialisation.		
46	Understand the significance of biomarkers as an integral part of the development process and economic evaluation of biopharmaceuticals	3.0	3.2

Bold: median for competence greater than global median of 3 (n = 4915 responses for industrial employees, =1305 responses for academics) ($p < 0.05$, Wilcoxon signed rank test) *Italics*: median less than global median ($p < 0.05$, Wilcoxon signed rank test). Grey coloured boxes refer to those competences in which at least one of the 2 scores was greater than the global median.

References

1. Competences for industrial pharmacy practice in biotechnology (PHAR-IN). PHAR-IN is funded by the European Commission *via* its Education, Audio-visual and Culture Agency; the EU reference is 538252-LLP-1-2013-1-BE-ERASMUS-EKA. Available online: http://www.phar-in.eu/ (accessed on 23 July 2015).
2. European Industrial Pharmacists' Group (EIPG). Available online: http://www.eipg.eu/. (accessed on 23 July 2015).
3. European Federation of Pharmaceutical Industries and Associations, (EFPIA). Available online: http://www.efpia.eu/ (accessed on 23 July 2015).
4. European Association of Faculties of Pharmacy (EAFP). Available online: http://www.eafponline.eu/ (accessed on 23 July 2015).

5. European Federation for Pharmaceutical Sciences (EUFEPS). Available online: http://www.eufeps.org/ (accessed on 23 July 2015).
6. Atkinson, J.; Nicholson, J.; Rombaut, B. Survey of Pharmaceutical Education in Europe Pharmine—Report on the integration of the industry component in pharmacy education and training. *European Industrial Pharmacy* **2012**, *13*, 17–20. Available online: http://eipg.eu/wp-content/uploads/2013/11/eip13-jun12.pdf#page=17 (accessed on 23 July 2015).
7. International Pharmaceutical Federation (FIP). Global pharmacy workforce report. 2012. Available online: http://www.fip.org/humanresources (accessed on 23 July 2015).
8. Rusu, A.; Kuokkanen, K.; Heier, A. Current trends in the pharmaceutical industry—A case study approach. *Eur. J. Pharm. Sci.* **2011**, *44*, 437–440. Available online: http://www.sciencedirect.com/science/article/pii/S0928098711002314 (accessed on 23 July 2015).
9. Atkinson, J.; Rombaut, B. The PHARMINE paradigm—Matching the supply of pharmacy education and training to demands. *Eur. Ind. Pharmacy* **2010**, *6*, 4–7. Available online: http://eipg.eu/wp-content/uploads/2013/11/eip6-jun10.pdf#page=4 (accessed on 23 July 2015).
10. Bjerrum, O.J. Excellence in education and training advances competitiveness of the pharmaceutical industry in Europe. *Eur. J. Pharmaceutical Sci.* **2011**, *44*, 174–175. Available online: http://www.sciencedirect.com/science/article/pii/S0928098711002296 (accessed on 23 July 2015).
11. Stupans, I.; McAllister, S.; Clifford, R.; Hughes, J.; Krasse, I.; March, G.; Owen, S.; Woulf, J. Nationwide collaborative development of learning outcomes and exemplar standards for Australian pharmacy programmes. *Int. J. Pharmacy Pract.* **2014**, 1–9, doi:10.1111/ijpp.12163. Available online: http://onlinelibrary.wiley.com/advanced/search/results (accessed on 23 July 2015).
12. Wu-Pong, S.; Gobburu, J.; O'Barr, S.; Shah, K.; Huber, J.; Weiner, D. The Future of the Pharmaceutical Sciences and Graduate Education: Recommendations from the AACP Graduate Education Special Interest Group. *Am. J. Pharm. Educ.* **2013**, *77*, 1–8. Available online: http://www.ncbi.nlm.nih.gov/pmc/journals/383/ (accessed on 23 July 2015).
13. Hsu, C.C.; Sandford, B.A. The Delphi Technique: Making Sense of Consensus. *Pract. Assess. Res. Eval.* **2007**, *12*, 1. Available online: http://pareonline.net/getvn.asp?v=12&n = 10 (accessed on 23 July 2015).
14. The TUNING network. Competences: Nursing practice and clinical decision making. Available online: http://www.unideusto.org/tuningeu/competences/specific/nursing.html (accessed on 23 July 2015).
15. The TUNING network. Competences: Medical doctors. Available online: http://www.unideusto.org/tuningeu/subject-areas/medicine.html (accessed on 23 July 2015).
16. Scott, D.G.; Washer, B.A.; Wright, M.D. A Delphi study to identify recommended biotechnology competences for first-year/initially certified technology education teachers. *J. Technol. Educ.* **2006**, *17*, 43–55. Available online: http://scholar.lib.vt.edu/ejournals/JTE/v17n2/pdf/scott.pdf (accessed on 23 July 2015).
17. Wells, J.G. Establishing a taxonometric structure for the study of biotechnology in secondary school technology education. *J. Technol. Educ.* **1994**, *6*, 1–7. Available online: http://scholar.lib.vt.edu/ejournals/JTE/v6n1/pdf/wells.pdf (accessed on 23 July 2015).
18. Innovative Medicines Initiative (IMI). Available online: http://www.imi.europa.eu/ (accessed on 23 July 2015).

19. Surveymonkey®. The PHAR-IN survey is given in the annex. Available online: https://www.surveymonkey.com/ (accessed on 23 July 2015).
20. Likert scales. Available online: http://www.socialresearchmethods.net/kb/scallik.php (accessed on 23 July 2015).
21. Leik, R.K. A measure of ordinal consensus. *Pac. Sociol. Rev.* **1966**, *9*, 85–90. Available online: http://www.jstor.org/stable/1388242 (accessed on 23 July 2015).
22. Graphpad®. Available online: http://www.graphpad.com/ (accessed on 23 July 2015).
23. De Villiers, M.R.; de Villiers, P.J.T.; Kent, A.P. The Delphi technique in health sciences education research. *Med. Teacher* **2005**, *27*, 639–643. Available online: http://informahealthcare.com/doi/pdf/10.1080/13611260500069947 (accessed on 23 July 2015).
24. Goodman, C.M. The Delphi technique: A critique. *J. Adv. Nurs.* **1987**, *12*, 729–734. Available online: http://onlinelibrary.wiley.com/doi/10.1111/j.1365-2648.1987.tb01376.x/abstract (accessed on 23 July 2015).
25. Marz, R.; Dekker, F.W.; van Schravendijk, C.; O'Flynn, S.; Ross, M.T. Tuning research competences for Bologna three cycles in medicine: Report of a MEDINE2 European consensus survey. *Perspect. Med. Educ.* **2013**, *2*, 1–15. Available online: http://www.ncbi.nlm.nih.gov/pmc/issues/222987/ (accessed on 23 July 2015).
26. CoDEG: Competency development and evaluation group. The general level framework. Available online: http://www.codeg.org/frameworks/general-level-practice/ (accessed on 23 July 2015).
27. Joint FIP/WHO guidelines on good pharmacy practice: Standards for quality of pharmacy services. Available online: http://www.fip.org/good_pharmacy_practice (accessed on 23 July 2015).
28. APEL: Accreditation of Prior Experiential Learning. Available online: http://www.city.ac.uk/" courses/cpd/accreditation-of-prior-experiential-learning-apel-claim (accessed on 23 July 2015).

7

Posaconazole: An Update of Its Clinical Use

Simon Leung [1], Mara N. Poulakos [2] and Jade Machin [3,*]

1 Memorial Regional Hospital, Hollywood, FL 33021, USA; E-Mail: sleung@mhs.net

2 Gregory School of Pharmacy, Palm Beach Atlantic University, West Palm Beach, FL 33416; USA; E-Mail: mara_poulakos@pba.edu

3 Boca Raton Regional Hospital, Boca Raton, FL 33486, USA; E-Mail: jmachin@brrh.com

* Author to whom correspondence should be addressed; E-Mail: mara_poulakos@pba.edu

Academic Editor: Yvonne Perrie

Abstract: Posaconazole (PCZ) is a relatively new addition to the azole antifungals. It has fungicidal activities against *Aspergillus fumigatus*, *Blastomyces dermatitidis*, selected *Candida* species, *Crytopcoccus neoformans*, and *Trichosporon*. PCZ also has fungistatic activities against *Candida*, *Coccidioides*, selected *Fusarium* spp., *Histoplasma*, *Scedosporium* and *Zygomycetes*. In addition, combining the drug with caspofungin or amphotericin B results in a synergistic interaction against *A. fumigatus*, *C. glabrata* and *C. neoformans*. The absorption of PCZ suspension is enhanced when given with food, nutritional supplements, and carbonated beverages. Oral administration of PCZ in divided doses also increases its bioavailability. PCZ has a large volume of distribution and is highly protein bound (>95%). The main elimination route of PCZ is fecal. PCZ is an inhibitor of the CYP3A4 enzyme; therefore, monitoring for drug-drug interactions is warranted with other CYP3A4 substrates/inhibitors/inducers. The most common adverse effects include headache, fatigue, nausea, vomiting and elevated hepatic enzymes. PCZ, with its unique antifungal activities, expands the azole class of antifungal agents. Because of its limit in formulation, PCZ oral suspension is recommended in immunocompromised patients with functional gastrointestinaltracts who fail conventional antifungal therapies or who are suspected to have a breakthrough fungal infection. However, a delayed-release tablet formulation and intravenous (IV) injection became available in 2014, expanding the use of PCZ in other patient populations, including individuals who are unable to take oral formulations.

Keywords: posaconazole; pharmacokinetics; pharmacodynamics; *crytococcus neoformans*; *Candida*; *aspergillus*; fusariosi; neutropenia; candidiasis; graft-*versus*-host

1. Introduction

Posaconazole (PCZ) oral suspension (Noxafil™, Schering-Plough Corporation) has received approval from the U.S. Food and Drug Administration (FDA) for prophylaxis against invasive aspergillosis and candidiasis in immunocompromised patients, 13 years of age and older [1,2]. PCZ is considered an extended-spectrum antifungal agent due to its unique spectrum of activity against various fungi, including the majority of yeasts, filamentous fungi and azole resistant *Candida* species (spp.) [3]. The patterns of *Candida* infections have shifted from the previous most common fluconazole (FCZ) sensitive *C. albicans* to other FCZ dose-dependent sensitive and FCZ resistant *Candida* species since the year 2000 [4]. These *Candida* species include, but are not limited to, *C. glabata*, *C. parapsilosis* and *C. tropicalis.* To complicate the treatment of fungal infections further, the emergence of breakthrough fungal infections (*i.e., fusarium*, *scedosporium* and *zygomycosis*) has occurred secondary to the use of potent immunosuppressive agents and a lack of antifungal activity against these pathogens from current antifungals [5]. Therefore, novel additions to the antifungal armamentarium are needed. Because of its extended-spectrum against a broader range of pathogens, PCZ offers a promising role in treating refractory fungal infections. The focus of this article is to review and provide updated information on the unique characteristics of PCZ.

2. Chemical Structure

PCZ (MW 700.8, pKa 3.6 and 4.6) is highly lipophilic with a triazole structure similar to itraconazole (ICZ) (Figure 1) [6]. The chemical structure of PCZ is an enantiomerically pure RRSS isomer with four chiral centers. PCZ's structure consists of a classic triazole and difluoro phenyl rings with common orientations characteristic of other azoles. The tetrahydrofuran oxygen of PCZ overlaps the hydroxyl oxygen component of FCZ [7]. The long side chain of PCZ mounts securely inside the space formed by the various structural domains of lanosterol 14α-demethylase, a cytochrome P450 (CYP450) enzyme, which contains helix A′, a β turn connecting strands β4-1 and β4-2, an FG loop, helix B′ and β-strands, β1-4 [7].

3. Mechanism of Action

PCZ exerts its activity by inhibiting fungal ergosterol biosynthesis. PCZ binds to the heme cofactor situated on the target site of lanosterol 14α-demethylase, which is a CYP450 dependent enzyme [7,8]. This enzyme is the product of CYP51A gene expression (ERG11). The integrity of the fungal cell membrane is maintained by ergosterol. PCZ prevents demethylation of ergosterol at C-14 and/or C-4 positions. The altered structure of ergosterol interferes with plasma membrane function, resulting in fungal cell death.

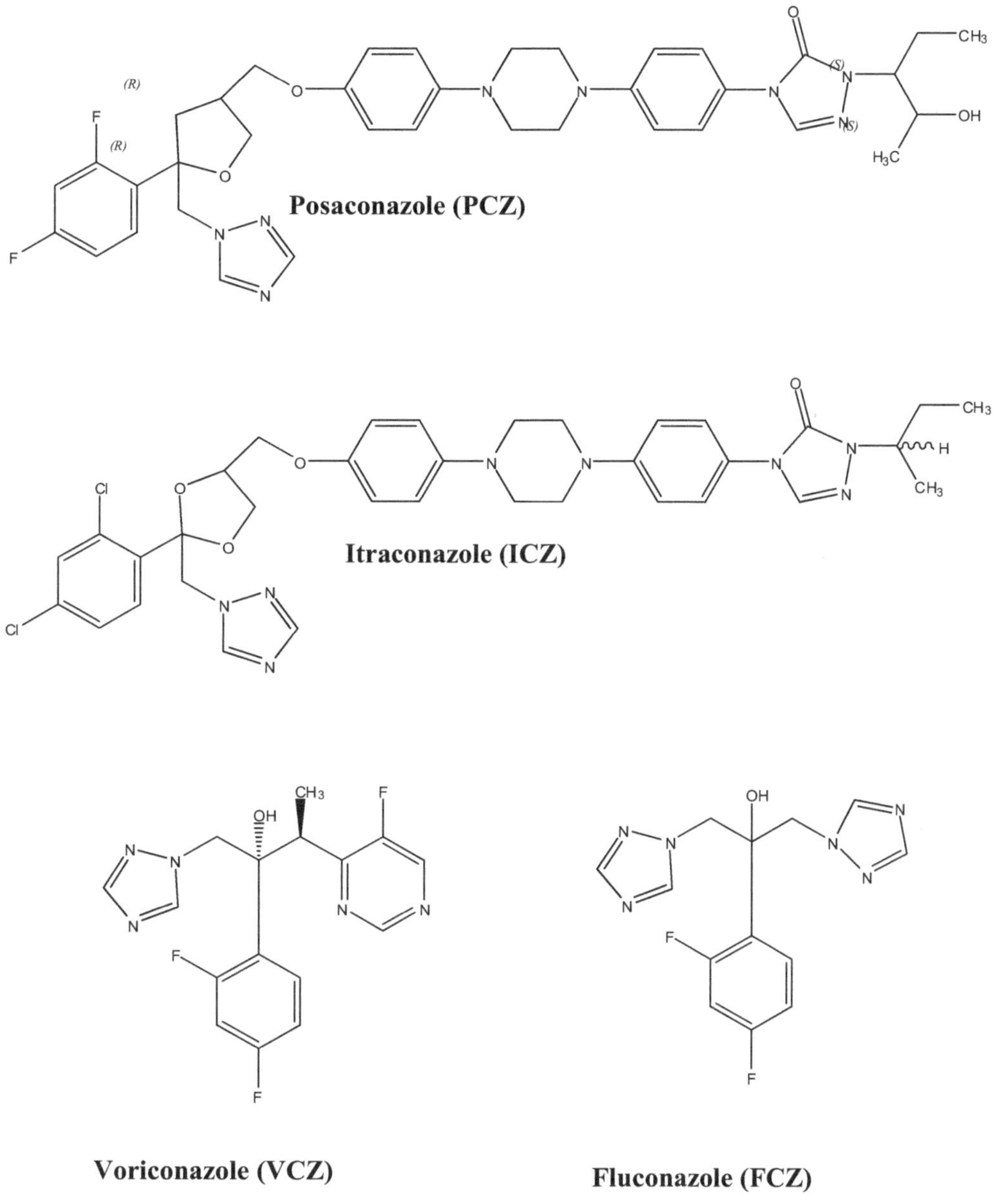

Figure 1. Structures of selected triazole antifungal agents.

Several *in vitro* studies have confirmed the antifungal mechanism of PCZ with liquid chromatography techniques [9,10]. Heimark *et al.* reported that *in vitro* PCZ depletes the production of ergosterol in *C. albicans* by inhibiting the enzyme lanosterol 14α-demethylase [9]. Similar studies have also demonstrated the depletion of ergosterol in both azole susceptible and resistant *C. albicans* when incubated with PCZ [minimum inhibitory concentrations, (MICs) ≤ 0.5 mcg/mL] [10]. Dose dependent inhibition of ergosterol and ergosterol-like compounds (*i.e.*, ergosta-5,8,22-trien-3-ol) was also observed in most *C. glabrata* strains and strain C110 respectively, when exposed to PCZ (MICs ≤ 4 mcg/mL). Exposure of *Aspergillus fumigatus* and *A. flavus* to PCZ (MICs ≤ 0.06 mcg/mL) also resulted in the inhibition of ergosterol synthesis.

4. Spectrum of Activity

PCZ has an extended spectrum of antifungal activity, as illustrated in Table 1 [11]. It has shown to have fungicidal activity *in vitro* and *in vivo*, against *Cryptococcus neoformans*, *Aspergillus (fumigatus, flavus*, and *terreus*), *Blastomyces dermatitidis*, *Trichosporon* and specific *Candida* spp. (*i.e.*, *C. krusei*, *C. parapsilosis*, *C. lusitaniae* and *C. inconspicua*) [11]. PCZ also has fungistatic activity against most other *Candida* spp., *Scedosporium*, *Coccidiodes*, *Zygomycetes* and specific *Fusarium* strains (*i.e.*, *F. oxysporum* and *F. moniliforme*) [12]. However, unlike antibacterials, *in vitro* and *in vivo* activities of antifungal agents do not relate with clinical outcomes.

5. Pharmacodynamics

The *in vitro* activity of PCZ was compared with that of amphotericin B (AMB), FCZ and ICZ against isolates of *C. neoformans*. Yeasts were inhibited and killed at lower concentrations of PCZ (MICs, ranged from 0.063 to 0.25 mcg/mL) than those of AMB (MICs ranged from 0.25 to1 mcg/mL). Inhibition was also noted at concentrations at least ten fold lower than those of FCZ (MICs ranged from 0.5 to16 mcg/mL) but not for ICZ (MICs ranged from 0.008 to 0.031 mcg/mL). In the three isolates used, which were clinical strains of *C. neoformans* (T-1, DUMC 133.95, and 89–610), growth was inhibited at high MIC values of FCZ (8–16 mcg/mL) in contrast to low MIC values of PCZ (0.125 to 0.25 mcg/mL). The *in vivo* activities of PCZ when compared to FCZ were similar in terms of reducing yeast counts in the cerebrospinal fluid of a rabbit model [13]. Barchiesi *et al.* demonstrated that PCZ, when compared to AMB, was effective in prolonging survival of mice infected with *C. neoformans*. In fact, PCZ was superior to AMB at reducing fungal burden in the brains of mice infected by two *Cryptococcal* isolates [14].

An *in vitro* study of voriconazole (VCZ), FCZ and PCZ against isolates of *Candida* and *C. neoformans*, found that both VCZ and PCZ had greatest activity against *C. albicans*, *C. parapsilosis*, *C. krusei* and *C. lusitaniae*, *C. tropicalis*, *C. dubliniensis*, and *C. kefyr* [15]. Moreover, 97%–98% of *Candida* spp. were susceptible at MICs ≤ 1 mcg/mL. Both PCZ and VCZ were less active against *C. glabrata* (80% susceptible at MICs ≤ 1 mcg/mL) and PCZ was less active against *C. pelliculosa* (44% susceptible at MICs ≤ 1 mcg/mL). FCZ was most active (≥95% susceptible at MICs ≤ 8 mcg/mL) against *C. albicans* (99% susceptible), *C. parapsilosis* (95%), *C. lusitaniae* (98%), *C. tropicalis* (98%), and *C. pelliculosa* (100% susceptible) and least active against *C. glabrata* (57%) and *C. krusei* (1%). Both VCZ and PCZ were highly active against *C. neoformans* (98%–100% susceptible at MICs ≤ 1 mcg/mL) when compared to FCZ (98% of *C. neoformans* susceptible at MICs ≤ 8 mcg/mL) [15].

A clinical study compared the activities of PCZ, ICZ and FCZ against 3312 clinical isolates of *Candida* and 373 isolates of *C. neoformans*. PCZ was shown to be more active (97% of the *Candida* spp. and 100% of *C. neoformans* were inhibited at MIC ≤ 1 mcg/mL) than both triazole antifungals. Only 78% of *C. neoformans* isolates were inhibited by FCZ (MICs ≤ 8 mcg/mL) compared to 96% by PCZ and 68% by ICZ (MICs ≤ 0.25 mcg/mL). Furthermore, *C. albicans*, *C. parapsilosis*, *C. krusei*, *C. lusitaniae*, *C. tropicalis*, *C. dubliniensis*, *C. guilliermondii* and *C. famata* were found to be most susceptible to PCZ (99%–100% of isolates susceptible at MICs ≤ 1 mcg/mL) whereas *C. glabrata* was least susceptible (80% susceptible at MIC ≤ 1 mcg/mL) [16]. Barchiesi *et al.* compared the *in vitro* activities of FCZ, ICZ, PCZ, AMB and 5-fluorocytosine against 56 clinical isolates of *Candida*. All *Candida* strains were susceptible to PCZ (MIC range ≤ 0.007–0.125 mg/L) and AMB (MIC range ≤ 0.03–0.5 mg/L) compared to 97% and 95% of the isolates susceptible to FCZ (MIC range ≤ 0.125–32 mg/L) and ICZ (≤0.007–1 mg/L), respectively [17].

Table 1. Comparative *in vitro* activities of posaconazole (PCZ), itraconazole (ICZ), voriconazole (VCZ) and amphotericin B (AMB) against molds and yeasts collected from 200 medical centers worldwide over a 10-year period [11]

		PCZ		ICZ		VCZ		AMB	
MIC (mcg/mL)		**50%**	**90%**	**50%**	**90%**	**50%**	**90%**	**50%**	**90%**
Organisms	**n**								
All *Aspergillus* spp.	1423	0.125	0.5	0.5	2.0	0.25	0.5	0.5	1.0
A. flavus	89	0.25	0.5	0.5	1.0	0.5	1.0	1.0	2.0
A. famigatus	1119	0.125	0.5	0.5	1.0	0.25	0.5	0.5	1.0
A. niger	101	0.25	0.5	1.0	2.0	0.5	2.0	0.125	1.0
A. terreus	22	0.25	0.25	0.5	0.5	0.25	0.5	2.0	2.0
All *Zygomycetes*	86	0.5	4.0	1.0	32.0	16.0	128.0	0.25	2.0
Rhizopus spp.	32	1.0	8.0	4.0	32.0	16.0	128.0	1.0	2.0
Mucor spp.	18	1.0	16.0	2.0	32.0	64.0	128.0	0.25	1.0
Absidia spp.	16	0.125	0.25	0.125	0.5	16.0	128.0	0.25	0.5
Cunninghamella spp.	6	0.031–1	0.031–1	0.125–2	0.125–2	8–128	8–128	0.125–2	0.125–2
Apophysomyces	5	0.031–4	0.031–4	0.031–8	0.031–8	16–128	16–128	0.031–4	0.031–4
Saksenaea spp.	4	0.016–2	0.016–2	0.016–0.125	0.5–4	0.5–4	0.5–4	0.063–0.5	0.063–0.5
Rhizomucor spp.	3	0.016–0.25	0.016–0.25	0.016–0.25	0.016–0.25	2–16	2–16	0.063–0.125	0.063–0.125
Cokeromyces spp.	2	0.25–4	0.25–4	0.25–8	0.25–8	16–64	16–64	0.125–0.5	0.125–0.5
All *Fusarium* spp.	67	16	32	16	32	16	32	8.0	32
F. solani	39	32	32	ND	ND	16	32	16	32
F. oxysporum	12	2.0	4.0	ND	ND	4.0	32	8.0	16
F. moniliforme	2	1.0	1.0	ND	ND	1.0	1.0	1–4	1–4
Other *Fusarium* spp.	14	16	16	ND	ND	4.0	16.0	1.0	2.0
All *Candida* spp.	6965	0.063	1.0	0.125	1.0	0.031	0.5	1.0	1.0
C. albicans	3525	0.031	0.063	0.063	0.25	0.008	0.063	1.0	1.0
C. glabrata	1218	1.0	2.0	1.0	4.0	0.25	2.0	1.0	1.0
C. parapsilosis	970	0.063	0.25	0.5	0.5	0.031	0.125	1.0	1.0
C. tropicalis	719	0.063	0.125	0.5	0.5	0.063	0.5	1.0	1.0
C. krusei	189	0.5	1.0	1.0	1.0	0.25	0.5	1.0	2.0

Table 1. *Cont.*

		PCZ		ICZ		VCZ		AMB	
MIC (mcg/mL)		**50%**	**90%**	**50%**	**90%**	**50%**	**90%**	**50%**	**90%**
C. lusitaniae	84	0.063	0.25	0.25	2.0	0.031	0.063	1.0	2.0
C. guillermondii	26	0.25	1.0	0.5	4.0	0.063	8.0	0.5	1.0
C. dubliniensis	164	0.031	0.125	0.063	0.5	0.016	0.125	0.5	1.0
Other *Candida*	60	0.25	2.0	0.5	1.0	0.063	0.25	1.0	1.0
Other Organisms									
Cryptococcus spp.	271	0.125	0.5	0.125	0.5	0.063	0.125	1.0	1.0
Scedosporium prolificans	80	16.0	32	64	64	ND	ND	16	32
Scedosporium apiospermum	26	0.25	1.0	1.0	32	ND	ND	2.0	8.0
Coccidioides spp.	25	0.125	0.25	0.125	0.25	ND	ND	0.5	0.5
Blastomyces	38	0.063	0.125	0.031	2.0	ND	ND	0.125	0.5
Histoplasma	53	0.019	0.25	0.019	0.063	ND	ND	0.25	0.5
Pseudallescheria	41	0.25	1.0	0.5	1.0	ND	ND	2.0	4.0

A 50% and 90% are minimum inhibitory concentrations (MIC) at which the growth of 50% and 90%, respectively, of the isolates were inhibited; b When $n < 10$, MIC ranges are given. ND, not determined.

6. *Cryptococcus neoformans*

An *in vitro* study by Barchiesi *et al.* investigated the effects of the interaction of PCZ and flucytosine (FC) against *C. neoformans* [18]. Synergy and additivism were observed in 33% and 67% of isolates, respectively. Indifference and antagonism were not observed. Even when synergy was not reached, the geometric mean MICs of both drugs dropped significantly when they were given in combination (MIC for FC dropped from 1.26 to 0.39 mcg/mL and MIC for PCZ dropped from 0.13 to 0.02 mcg/mL, $p = 0.0001$) [18]. The beneficial interaction was also demonstrated by a reduction in the numbers of colony forming units (CFU) of *C. neoformans* isolates. Combination therapy of PCZ and FC at subinhibitory concentrations, eight fold lower than the respective MICs, significantly reduced the counts below those observed with each drug alone ($p = 0.0001$) [18]. The same study investigated the *in vivo* effects of this combination therapy, and found that it was not significantly more effective than each drug alone in terms of survival [18]. However, tissue burden studies showed that combination therapy reduced the counts significantly below that with each drug used alone. It should be noted that this study only utilized one clinical isolate of *C. neoformans*. In conclusion, because of the genetic variations that exist among these isolates, further investigation of combination therapy using multiple strains is needed.

Another study examined the *in vitro* interaction of AMB with triazoles against *Cryptococcus neoformans*. Synergy was observed in 33% of the isolates for PCZ-AMB combination, compared to 7% for FCZ-AMB and ICZ-AMB combinations [19]. Additivism was noted in 53%, 67% and 73% of the isolates for PCZ-AMB, FCZ-AMB and ICZ-AMB interactions, respectively [19]. Indifference was observed in 14%, 20% and 26% of the isolates for PCZ-AMB, ICZ-AMB and FCZ-AMB combinations, respectively [19]. Antagonism was not observed. This study also investigated the *in vivo* interaction of FCZ-AMB combination and compared it to FCZ and AMB therapy alone. Survival and tissue burden studies revealed that combination therapy was more effective than FCZ therapy ($p = 0.0001$), and equally or more efficacious than AMB therapy alone. *C. neoformans* grown in a medium containing FCZ, with subsequent exposure to AMB, lead to an increase in AMB resistance. However, this antagonism was not observed *in vivo*, and in fact, a positive interaction occurred [19]. This *in vivo* study only used one clinical isolate of *C. neoformans*, and for this reason further studies of this combination treatment with multiple strains should be explored.

7. *Candida glabrata*

Terbinafine (TBF) combinations with four triazoles (*i.e.*, FCZ, ICZ, VCZ and PCZ) were examined *in vitro* against weakly susceptible strains of *C. glabrata* to azoles [20]. Synergy was observed in 17% of the TBF-FCZ combinations, 21% of the TBF-ICZ combinations, 33% of the TBF-VCZ combinations, and 12% of the TBF-PCZ combinations [20]. Combinations where synergy was not observed revealed a decrease in the MIC of one or both drugs when given in combinations [20]. Another study evaluated the *in vitro* interaction of PCZ with caspofungin against *C. glabrata* [21]. Synergy was observed in 18% of all the isolates ($n = 119$) including 4% of the isolates resistant to FCZ ($n = 26$) [21]. No antagonism was observed between these drugs. *Candida* resistance has been reported with the older azoles (*i.e.*, FCZ and ICZ) and is now being reported with caspofungin. PCZ and caspofungin may have a role in relapsing

Candida infections and for FCZ-resistant isolates with high PCZ MICs. Studies are warranted to explore the *in vivo* benefits of this combination therapy.

8. *Aspergillus* and *Candida* spp.

The activity of PCZ was tested *in vitro* and *in vivo* against *Aspergillus* and *Candida* strains. Overall, PCZ (MICs ranged from ≤0.002 to 0.5 mcg/mL) was more active than ICZ (MICs ranged from ≤0.008 to 1 mcg/mL) against 39 strains of *Aspergillus* [22]. PCZ was also more active (MICs of PCZ ranged from≤ 0.004 to 16 mcg/mL) than FCZ (MICs ranged from ≤0.062 to >64 mcg/mL) against 275 strains of *Candida* and nine strains of *C. neoformans* [22]. Pfaller *et al.* compared the *in vitro* activities of PCZ, ravuconazole (RCZ) and VCZ to ICZ and AMB against 239 isolates of *Aspergillus* and other filamentous fungi. PCZ was most active, inhibiting 94% of isolates at MIC ≤1 mcg/mL, followed by VCZ (91%), AMB (89%), RCZ (88%) and ICZ (70%) [23]. Another study by Manavathu *et al.* expanded these findings and found that the geometric mean MICs of PCZ against *Aspergillus fumigatus* (0.17 ± 0.11) and *non-Aspergillus fumigatus* (0.16 ± 0.28) were significantly lower ($p \leq 0.05$) than AMB, ICZ and VCZ. AMB-resistant *Aspergillus* strains were susceptible to PCZ. ICZ- and VCZ-resistant strains showed low level (2 to 3 fold increase in MIC) cross-resistance to PCZ. Time-kill studies against *Aspergillus* demonstrated that the fungicidal activity of PCZ is dependent on time and concentration. This highlights the fact that PCZ is more active than ICZ and VCZ [24].

9. *Aspergillus fumigatus*

A study by Manavathu *et al.* evaluated drug combinations of caspofungin with triazoles against *A. fumigatus* [24]. Synergy was observed *in vitro* with PCZ (FICI = 0.32 ± 0.09) and ICZ (FICI = 0.49 ± 0.04) [24]. In contrast, when caspofungin was combined with RCZ (FICI = 0.61 ± 0.31) and VCZ (FICI = 1.61 ± 0.42) there was no interaction [24]. No antagonism was observed. Animal studies are needed to investigate the combination of caspofungin with PCZ or ICZ.

10. *Blastomyces dermatitidis*

The activity of PCZ was tested *in vitro* and *in vivo* against *Blastomyces dermatitidis*. PCZ was more active when compared to AMB, ICZ and FCZ [MIC_{90} of 0.06 mcg/mL and minimal fungicidal concentration (MFC_{90}) of 4 mcg/mL] [25]. The potency of PCZ treatment was confirmed in a murine model with pulmonary blastomycosis. Survival in mice was prolonged at all PCZ doses (25, 5, or 1 mg/kg) and sterilization of lungs was achieved with AMB (1 mg/kg) and PCZ (only with the 25 mg/kg/day dosing regimen) but not with ICZ (150 mg/kg/day) and FCZ. The potency of PCZ was further exemplified at low doses (1 mg/kg/day) where it was shown to be more effective than ICZ (150 mg/kg/day) in prolonging survival of mice infected with *Blastomyces dermatitidis* [25]. Further studies with human subjects are needed to explore the roles of PCZ in the treatment of *Cryptococcus*, *Aspergillus*, *Candida* and *Blastomyces* infections.

11. *Trichosporon* spp.

The activities of AMB, PCZ, ICZ, FCZ, VCZ and RCZ were tested against *Trichosporon* spp. *in vitro* [26]. The fungicidal activities against *Trichosporon* with PCZ, VCZ and RCZ were more active than AMB and FCZ, but similar to ICZ [26]. Further *in vivo* studies to determine the role of PCZ in the treatment of *Trichosporon* are needed.

12. *Scedosporium* spp.

Meletiadis *et al.* compared the *in vitro* activities of the azoles [miconazole (MCZ), ICZ, VCZ and PCZ] to the polyenes (AMB and nystatin) and terbinafine against 13 clinical isolates of *Scedosporium apiospermum* and 55 clinical isolates of *Scedosporium prolificans* [27]. *S. apiospermum* isolates were most susceptible to VCZ (MIC_{90} of 0.5 mcg/mL) followed by MCZ (MIC_{90} of 1 mcg/mL), PCZ (MIC_{90} of 2 mcg/mL) and ICZ (MIC_{90} of 4 mcg/mL). The MIC_{90} values of AMB (16 mcg/mL), nystatin (32 mcg/mL) and terbinafine (>32 mcg/mL) were high. *S. prolificans* isolates were less susceptible (MIC_{90} for all drugs were high (>16) except VCZ, which had a value of 4 mcg/mL). Cross-resistance was observed among all the azoles except PCZ [27]. Another study compared the *in vitro* activities of triazoles (MCZ, VCZ, RCZ, PCZ and UR-9825) to conventional antifungals (AMB, ketoconazole, ICZ and nystatin) against 11 clinical isolates of *S. apiospermum* and 33 clinical isolates of *S. prolificans* [28]. The latter group was ineffective against both spp. (MIC_{90} values were >16 mcg/mL), whereas the triazoles showed activity against *S. apiospermum*. RCZ was more active (MIC_{90} of 0.125 mcg/mL) than PCZ or VCZ (MIC_{90} values of 0.25 mcg/mL). Similar to the prior study, *S. prolificans* isolates were less susceptible (MIC_{90} values were 16 for PCZ and RCZ and 4 mcg/mL for VCZ) [28]. Further studies in animal models are needed in an attempt to correlate these important *in vitro* results with *in vivo* data.

13. *Coccidioides immitis*

PCZ displayed similar *in vitro* activity to ICZ (MIC range for PCZ was 0.25 to 1 mcg/mL, and for ICZ was 0.125 to 0.5 mcg/mL); however, it was more effective against *Coccidioides immitis in vivo* [29]. Cultures of whole spleens and livers from mice treated with PCZ (10 mg/kg/day) showed ≥70% sterilization, whereas no sterilization was seen with ICZ, even at the higher dose of 30 mg/kg three times daily [29].

14. *Mucor* spp.

The *in vivo* activities of PCZ (at doses of 5, 15, and 30 mg/kg twice daily), ICZ (at a dose of 30 mg/kg three times daily), and AMB (at a dose of 1 mg/kg once daily) against *Mucor* spp. were compared in immunocompromised mice [30]. PCZ at doses of 15 and 30 mg/kg twice daily prolonged survival and reduced fungal tissue burden, while ICZ did not. PCZ given at 30 mg/kg twice daily (total daily dose of 60 mg/kg/day) was as potent as AMB [30]. The activity of PCZ is effective in immunocompromised mice; however, further studies are needed to determine its role in the treatment of human coccidioidomycosis and *zygomycosis*.

15. *Pseudallescheria boydil*

An *in vitro* study by Gonzalez *et al.* demonstrated that PCZ (MIC_{90} of 1 mcg/mL) was more active against *Pseudallescheria boydil* than ICZ (MIC_{90} of 4 mcg/mL) and FCZ (MIC_{90} of >64 mcg/mL) [31]. Furthermore, there were no statistically significant differences ($p > 0.05$) on survival between treatment with PCZ (at doses of 0.5, 1, 5 and 10 mg/kg once daily) and ICZ (at doses of 30 mg/kg three times daily). However, PCZ was more effective in preventing death (70%–75% survival) at the higher doses (30 or 50 mg/kg once daily and 25 mg/kg twice daily), than FCZ (50% survival at a dose of 20 mg/kg twice daily). This study confirms the relative resistance of PCZ to *Pseudallescheria boydil* [31].

16. Dermatophytes

PCZ was considered equally efficacious *in vitro* against dermatophytes when compared to ICZ (MIC_{90} values of 0.5 and 1 mcg/mL, respectively). However, PCZ (MFC_{90} of 1 mcg/mL) showed a higher fungicidal activity than ICZ (MFC_{90} of 2 mcg/mL) against isolates of the *Microsporum* genus ($p = 0.03$). *In vivo* studies are needed to investigate the potential clinical use of PCZ in the treatment of dermatophytes [32].

17. Synergy

Studies have investigated the interaction of PCZ with other antifungal regimens against *C. neoformans*, *C. glabrata*, and *A. fumigatus* [18–21,33]. In these studies, synergy is defined as fractional inhibitory concentration index (FICI) of ≤0.5, additivism as FICI > 0.5 to 1, indifference as FICI > 1 to ≤2, and antagonism as FICI > 2. PCZ has been shown to have synergistic and additivistic activities with other antifungals. These combinations may help avoid the emergence of drug resistance, decrease drug related toxicities with the use of lower doses, expand the spectrum of activity and shorten duration of treatment.

18. Postantifungal Effect

Postantifungal effect (PAFE) is defined as fungal growth suppression that persists after exposure to an antifungal drug. It reflects the time it takes for an organism to recover from the exposure to the drug and resume normal growth. This effect varies depending upon the pharmacodynamic interaction between the microorganism and the antifungal agent. In general, fungistatic drugs are expected to produce shorter PAFE compared to fungicidal agents. This is due to the fact that fungistatic drugs, unlike the fungicidal agents, do not cause permanent injury to the fungal cell wall which recovers as soon as the drug is removed.

A comparative study has shown that PCZ produced a short PAFE against *A. fumigatus* (0.75 ± 0.35 h) and *C. albicans* (≤0.5 h) compared to the long PAFE of AMB (7.5 ± 0.7 h and 5.3 ± 1.15 h, respectively) [34]. Although PCZ has fungicidal activity against *Aspergillus*, it has a short PAFE. The fungicidal activity of triazoles is slow (12–24 h for ≥90% killing of cells) due to the prolonged time required for the depletion of lanosterol in the fungal cell by inhibition of CYP450 dependent lanosterol 14α-demethylase. The PAFE is defined on the basis of short exposure (2 h in this study) of the cells to the drug instead of long exposure. The slow fungicidal effect of PCZ explains the short PAFE, in contrast to the rapid fungicidal activity and the long PAFE of AMB [34].

19. Pharmacokinetics

Animal Studies

The pharmacokinetics (PK) of PCZ have been measured in animals (*i.e.*, mice, rats, dogs, monkeys, and rabbits) [35]. After an 18-h overnight fast, these animals were randomly assigned to receive either a single intravenous (IV) or oral (PO) dose of PCZ (20 mg/kg) as a solution or suspension. The IV dose of PCZ was prepared with a 40% aqueous hydroxypropyl-β-cyclodextrin (HPβCD) solution, whereas the PO dose of PCZ was manufactured to either a solution in HPβCD or a suspension containing 0.4% methylcellulose, 0.5% polysorbate 80, and 0.9% sodium chloride (MPS). Blood from research animals were collected according to the study protocol [35]. PCZ concentrations were analyzed by high performance liquid chromatography (HPLC). The results of this study demonstrated that PCZ PO in mice was 100% bioavailable from the HPβCD solution; however, its systemic exposure was 47% from the MPS suspension [35]. The mean area under the concentration time curve ($AUC_{0-\infty}$, mcg·h/mL) values between IV and PO HPβCD solutions were 137 and 143, respectively [35]. Conversely, the mean $AUC_{0-\infty}$ for the PO MPS suspension was 64. The bioavailability values of PCZ in MPS suspension and HPβCD solution in rats were approximately 48% and 66%, respectively [35]. Similar results were reported in dogs (37% and 72%, respectively) and monkeys (14% and 52%, respectively). The half-life ($t_{½}$) values of IV PCZ HPβCD solution were the same at 7 h among mice and rats and were longer among the rabbits ($t_{½}$ = 9 h), dogs ($t_{½}$ = 15 h) and the monkeys ($t_{½}$ = 23 h) [35]. Based on these results, PCZ demonstrated good bioavailability in the animals tested. Results suggest that PCZ PO formulated in the HPβCD solution had a higher gastrointestinal absorption than PCZ formulated in the MPS suspension, suggesting no precipitation had occurred. The authors concluded PCZ may be administered once daily. This dosing is based on the fact that the plasma concentrations of PCZ at 24 h were maintained above the MICs and minimal fungicidal concentrations. However, the above information was not shown in the article.

Various doses of PCZ PO suspensions ranging from 20 to160 mg/kg were given to mice and 10 to 120 mg were administered to rats after feeding [35]. At determined time points, animals (n = 3 from each group) were sacrificed and plasma PCZ concentrations were measured by HPLC. Results show a relative dose-dependent effect in the systemic exposure of PCZ PO suspension. This effect was seen at doses of up to 80 mg/kg, in which maximum plasma concentration (C_{max}, mcg/mL) and $AUC_{0-\infty}$ (mcg·h/mL) were achieved [35]. Furthermore, as doses increased, C_{max} increases were less than $AUC_{0-\infty}$ increases, suggesting that absorption rates reached a plateau at higher doses.

A parallel study conducted by Nomeir and colleagues in fed and unfed dogs demonstrated that food significantly improved the relative systemic absorption (a relative 4-fold increase in C_{max} and $AUC_{0-\infty}$) of a single PO dose of PCZ in MPS suspension (at a doses of 10 mg/kg) [35]. A crossover study was subsequently conducted in fed dogs to assess the effect of various PCZ PO doses on plasma concentrations [35]. Each dosing phase (10, 40, 80, and 120 mg/kg) was separated by a 2-week washout period. Similar to the results seen in mice and rats, there was a relative dose related increase in C_{max} and $AUC_{0-\infty}$ at doses of up to 80 mg/kg and 120 mg/kg, respectively [35].

Another multiple dosing study was also conducted in fed dogs to investigate the PK of PCZ at 40 mg/kg daily for 8 consecutive days [35]. All blood samples were collected up to 13 days and the plasma PCZ concentrations were measured by HPLC. The authors reported an accumulation index of

2.6 for PCZ PO in MPS suspension. This was based on the mean C_{max} (percent of coefficient of variation, %CV) of 5.6 mcg/mL (43) and 2.1 mcg/mL (31) on days 8 and 1, respectively. However, the mean $AUC_{0-\infty}$ values (%CV) remained similar between the two days (107 mcg·h/mL (47) *vs.* 105 mcg·h/mL (30), respectively) [35]. As a result, the authors suggested that significant accumulation of PCZ was unlikely to occur in multiple daily dosing regimen in fed dogs.

Although the results of these preclinical studies demonstrated the PK of PCZ in animals, it is difficult to extrapolate this data to humans. Furthermore, research on PK, efficacy and safety of PCZ in humans would supplement our knowledge of this agent.

20. Dosing Studies of PCZ

The PK of PCZ are summarized in Table 2 and the PK of PCZ from the following studies are displayed in Tables 5a,b. The PK of various PO dosing regimens of PCZ were investigated in two independent, randomized, double-blind, placebo controlled and parallel clinical trials conducted in adult healthy volunteers [36]. The first study was designed in a single dose escalation approach, whereas the latter was conducted in a multiple dosing manner. The study participants (single dose study: $n = 36$, PCZ group and $n = 18$, placebo group; multiple dose study: $n = 36$, PCZ group and $n = 12$, placebo group) remained in the research facility for up to 48 h after the final PCZ dose in the single dose study and the morning dose of PCZ in the multiple dose study. All subjects were followed on an outpatient basis for another 72 h. A series of time specific blood sample collections were performed up to 120 h after PCZ administration in the single dose study, and up to 24 h post-dosing of PCZ on days 1 and 14 in the multiple dosing study according to the research protocol [36]. Plasma PCZ concentrations were measured by HPLC and the PK parameters of PCZ were analyzed by model independent methods. The mean age (range) of both treatment and placebo groups in this study was 23 (18–44) years and the subjects were within 15% of ideal body weight. Except for two females recruited in the multiple dosing study, the rest were males. The race was not specified in both studies.

In the single dose escalation study, PCZ tablets were administered orally in a single dose from 50 mg up to 1200 mg in the morning after a standardised high fat content breakfast. The mean C_{max} (%CV) (ng/mL) of PCZ increased proportionally with the single PO dosing regimen of 50 mg to 800 mg (113 (52) to 1320 (343), respectively). whereas the mean C_{max} of the 1200 mg dose did not show any more increase from the previous levels. Therefore, saturation of PCZ PO absorption was reached at the single 800 mg dose [36]. This observation was also confirmed when comparing PCZ $AUC_{0-\infty}$ values (%CV) (ng·h/mL) with a single dose of 800 mg *vs.* 1200 mg (49,841 (21,431) *vs.* 45,260 (19,914), respectively) [36]. The mean times to reach PCZ C_{max} values (T_{max} (%CV), h) ranged from 6.3 (3.2) to 6.2 (2.9) with single dose range of 50 to 800 mg, respectively [36]. PCZ had a large mean apparent volume of distribution (V/F (%CV), liters) ranging from 431 (86) to 781 (383) for doses of 100 mg to 400 mg, suggesting significant tissue distribution. However, there was no predictable pattern between tissue distribution and the various doses (Table 5a). Overall, a single dose PCZ tablet is well absorbed systemically but the rate of absorption is relatively slow.

According to these authors, a dose dependent clearance (CL/*F)* was observed with single PCZ doses (50–1200 mg) ranging from 4.1 to 6.6 mL/min/kg [36]. The t½s (%CV, hours) of PCZ ranged from 15.9 (2.9) for the 50 mg to 28.5 (7.4) for the1200 mg doses. These results were similar to those reported in other animal studies [35]. Moreover, the lower doses (*i.e.*, 50- and 100 mg) appeared to have a much shorter t½s than the higher doses (*i.e.*, 200-, 300-, 800- and 1200 mg) [36]. Based on this data, the authors concluded that PO PCZ tablet can be administered in a once or twice daily interval depending on the dosing regimen.

Table 2. Mean pharmacokinetics (PK) of Posaconazole (PCZ) after a single oral (PO) dose of 400 mg susp and 400 mg twice daily in healthy volunteers at steady state [2].

	Single Dose	Steady State
Parameter	**Value**	**Value**
Maximum concentration (ng/mL)	555	
Average concentration (ng/mL)		723
Time to reach maximum concentration (hours)	5.5 *	5 *
Serum protein binding (%)	98.5	
Volume of distribution (Liters)		3088
AUC_{0-X} (ng·h/mL)	11295 [a]	9093 [b]
Systemic clearance (L/hr)	43	76.1
Half-life (h)	24.1	31.7
Urinary excretion (%)	14	
Dialyzable	No	
Food or nutritional supplement enhance GI absorption	Yes	

* Data is presented as median; PK = pharmacokinetics; PCZ = posaconazole; PO = oral; susp = suspension; mg = milligram; AUC = area under the concentration time curve from time zero to time X; a = 0 to infinity; b = 0 to 12 h.

The results from the single dose escalation study suggest that frequent administration of PCZ by dividing the dose may lead to improved systemic drug exposure. The authors examined the effects of multiple PCZ dosing in a randomized, placebo controlled study [36]. PCZ was administered at multiple dosing regimens of 50 100, 200, and 400 mg tablets every 12 h for 14 days. The T_{max} after the first and second dose ranged from 5 to 6 and 9 to 11 h and the C_{max} (%CV, ng/mL) ranged from 457 (38) to 4150 (20) and from 371 (30) to 3239 (19), respectively. These results were comparable to those of a single dose regimen (Table 5b) [36]. Steady state of PCZ was reached at day 10 of the study. Accumulation of PCZ was noted with the ratio ranging from 6.6- to 8.3-fold between days 1 and 14 [36].

PCZ appeared to be well tolerated in both single and multiple dosing studies. The most common (≥10%) adverse events reported in the single dose PCZ study included headache, somnolence, and dizziness which were also noted in the placebo group [36]. The frequency of these adverse effects did not increase as the dose of PCZ increased. It should be noted that fatigue (11%) only occurred in the PCZ group. Adverse effects in the multiple dosing study included headache, dry mouth, somnolence, dizziness, fatigue and constipation. Similar findings were reported in the placebo group [36]. Most of the laboratory and diagnostic results, as well as physical examinations, did not change from baseline, with the exception of a few incidents of alterations in liver enzymes. Therefore, the authors concluded that PCZ was safe, well tolerated and could be administered once or twice daily due to its long t½.

21. Effects of Empty Stomach

Ezzet *et al.* conducted a randomized, open label, three way crossover study in healthy volunteers ($n = 18$) evaluating the PO bioavailability of PCZ administered at three different dosing regimens [37]. After at least a 12 h overnight fast, subjects who qualified for the study were randomized to receive PCZ suspension either as a single dose of 800 mg (regimen A) or as two doses of 400 mg every 12 h (regimen B), or four doses of 200 mg every 6 h (regimen C). No food was allowed for 24 h after the initial PCZ dose. Instead, 1400 mL IV fluid (5% dextrose in water with 0.45% saline) was administered at 100 mL/hour for caloric and fluid supplementation. Subjects were confined to the research facility for 48 h after the initial PCZ dose until the completion of the last blood sample. Blood samples were collected up to 22, 48, and 36 h after the first dose for regimens A, B and C, respectively, and plasma PCZ concentrations were analyzed by HPLC [37]. Safety and tolerability were monitored throughout the entire research study.

There were eighteen healthy subjects (thirteen black and five white) with a mean age (range) of 36 (26 to 44) years and mean weight (range) of 82 (64 to 100) kilograms [37]. The results of this study showed that regimen C had the highest mean ± standard deviation (SD) C_{max} (405 ± 280 mcg/L), T_{max} (24.2 ± 32 h) and C_{min} (189 ± 135 mcg/L) values measured at 48 h after the initial PCZ dose. Regimen B had the modest mean ± SD C_{max} (225 ± 115 mcg/L), T_{max} (16.6 ± 3.9 h), and C_{min} (96 ± 46 mcg/L) values. Regimen A had the lowest of those values (137 ± 90 mcg/L, 7.8 ± 4.7 h 50 ± 26 mcg/L, respectively) [37]. In this study, the authors were able to characterize PCZ PK parameters in a one compartment PO model using the "goodness of fit approach" [37]. PCZ's absorption rate constant, absorption t½, elimination rate constant, and terminal elimination t½ were 0.197 h^{-1}, 3.5 h, 0.048 h^{-1} and 15 h, respectively [37]. The intersubject coefficients of variation in the absorption rate constants were 18, 60 and 70 for regimens A, B, and C, respectively [37]. Data also demonstrated that the relative bioavailabilities of PCZ 800 mg suspension increased by 98% and 220% with regimens B and C (*i.e.*, 400 mg every 12 h and 200 mg every 6 h), respectively, when PCZ was given under fasting conditions. In addition, minimal adverse effects were reported with all three regimens. The authors concluded that dividing daily administration doses (every 12 and 6 h) significantly increased PCZ exposure under fasting conditions. These results corroborated with the findings from previous studies [36]. Splitting the total 800 mg daily dose of PCZ had better overall absorption as shown by the increased soluble fraction of PCZ and increased gastrointestinal residence time.

22. Effects of Food

For optimal absorption, PCZ suspension should be administered with food or a nutritional supplement that contains fat. The effects of a fed state on the relative bioavailability of PCZ was examined in several phase I clinical studies [6,38–40]. Courtney *et al.* conducted a randomized, open label, four way crossover PK study in healthy volunteers ($n = 20$) evaluating the effect of food on PCZ PO bioavailability [6]. The dose and formulations of PCZ used in this study were 200 mg/5 mL suspension and 200 mg tablet (two 100 mg tablets). After a 10-h overnight fast, subjects were randomized to receive four different regimens of either a single dose PCZ suspension with or without a high fat (841 calories, 52% fat) or nonfat (461 calories, 0% fat) breakfast or a single dose PCZ tablet with the high fat content breakfast. All meals were consumed within a 20-min period and the assigned treatments were initiated 5 min after. Water was the only fluid allowed as needed during the fasting phase. All subjects were required to complete all four regimens at various time periods and to stay in the research center for 48 h according to the study protocol [6]. Blood samplings were performed at designated periods and the last sample was collected at 72 h post-PCZ administration. Plasma PCZ concentrations and PK of PCZ were analyzed by HPLC and model independent methods, respectively. Safety and tolerance were also monitored throughout the study.

All subjects were 22 to 45 year old, healthy male Caucasians who resided in Germany. The results of this study demonstrated that the mean (%CV) C_{max} (ng/mL) were significantly higher when PCZ suspensions were administered with a high-fat meal than when administered in a fasting state ($p < 0.001$) or PCZ tablets with a high fat meal ($p < 0.004$) [6]. These values in descending order were 512 (34) > 413 (33) > 132 (50), respectively [6]. The mean (%CV) C_{max} of PCZ suspension administered with a nonfat meal was 378 (43), which was also significantly higher than the same formulation administered under a fasting state ($p < 0.001$) [6]. The mean (%CV) $AUC_{0-72\ h}$ values (ng·h/mL) of PCZ suspension varied among the three controlled conditions as follows: High fat meal *vs.* nonfat meal *vs.* fasted state (13,885 (41) *vs.* 9511 (38) *vs.* 3553 (36)) respectively [6]. Clearly, PCZ is absorbed three to five times greater when administered with meals. The mean $AUC_{0-72\ h}$ (%CV) value (ng·h/mL) of PCZ tablets when administered with a fatty meal was 10,304 (41), which was significantly lower than the PCZ suspension given with a high fat meal ($p = 0.001$) [6]. Finally, times to reach maximum PCZ concentration (T_{max}, h) and t½s (h) were similar for both suspension and tablet formulations ranging from 4.1 (21) to 5.5 (32) and 21 (15) to 23.5 (25), respectively [6].

Headache and fatigue were the two most reported adverse effects with PCZ [6]. This study is limited because subjects were all male and healthy Caucasians less than 45 years. It may be difficult to extrapolate these data to the female gender, other age groups, such as children and elderly, and other races including African Americans and Hispanics. The findings from this study may not be applied to patients with other disease states (*i.e.*, obesity, diabetes mellitus, and HIV/AIDS infection) and patients on medications that alter gastric acid secretion (*i.e.*, antacids, H2 receptor antagonists and proton pump inhibitors). In these situations, multiple dosing PK of PCZ is needed. Moreover, clearance and volume of distribution of PCZ were not determined. The authors concluded that for optimal absorption, PCZ should be administered with food based on bioavailabilities of 168% (2.6 fold) *vs.* 290% (4 fold) with nonfat and high-fat meals, respectively.

The PK parameters of PCZ in the fasted state and after a high-fat meal were also studied by Xu *et al.* in an open-label, randomized, 2 × 2 crossover study that had a washout period of 14 days [38]. A LC-MS method, which was precipitated with 0.6 mL of acetonitrile, was developed in order to measure the PCZ concentrations in human plasma. The lower limit of detection was set to 2 ng/mL. A total of 12 participants were enrolled and were administered 5 mL of PCZ suspension (200 mg) in the fasted state and with a high-fat meal [38]. The study subjects were given a light snack more than 10 h before each treatment on day-1. In the fasting period, food intake was withheld 4 h after the administration of the drug. In the fed phase, a standardised high-fat breakfast was served half an hour before administration of PCZ. Blood samples were drawn pre-administration and at 30 min intervals up to 120 h post-dose [38].

The C_{max} of PCZ ranged between 62.46 and 528.39 ng/mL [38]. In the fasted state, the mean C_{max} was 128.02 ± 92.21 ng/mL compared to 354.29 ± 82.02 ng/mL in the fed state ($p < 0.05$). The corresponding T_{max} levels were 3.88 ± 1.11 and 7.38 ± 2.87 h, respectively ($p < 0.05$). Mean AUC_{0-t} was reported to be 3075.27 ± 1917.00 ng·h/mL and 12229.08 ± 2923.37 ng·h/mL in the in the fasted and fed states, respectively ($p < 0.05$). The half-life was 22.11 ± 3.02 h in the fasted state compared to 21.39 ± 5.34 h in the fed state. The results demonstrated that the ingestion of a high-fat meal increases the absorption and bioavailability of PCZ without affecting its elimination [38]. This suggests that simultaneous administration of food can lead to higher plasma concentrations of PCZ and, potentially, more effective antifungal activity. This study was limited in that it only included Chinese subjects, which limits the extrapolation of the results to a broader population of patients. Additionally, compliance and the use of concomitant medications were not addressed. It would also be important to determine how the high plasma concentration levels of PCZ translate into better efficacy of the antifungal in future clinical studies.

The effects of food on the PK of PCZ were further evaluated by Lin *et al.* in a phase I, randomized, 3-way crossover study [39]. The objective of the investigation was to analyze the PK parameters of a single dose of 400 mg of PCZ oral suspension given under fasting and fed conditions in healthy male Taiwanese subjects. Study participants ($n = 16$) were administered PCZ 400 mg oral suspension following an overnight fast, or right after a normal-fat meal (700–800 calories; 30% fat), or after a high-fat breakfast (800–1000 calories; 50% fat). There was a washout period of 1 week between each treatment. Blood samples were collected at 0, 1, 2, 3, 4, 4.5, 5, 5.5, 6, 8, 10, 12, 24, 48, 72, 96, and 120 h, and serum plasma concentrations were analyzed using HPLC [39].

A total of 14 participants completed the study and two subjects withdrew after experiencing an adverse event [39]. However, only 13 patients were included in the PK analysis; but the reasons were not stated. The results revealed that C_{max}, AUC_{0-t}, and $AUC_{0-\infty}$ of PCZ were higher after a normal- or high-fat meal than under fasting conditions. Fasting, normal-fat, and high-fat mean C_{max} values of PCZ were 279.00 ± 123.32 ng/mL, 662.46 ± 251.02 ng/mL, and 608.38 ± 183.22 ng/mL, respectively ($p < 0.0001$); mean AUC_{0-t} values under each condition were 6828.56 ng·h/mL, 662.46 ± 251.02 ng·h/mL, and 608.38 ± 183.22 ng·h/mL, respectively after a normal-fat meal (700–800 calories; 30% fatiepectively ($p < 0.0001$); and mean $AUC_{0-\infty}$ values under each condition were 7304.72 ± 3444.54 ng·h/mL 21,326.65 ± 8495.01 ng·h/mL and 21,626.08 ± 8193.31 ng·h/mL respectively ($p < 0.0001$) [39]. Under fasting conditions, the mean T_{max} was much shorter when compared to the T_{max} after a normal or high-fat meal (3.15 h *versus* 4.88 h, respectively; $p = 0.0178$). The mean $t_{½}$ was 22.0, 20.8, and 22.0 h for each condition, respectively [39]. After analyzing these results, the investigators of the study concluded that the systemic absorption of PCZ increases when administered with food compared to under fasting conditions, and that the parameters are similar when the medication is administered with a normal-fat *versus* a high-fat meal [39]. It is important to note that this study was performed on a small number of Taiwanese patients, limiting the ability to extrapolate the results. Moreover, the clinical relevance of the observed increase in C_{max} and AUC was not discussed.

23. Effects of Nutritional Supplements

Sansone-Parsons *et al.* conducted a randomized, open label and crossover study in healthy volunteers ($n = 23$) to evaluate the effects of a nutritional supplement (Boost plus ™) on PCZ exposure [40]. After an overnight fast, subjects were randomized to receive a single dose of PO PCZ (400 mg suspension), either alone or with 240 mL of Boost Plus™ (16% protein, 34% fat and 50% carbohydrate providing 1.5 calorie/mL). After a washout period of at least 14 days, subjects would crossover to receive the alternate treatment. In each study phase, subjects were not allowed to consume any food until 4 h after receiving PCZ and to leave the research center until after the last sample collection at 72-h post dose. A series of time sensitive blood sampling was performed and the plasma PCZ concentrations were measured by LC-MS. PK of PCZ were analyzed by a noncompartmental method. Safety and tolerance of PCZ were monitored during the study period [40].

This study used twenty-four subjects with a mean age (range) of 39.4 (24–53) years and a mean body mass index of 26.2 kg/m^2 [40]. One of the participants withdrew from the study due to personal reasons. The results of this study demonstrated that co-administration of a nutritional supplement (*i.e.*, Boost plus™) significantly enhanced the relative PO absorption of PCZ by 263% (90% confidence interval: 226–307) than when given alone. The mean (%CV) C_{max} (ng/mL) and AUC_{0-72} (ng·h/mL) values were 355 (43) and 9076 (42) *vs.* 121 (75) and 3552 (53), respectively [40]. The T_{max} and $t½$ values were no different between the two treatment phases. The mean (%CV) total body clearance (CL/F, liters/h) and apparent volume of distribution (V/F, liters) values were lower when PCZ was administered with Boost plus™ (42.6 (56) *vs.* 91.2 (40) and 1573 (51) *vs.* 3674 (51), respectively) [40]. These observations were similar to the data published in previous studies [6,36–39]. No adverse events were reported. The authors concluded that PCZ taken with any type of food shows enhanced bioavailability (a 2.6 fold increase). As compared to previous trials, there were more Hispanics (16 out of 23) and female subjects ($n = 12$) recruited in this study [6,36–39].

24. Effects of pH and Comedication

Abnormal pH levels have been associated with changes in PK, leading to unpredictable bioavailability and subtherapeutic concentrations of certain medications. Walravens *et al.* performed a crossover study on five healthy subjects in order to determine the impact of pH on the absorption of PCZ and investigate the mechanisms of increased intestinal absorption when an acidic carbonated beverage is coadministered [41]. Study subjects received a single dose of 10 mL of PCZ suspension (40 mg/mL) in four different conditions: With 330 mL of water, with 330 mL of a cola beverage (Coca-Cola), with 330 mL of water after the administration of esomeprazole 40 mg once a day for 3 days, or with 330 mL of Coca-Cola after the administration of esomeprazole 40 mg once a day for 3 days [41]. Blood and gastrointestinal samples were taken at different intervals during the study in order to measure PCZ concentrations and investigate the gastric and intestinal behavior of the antifungal [41].

After analyzing the data, it was shown that administering PCZ with Coca-Cola did not affect the pH of the intraluminal environment when compared to water; however, it did lead to an increase in PCZ gastric concentrations by 102% ($p = 0.001$) and systemic exposure by 70% ($p < 0.05$) [41]. The investigators attributed this effect to a probable increase in PCZ solubility in Coca-Cola and a prolonged gastric residence. Concomitant use of esomeprazole was shown to increase the gastric pH and lead to decreased absorption of PCZ with a drop of 37% and 84% in the mean plasma and gastric AUC values, respectively. Administration of Coca-Cola was not sufficient to compensate for the increase in gastric pH induced by the esomeprazole, since the mean plasma and gastric AUC values were still decreased by 19% and 73%, respectively, when the study participants were given PCZ with both esomeprazole and Coca-Cola. There was a strong correlation between the gastric and plasma concentrations of PCZ ($r = 0.8165$; $p < 0.0001$) showing that dissolution in the stomach is important for the absorption of PCZ [41]. Based on these results, the authors concluded that coadministration of Coca-Cola could serve to increase the bioavailability of PCZ in the fasted state. Nevertheless, they labeled it as only a "partially efficient strategy" for patients that have inadequate food intake and abnormal pH levels due to concomitant use of acid-suppressive agents [41]. Further studies would serve to confirm the impact of pH on the serum concentrations and efficacy of PCZ. However, it is important to note that the PCZ package insert currently recommends the oral administration of PCZ during, or within 20 min, of a meal, with a liquid or nutritional supplement, or with an acidic carbonated beverage [2].

25. Protein Binding

PCZ is greater than 98% protein bound to serum albumin [2,36,42]. Protein binding of PCZ was not affected in patients with various stages of chronic kidney disease or in patients with conventional hemodialysis [42]. These values were consistently greater than 98% [42].

26. Disposition Studies

Krieter *et al.* conducted a small open label PK study in healthy volunteers (n = 8) to examine the absorption, metabolism and excretion of radiolabeled [^{14}C] PCZ [43]. Healthy subjects with a mean age of 28 years underwent an overnight fast and received a single dose of radiolabeled [^{14}C] PCZ (400 mg suspension, 82 mcCi). PCZ was administered 5 min after the consumption of a standardised high fat breakfast. All subjects remained at the research site for blood, urine and stool sampling and were released after 90% of the administered radioactive dose was excreted and recovered. Recovery times after [^{14}C] PCZ administration ranged from 168 h to 14 days post PCZ dose. PCZ was quantified and its metabolites in blood and urine samples were measured by HPLC and LC-MS. The amount of radioactivity from the [^{14}C] was assessed by liquid scintillation technique. The PK of PCZ were characterized by model independent methods. Safety and tolerance were monitored during the study period [43].

The PK of PCZ reported in this study were comparable to previous studies [36,41]. The mean (%CV) C_{max} (ng/mL), $t_{1/2}$ (hours), CL/F (Liters/hours), V/F (Liters) and CL_R (mL/min) were 654 (19), 20 (19), 16.3 (30), 465 (31) and 0.0114 (76), respectively [42]. The median (range) T_{max} (hours) was 9.25, whereas the mean (%CV) $AUC_{0-\infty}$ (ng • h/mL) was 26100 (26) [43].

The pooled amounts (%) of radioactivity expressed as mean (%CV) in feces and urine were 76.9 (12) and 14 (11), respectively [43]. After 24 h, the pooled amounts of PCZ and its glucuronide metabolites (M8, M5, and M2) in plasma were 65.7%, 17.5%, 8.97% and 7.88%, respectively [43]. M5 and M2 were diglucuronide conjugates of PCZ, whereas M8 was monoglucuronide. All metabolites of PCZ were inactive. Urinary metabolites (*i.e.*, M8, M9, a monoglucuronide, and M5) accounted for no more than 2% of the administered dose of PCZ. Fecal metabolites contributed up to 94% of the pooled amount of radioactivity which translated into 66.3% of the administered dose. These data suggested that PCZ had minimal interaction with the cytochrome P450 system. Furthermore, PCZ's metabolism is mediated predominantly through phase II UDP-glucuronosyltransferase (UGT) enzyme pathway, especially UGT1A4 [44].

27. P-glycoprotein

The manufacturer database categorizes PCZ as a substrate and inhibitor of P-glycoprotein (P-gp). Sansone Parsons *et al.* conducted a pharmacogenetic study to evaluate the effect of MDR1 gene and its product, P-gp, on systemic exposure of PCZ between black and white subjects [45]. The procedures for the MDR1 single nucleotide polymorphism (SNP) and MDR1 mRNA expression were described in detail in the report. The results of this study showed that the distribution of MDR1 genotypes among the black and white study subjects was similar to the general population [45]. Furthermore, no direct association was observed between any MDR1 single nucleotide polymorphism and the AUC of PCZ. Thus, P-gp did not have a significant influence on the PK of PCZ. Further studies are required to determine the role of other drug transport proteins on the systemic exposure of PCZ.

28. Newer Solid Oral Tablet Formulation

Krishna *et al.* investigated the rising single- and multiple-dose PK of PCZ for a new oral tablet formulation in a phase I, randomized, single-center, placebo- controlled study on healthy subjects [46]. The safety and tolerability of the tablet formulation was also evaluated. The study was conducted from 19 March 2009 to 20 May 2009. A total of 25 participants were included in the study and were randomized into two cohorts via a computer-generated sponsor-provided randomization code. Group 1 was administered PCZ 200 mg (n = 9) or a matching placebo (n = 3) with the following schedule: A single morning dose on day 1, twice daily on day 6, once a day on day 7–14, and twice a day on days 15–22. Group 2 was given PCZ 400 mg (n = 9) or a matching placebo (n = 3) with the following schedule: A single morning dose on day 1, twice a day on day 6, once a day on days 7–14, but not the 400 mg twice a day on days 15–22 to avoid exceeding the PCZ exposure range that is considered to be safe. Blood samples were collected for both groups on day 1 at 0 h (pre-dose), and at 2, 3, 4, 5, 6, 8, 12, 24, 48, 72, and 120 h post-dose. On day 6, blood samples were taken at 2, 3, 4, 5, 6, 8, 12, 24, and 48 h post-dose. Pre-dose samples were taken on days 12 and 13 of the study. Additional samples were taken for Group 1 on days 14 and 22, and on day 14 for Group 2. The samples were analyzed using liquid chromatography with tandem mass spectrometric (LC-MS) detection with a calibrated range of 5–5000 ng/mL. Safety was addressed via assessment of vital signs, physical examination, electrocardiogram (ECG), clinical laboratory tests and incidence of adverse events throughout the study [46].

Inclusion criteria included male and female between the ages of 18 to 65 years with a BMI of 19 to 35 kg/m^2. They were required to have blood chemistry, hematology, and urinalysis laboratory test results within normal limits. Female participants had to be post-menopausal, surgically sterilized, or using an accepted method of contraception, and male participants had to be using an accepted method of contraception, or agree to abstain from sexual intercourse during the study and up to 1 month after. Exclusion criteria included a history of an infectious disease occurring 4 weeks prior to the initiation of the study, a positive hepatitis B, hepatitis C, or HIV test, use of medications with a high potential for drug abuse, history of alcohol or drug abuse in that past two years, among many others [46].

The results of this intention-to-treat analysis included 13 subjects in Group 1 (including a replacement subject) and 12 participants in Group 2. They were aged between 31 to 59 years with a mean of 45.9 years and were white and of Hispanic or Latino ethnicity. The analysis revealed that exposure to PCZ is increased in a dose-related manner after both single and multiple oral dose administration of PCZ tablets (200 and 400 mg); mean C_{max} for Group 1 was 778 ng/mL and 1290 ng/mL for Group 2 after single dose administration; and 1800 ng/mL (200 mg QD; Group 1), 2980 ng/mL (200 mg BID, Group 1), and 2940 ng/mL (400 mg QD, Group 2) after multiple dose PO administration. After single administration, mean t½ values were 25 and 26 h for the 200 and 400 mg doses, respectively; C_{max} were reached at a mean T_{max} of 4 and 5 h for the 200 and 400 mg doses, respectively. After multiple dose administration, the accumulation ratio of PCZ in a period of 8 days was approximately 3 for the 200 and 400 mg dose, and around 5 for the 200 mg BID dose. Safety results demonstrated the oral tablet formulation to be generally safe and well-tolerated. A total of 12 study participants (48%) reported at least one treatment-related adverse event. These included elevated hepatic enzymes, diarrhea, headache, dizziness, dry mouth, and nausea; however, none of these adverse events had any clinical sequelae [46].

The authors concluded that the exposure of PCZ from the new oral tablet formulation increased in a dose-related manner with a steady-state C_{avg} exceeding the dose that has been previously considered to be effective against invasive fungal infections (IFIs). They also stated that PCZ tablet is generally safe and well tolerated in healthy individuals [46]. Nevertheless, it is important to consider that the sample size of this study was very small and differential statistics were not employed. Therefore, no p values were reported for any of the data. Also, the study population only included healthy patients of Hispanic or Latino ethnicity, limiting the ability to extrapolate the results to unhealthy patients of other ethnicities.

29. Prophylaxis in Neutropenia

Patients with neutropenia resulting from chemotherapy for hematologic cancers and for myelodysplastic syndrome are at risk for invasive and fatal fungal infections. FCZ and ICZ prophylaxis have been the standard of care in order to reduce the incidence and mortality of these infections. FCZ is effective for preventing *Candida* infections but lacks efficacy against filamentous fungi. ICZ has a wider spectrum of activity than FCZ and includes activity against *Aspergillus*, but its use has been limited by the poor tolerability of the oral solution, the erratic bioavailability of the oral capsule and the greater toxicity.

Cornely *et al.* conducted a randomized, multicenter study comparing the efficacy and safety of PCZ ($n = 304$) with those of FCZ ($n = 240$) or ICZ ($n = 58$) prophylaxis in patients with prolonged neutropenia from chemotherapy for acute myelogenous leukemia or myelodysplastic syndrome [47]. Patients were randomly assigned to receive prophylaxis with PCZ (200 mg PO suspension three times daily), FCZ (400 mg PO suspension daily) or ICZ (200 mg PO solution twice daily). Drug prophylaxis was given with each chemotherapy cycle until recovery from neutropenia and complete remission, occurrence of invasive fungal infection or for up to 12 weeks from randomization, whichever came first. Patients who were unable to tolerate the oral study drug were given IV prophylaxis for 3 days or less per chemotherapy. In the PCZ group, the IV drug was AMB deoxycholate (0.3–0.5 mg/kg of body weight), and in the FCZ or ICZ group, the IV prophylaxis was the same dose of the PO drug [47].

The primary end point was the incidence of proven and probable IFIs during the treatment phase, defined as the period from randomization to 7 days after the last dose of the study drug administered during the last chemotherapy cycle [47]. PCZ (2%) was found to be superior in terms of the primary endpoint as compared to the FCZ or ICZ group (8%). Absolute reduction in the PCZ group was −6% with a 95% CI −9.7 to −2.5%, $p < 0.001$ [47]. The secondary end points included the incidence of invasive aspergillosis, mortality from any cause and time to death related to fungal infections. The PCZ compared to the FCZ or ICZ group had significantly fewer patients with invasive aspergillosis (1% *versus* 7%, $p < 0.001$), displayed lower mortality (16% *versus* 22%, $p < 0.048$) and showed a significant benefit ($p = 0.01$) in the analysis of time to death [47]. Serious adverse events, possibly, or probably, related to treatment were reported in 6% of the PCZ compared to 2% of the FCZ or ICZ group ($p = 0.01$). Serious events included QT prolongation, atrial fibrillation, a decreased ejection fraction, and torsades de pointes [47].

The authors mentioned that most of the probable aspergillosis cases were based on a positive *Aspergillus* galactomannan antigen test and not on positive cultures. If these probable cases were removed from the study, PCZ may not have shown to be superior to FCZ or ICZ [48]. There are concerns of *Aspergillus*-resistant strains and cross-resistance with other azoles developing from the use of a broad spectrum drug such as PCZ. This may also translate to the lack of fungicidal activity of VCZ in the treatment of *Aspergillus* infections. It is unknown as to whether aspergillosis occurred as a result of PCZ resistance or other factors, including suboptimal PCZ levels [49]. Sixty-five patients received ICZ, compared to 240 who received FCZ. In lieu of this fact, there may not have been adequate statistical power in this study to conclude that PCZ was better than ICZ [50]. PCZ prophylaxis should probably be reserved for the high-risk patients with hematologic cancers [49].

30. Persistent Febrile Neutropenia and Invasive Fungal Infections

Ullmann *et al.* conducted a computer assisted, randomized and open label clinical trial in patients with febrile neutropenia ($n = 66$) or refractory IFIs ($n = 32$) [51]. This study evaluated the PK, safety and tolerability of various dosing regimens of PCZ PO suspension. Most patients in the refractory invasive fungal infection group had experienced treatment failure with caspofungin and/or AMB. The study regimens included PCZ 200 mg four times daily for nine doses, followed by 400 mg twice daily (Group 1); PCZ 400 mg four times daily for nine doses, followed by 600 mg twice daily (Group 2); and PCZ 800 mg twice daily for five doses, followed by 800 mg daily (Group 3). The PK phase of the study was completed after 10 days of treatment, whereas the clinical phase continued up to 6 months in patients with refractory invasive fungal infection or until neutrophil recovery in patients with febrile neutropenia. PCZ concentrations from blood samples in the PK phase were collected on days 3 and 10. On day 10, blood samples were taken at 0 and up to 12-h post dose for all treatment groups. An additional 24-h post dose was done for groups 1 and 2. All plasma PCZ concentrations were determined by LC-MS and PK of PCZ was characterized by compartmental modeling. The efficacy of PCZ was evaluated by clinical response defined by the study criteria [51].

Sixty-nine patients (70%) were assessed for PK analysis on day 3 following the initial high PCZ doses and sixty-one (62%) were assessed on day 10. The results showed that steady state PCZ plasma concentrations among the three dosing groups were not reached on day 3 due to the mean long half-life of PCZ (35 h). On day 10, plasma PCZ steady state concentrations were reached in all three groups. The mean (%CV) systemic exposure (*i.e.*, AUC_τ, ng • h/mL; C_{max}, ng/mL; C_{min}, ng/mL; and C_{av}, ng/mL) and log-transformed values (NAUC, ng • h/mL) of PCZ in group 1 were the highest compared to those of Groups 2 and 3 [51]. The exposure of PCZ in bone marrow transplant (BMT) recipients was 52% lower than in patients with no history of BMT (191 *versus* 402, ng/mL, $p < 0.003$). The authors explained that this phenomenon might be due to the small sample of BMT patients ($n = 12$). The mean (%CV) apparent clearance (CL/F, liters/h) values were similar among all three groups (283 (354), 179 (82) and 215 (81), respectively) [51].

The baseline characteristics were similar among all the groups with a co-morbid condition of hematologic malignancy ($n = 89$) or BMT ($n = 32$). The percent of refractory invasive fungal infection responders, defined as all randomized subjects who had complete and partial responses, at the end of PCZ treatment were 50%, 10% and 40% in groups 1 ($n = 12$), 2 ($n = 10$) and 3 ($n = 10$), respectively [51]. The success rates of PCZ treatment in febrile neutropenic patients were similar among all study groups (in all randomized patients at the end of therapy the rates were 61% ($n = 23$), 67% ($n = 21$) and 64% ($n = 22$) and, in efficacy evaluable patients after 7 days of therapy, the rates were 76% ($n = 17$), 82% ($n = 17$) and 85% ($n = 13$) for Groups 1,2, and 3, respectively) [51]. Regardless of the dosing regimens, adverse events were headache, edema and rigors (which accounted for 7%), nausea (4%), diarrhea (4%) and vomiting (6%). Adverse effects involving subcutaneous tissue included rash, pruritus, and fissures among all study groups ($n = 98$). Predictable adverse effect patterns were not observed in all study groups with the exception of nausea frequently reported in Group 1 regimen. The overall mortality rate was 22% for all randomized patients with a total of 47% and 11% deaths in the refractory IFIs and the febrile neutropenia groups, respectively [51].

Based on the results of this study, the authors concluded that PCZ was safe and well tolerated [51]. The recommended dosing regimen for PCZ PO suspension was 400 mg twice daily in persistent febrile neutropenia or refractory invasive fungal infection. A much larger and well controlled clinical trial is needed to confirm the clinical outcome of this study.

Several other clinical trials have explored the use of PCZ for the prevention and treatment of IFIs. In a study by Huang *et al.* the administration of PCZ oral suspension for the treatment of IFIs in patients that were refractory to, or intolerant to the first-line therapy, was investigated [52]. It was a multicenter, open label study that included a total of 63 patients [52]. Treatment with PCZ had a clinical response rate of 64.4%, and 52.9% of the patients showed eradication of the invasive fungal infection [52]. The authors reported that the adverse events that were observed were mild-moderate in severity and had a short duration. Therefore, they claimed that PCZ can be used as an alternative or salvage therapy for the treatment of IFIs [52]. Nevertheless, a comparative study would be necessary in order to determine how these clinical response rates compare to those of other antifungals currently used as salvage therapy for IFIs.

In another study, Shen *et al.* investigated the efficacy of PCZ in the prevention of IFIs in a Chinese population [53]. It was a randomized, multicenter study that was conducted in China on patients with acute myelogenous leukemia\and myelodysplastic syndrome who had persistent chemotherapy-induced neutropenia [53]. Administration of PCZ for prophylactic treatment was performed for a maximum of 12 weeks, or until the neutropenia was resolved with complete remission, or until an IFI occurred. Study participants were randomly assigned to receive PCZ oral suspension ($n = 129$) or FCZ ($n = 123$), but only 117 patients in each cohort were included in the statistical analysis. The primary endpoint of the study was the occurrence of proven, probable or possible IFI during the treatment with PCZ. Secondary endpoints included clinical failure rate, all-cause mortality, and the time to first systemic antifungal treatment [53].

The results of this study reported that 11 of 117 (9.4%) of the patients in the PCZ group *versus* 26 of 117 (22.2%) in the FCZ group had an incidence of proven, probable, or possible IFI ($p = 0.0114$) [53]. Moreover, the clinical failure rate was lower in the PCZ group (37/117 (31.6%; 95% CI; 23.3–40.9)) when compared to the FCZ group (49/117 (41.88%, 95% CI; 32.8–51.4)) ($p = 0.168$). Onset of first systemic antifungal treatment was also later in patients receiving PCZ *versus* FLU ($p = 0.0139$). The most commonly reported adverse event was abnormal liver enzymes which was seen in 11 (8.8%) patients in the PCZ group and 6 (5.0%) patients in the FCZ group ($p = 0.221$). The authors of this investigation concluded that PCZ proved to be efficacious and well tolerated in the prophylaxis of IFIs in high-risk neutropenic Chinese patients [53]. However, the results of this study can only be extrapolated to a Chinese population; a larger study with a broader population of patients is guaranteed in order to confirm the clinical relevance of this study.

A more recent study by Kaya *et al.* aimed to compare the efficacy of PCZ to FCZ when used as prophylactic agents in patients with hematological malignancies and high risk for IFIs) [54]. It was a 2 year, retrospective, observational study [54]. High risk for IFI was defined as a deep neutropenia (<100/mm^3) lasting more than one week. Its diagnosis was based on blood cultures, pulmonary high resolution computerized tomography (HRCT), serum galactomannan (GM) levels, and histopathological analysis. Positive GM levels were defined as >0.5 in two consecutive readings, or >0.7 in a single reading, and they were analyzed twice a week. Positive pulmonary fungal disease and invasive pulmonary aspergillosis (IPA) were diagnosed based on radiological findings, as well as GM positivity for the IPA. Patients with similar characteristics were administered either FCZ 400 mg/day PO ($n = 70$) or PCZ 3 × 200mg/day PO ($n = 35$); the specific PO formulation employed was not noted. Prophylaxis was continued until patients were no longer at high risk for IFIs. Prophylactic failure was defined as the occurrence of IPA or a documented fungal infection despite the use of antifungal prophylaxis, and/or the initiation of empiric antifungal therapy while the prophylaxis was being administered [54].

A total of 105 patients were included in the retrospective cohort with a mean age of 44.5 years; 64% were male and 36% were female [54]. A fungal infection was reported in 22 out the 70 (31%) patients receiving FCZ and 13 out of the 35 (37%) patients who were administered PCZ ($p = 0.827$). Similar results were seen in terms of incidence of IPA, where 21 out of 70 (31%) subjects in the FCZ group *versus* 9 out of 35 (26%) subjects in the PCZ group reported an event ($p = 0.705$). Initiation of empiric antifungal treatment was needed in 21% and 20% of patients in the FCZ and PCZ groups, respectively ($p = 0.932$). Mortality, which was defined as death due to any reason, was reported in 17 (24%) and 4 (8%) patients in the FCZ and PCZ groups, respectively ($p = 0.195$). Differences in frequency of adverse events were not statistically significant between the FCZ and PCZ groups ($p = 0.276$); the most commonly reported included nausea and vomiting. Based on these results, the authors concluded that incidence of IFIs and crude mortality are similar between FCZ and PCZ since no statistical significance was found [54]. They attributed the higher rates of fungal infection and initiation of empiric antifungal therapy in the PCZ group to poor absorption of the drug from the gastrointestinal tract due to nausea and vomiting. The investigators stated that both FCZ and PCZ can be successfully used for fungal infection prophylaxis in patients at high risk [54]. Nevertheless, it is important to note the small sample size of the study and difference in number of study subjects between the two groups that could have affected the results. Also, compliance, use of concomitant medications, and food intake with PCZ was addressed. The study was also conducted in Turkey, limiting its applicability to patients of other nationalities.

31. Prophylaxis in Severe Graft-*versus*-Host Disease

Recipients of hematopoietic stem-cell transplants are at increased risk for IFIs. FCZ prophylaxis has become a standard of care for antifungal prophylaxis in the post-transplant patient. An international, randomized, double-blind, multicenter trial conducted by Ullmann *et al.* compared PCZ with FCZ for prophylaxis against fungal infections in patients who had either acute graft-*versus*-host disease (GVHD), chronic extensive GVHD, or being treated with intensive immunosuppressive therapy [55]. Patients (n = 600) were randomized to receive PCZ (n = 301) PO suspension 200 mg three times daily plus placebo capsules once daily or FCZ (n = 299) 400 mg tablet once daily plus placebo oral suspension for a period of 112 days (treatment period). The primary endpoint was the incidence of proven or probable IFIs during the treatment period. Other end points were the incidence of proven or probable aspergillosis, the time to the occurrence of an invasive fungal infection, the overall mortality and the mortality due to fungal infection. The safety and tolerability of the study drugs were also monitored for a period of 24 weeks [55].

PCZ was found to be as efficacious as FCZ in preventing IFIs (incidence of 5.3% *vs.* 9%, respectively; $p = 0.07$) and superior in preventing proven or probable invasive aspergillosis (2.3% *vs.* 7%, respectively; $p = 0.006$) [55]. There was a delay in the onset of infections in the PCZ compared to the FCZ group (mean day 102 *vs.* mean day 88, respectively; $p = 0.048$). The number of overall deaths was similar between the two groups but mortality from IFIs was significantly lower in the PCZ group (1% *vs.* 4% in the FCZ group, $p = 0.046$) [55]. The frequency of drug discontinuation because of adverse effects (34% in the PCZ and 38% in the FCZ group), and the frequency of treatment-related adverse effects (36% in the PCZ and 38% in the FCZ) and serious adverse effects (13% and 10%, respectively) were similar [55].

This study failed to state that patients were excluded from the study if they were unable to take medications orally, since PCZ is only given by mouth. The low incidence of aspergillosis in the FCZ group may be explained by the unintentional selection of less sick patients. Factors such as compliance, diet (intake of a fatty meal can increase PCZ absorption) and serum concentrations were not reported, yet they can have an important impact on treatment success [55].

Provided invasive fungal disease is detected early, treatment is successful with the VCZ and liposomal AMB. For this reason, PCZ prophylaxis in patients with severe GVHD should be reserved for the medical centers that have a low incidence of invasive aspergillosis and have the facilities to pursue a preemptive approach [55].

Winston *et al.* also evaluated the efficacy, safety, and breakthrough infections that are related to long-term treatment with PCZ for the prevention of IFIs in patients with allogenic stem cell transplantation (SCT) [56]. Data was collected from a total of 106 SCT recipients who were administered PCZ as prophylactic treatment. The study was single-center and conducted from 1 January 2007 to 31 December 31 2008 [56]. Study participants were administered an oral suspension of PCZ 200 mg three times a day with meals, whenever possible, from day 1 after the SCT until day 100. For patients unable to take medications orally, itraconazole 200 mg IV q 24 h was temporarily substituted for the oral PCZ suspension. Voriconazole 6 mg/kg IV q 12 h on day 1, followed by 4 mg/kg IV q 12 h was given in place of itraconazole when it became unavailable in the US. Incidence of breakthrough infections was assessed through cultures of blood and other suspected sites of infections, CT scans of chest and abdomen, and *Aspergillus* galactomannan assays. Susceptibility of fungal isolates to PCZ was measured via a microbroth assay, and serum plasma concentrations of PCZ were analyzed by HPLC. Patients were taking several others concomitant medications for their health conditions including chemotherapy, cyclosporine, corticosteroids, methotrexate, mycophenolate, trimethoprim-sulfamethoxazole, atovaquone, maribavir, ganciclovir, and pantoprazole [56].

Results were reported for the 106 patients that were treated and evaluated. Their median age was 46 years and they had many of the factors associated with high risk for IFIs including hematologic disease (56%), unrelated donor (42%), high-dose corticosteroid use (76%), and acute GVHD (60%) [56]. A large percentage of these patients (85%) had oral mucositis during their neutropenic state after the transplantation procedure and before the engraftment, and most were taking pantoprazole during the study (>90%). Study subjects experienced neutropenia for a mean duration of 19.6 days, and prophylaxis with PCZ had a mean duration of 113 days with a range of 1–180 days. A total of 34 patients (32%) had to be changed temporarily to itraconazole or voriconazole during the course of the study due to severe oral mucositis or inability to take medications orally for a mean duration of 9.6 days. Eight of 106 patients (7.5%) had a breakthrough infection during the first 6 months after transplantation, and three other participants had an IFI within 53–66 days after finishing preventive treatment with PCZ; however, these patients were taking another systemic antifungal agent when the infection developed. The onset time for the 11 IFIs was 65 days after the transplantation procedure with a range of 2–162 days. The factors that were associated with the development of these infections included neutropenia (four cases), an infected central IV line (three cases), poor compliance (two cases), administration of PCZ via gastric tube (one case), and engraftment failure (one case). It is important to note that all patients who had an IFI were also taking pantoprazole, and eight of these patients had concurrent diarrhea or mucositis which could have reduced the serum concentrations of PCZ. The most common organisms causing the fungal infections were *Candida* species which was responsible for eight cases, *Aspergillus* species which affected two patients, and a combination of *Aspergillus* species with *Coccidioides immitis* in one patient. Out of the nine infecting isolates that were tested for susceptibility to PCZ, only two showed to be resistant with an MIC >1.0 μg/mL; both were *Candida glabrata*. PCZ plasma concentrations were not initially monitored since a target concentration of PCZ has not been established and a dose of 200 mg three times a day has been proven to be efficacious in previous studies; however, after the development of IFIs in several patients, peak and trough plasma levels of PCZ were measured on days 2, 8, and 15 after transplantation in 15, 14, and 10 patients with neutropenia, respectively. The plasma PCZ concentrations of these patients who developed IFIs were similar to those who did not experience an infection. The reported values of mean peak and trough concentrations were 168 ng/mL and 121 ng/mL on day 2 post-transplantation, 306 ng/mL and 276 ng/mL on day 8, and 257 ng/mL and 211 ng/mL on day 15, respectively. In terms of safety, PCZ was generally well-tolerated with a total of nine patients who experienced nausea and no other adverse events being associated with PCZ administration. After six months post-transplantation, the overall patient-survival was reported to be 65% and fungal-free survival was 62%. There were a total of 37 deaths, with four being associated to the development of an IFI. The most common causes were malignancy relapse, GVHD, and infection [56].

After analyzing these results, the authors concluded that long-term prophylaxis with PCZ after allogenic SCT is safe and associated with few incidences of IFIs [56]. Nevertheless, they expressed their concern with the development of breakthrough infections by PCZ-susceptible organisms even when the recommended prophylactic doses of PCZ were being used. Consequently, the investigators recommended different strategies to increase exposure to PCZ, such as the use of higher doses, administration with an acidic beverage, and limiting the concomitant use of proton pump inhibitors (PPIs) [56]. Future research employing these recommended strategies is warranted in order to determine their impact on the successful prevention of IFIs. Furthermore, it would also be important to determine the statistical and clinical significance of the incidence of IFIs while on PCZ treatment when compared to other antifungals that are currently used for the prevention of these infections.

32. Fusariosis

A retrospective analysis of three open label clinical trials included 21 patients with hematological malignancies and other related conditions to evaluate the effectiveness of PCZ in *Fusarium* infections [57]. PCZ was given as an oral suspension of 800 mg per day in 2 to 4 divided doses [57]. All patients had proven or probable invasive fusariosis refractory to (for at least 7 days) or intolerant of (defined as severe infusion-related toxicity, nephrotoxicity, or other organ dysfunction) AMB, which is the conventional antifungal treatment. These patients subsequently received PCZ. Successful response to PCZ therapy occurred in 48% of all patients, and 50% of patients with leukemia [57].

Although there are limitations to a retrospective study, these results show that PCZ is safe, well tolerated and can be used as an alternative to conventional AMB therapy for the treatment of invasive fusariosis [57]. A patient in this study with AMB and natamycin resistant *Fusarium solani* keratitis and endophthalmitis responded well to oral (200 mg PO four times daily) and topical (10 mg/0.1 mL) PCZ treatment. After 3 weeks of therapy, the ocular penetration of PCZ was confirmed by vitreous analysis at a concentration of 0.25 mcg/mL [58]. Another study looked at the *in vivo* effects of PCZ solution at doses of 10 to 100 mg/kg/day against *Fusarium solani* in immunocompetent mice [59]. The results show that treatment with higher doses (50 or 100 mg/kg of body weight/day) were not statistically different from those produced with AMB solution (1 mg/kg of body weight/day) in terms of survival and in reducing the numbers of CFU per gram of kidney and liver [59].

33. Oropharyngeal Candidiasis

A multi-center, randomized, investigator-blinded, active treatment study was conducted to compare the efficacy and safety of PCZ and FCZ in HIV/AIDS patients ($n = 350$) who presented with documented oropharyngeal candidiasis [60]. The mean ± SD CD4 cell counts (cells/mm^3) in both groups were 137 ± 170.5 and 132 ± 160.7, respectively. About 60%–70% of these HIV/AIDS patients were not receiving any antiretroviral medication and the majority (90.2%–92.3%) of isolated fungal cultures at baseline were *C. albicans*. In this study using a modified intent-to-treat analysis, 200 mg daily of PCZ PO suspension ($n = 178$) was found to have similar clinical success (cured and improved condition) as 200 mg on day 1 followed by 100 mg daily of FCZ PO suspension ($n = 172$) at days 7 and 14 of therapy (97% *vs.* 96.9% and 91.7% *vs.* 92.5%, respectively) [60]. In the modified intent-to-treat analysis, randomized participants received one or more doses of PCZ with cultures positive for *Candida* spp. at baseline. Clinical success was defined as resolution (absence of plaques or ulcers and no or minimal symptoms) or partial resolution of pretreatment signs and symptoms of candidiasis based on a scoring system [60]. Similar results were also observed in the per protocol analysis. Although the clinical relapse (defined as ≤20 CFU/mL of *Candida* spp. on day 14 and >20 CFU/mL on day 42) rate appeared to be lower in the PCZ group (31.5%) than in the FCZ group (38.2%), the difference was not statistically significant ($p = 0.24$) [60].

In this study, the rates of mycological success (defined as a quantitative yeast culture yielding ≤ 20 CFU/mL of *Candida* spp.) on days 7 and 14 were similar for both groups (49.7% *vs.* 45% and 60.4% *vs.* 58.1%, respectively) whereas the same rates on day 42 were significantly higher in the PCZ compared to the FCZ group (40.6% *vs.* 26.4%, respectively; $p = 0.038$) [60]. Furthermore, the rates of mycological eradication (defined as zero CFU/mL) were found to be similar in both groups (35.6% *vs.* 24.3%, respectively) with a trend favoring the PCZ group ($p = 0.084$). The discontinuation during treatment and follow up and adverse event rates were similar between both treatment groups. Overall, PCZ PO suspension 200 mg daily was as efficacious as FCZ PO suspension 200 mg on day 1 followed by 100 mg daily given for a total of 14 days for oropharyngeal candidiasis in HIV/AIDS patients [60]. Some of the limitations included small sample size, high risk immunosuppressed patients, changes in immunosuppression status over time, and no antiretroviral therapy and potential drug-drug interactions.

34. Invasive *Aspergillus*

Invasive aspergillosis is an infection that significantly affects patients with hematological disorders. According to guideline recommendations, voriconazole is the first-line therapy, and a change in antifungal agent is required as salvage therapy. Heinz *et al.* investigated if the use of PCZ is suitable for the treatment of invasive aspergillosis after voriconazole has failed [61]. It was a retrospective investigation conducted in four different hospitals in Germany [61]. Study subjects were administered sequential antifungal therapy with PCZ after they had received voriconazole. Response rates were measured at 30 and 60 days after initiating PCZ therapy and safety was addressed via measurement of liver enzymes and cholestasis parameters [61].

After analyzing the data, it was shown that PCZ had a success rate of 72.2%; 15 out of 36 (41.7%) patients had a complete response and 11 patients (30.6%) had a partial response at any point in time [61]. A total of eight patients failed treatment and two were not evaluable. Mean liver enzyme levels increased during voriconazole treatment when compared to PCZ treatment; there was an aspartate aminotransferase increase of 31.9 U/L with voriconazole *versus* a decrease of 19.6 U/L with PCZ; alanine aminotransferase was 32.4 U/L with voriconazole and 19.8 U/L with PCZ; gamma-glutamyl transferase levels were 124.2 U/L when compared to 152.3 U/L) with PCZ treatment; and alkaline phosphatase was 71.5 U/L compared to 40.3 U/L with voriconazole and PCZ, respectively. Moreover, there were no study withdrawals due to an adverse event. Based on these results, study investigators concluded that PCZ is both effective and safe as salvage therapy for invasive aspergillosis in patients that had prior administration of another triazole [61]. Nevertheless, it would be important to know if the success rate of PCZ is significant when compared to the success rate of other antifungals that are currently used as salvage therapy. A future study involving differential statistics and a larger sample size would be necessary to further establish the role of PCZ as salvage therapy for invasive aspergillosis.

35. Dosing and Administration

PCZ is available in the U.S. as a PO suspension (40 mg/mL). Table 3 summaries the dosing and administration of PCZ. For the treatment of oropharyngeal candidiasis in HIV/AIDS patients of 18 years of age or older, the recommended dose of PCZ is 200 mg PO on day 1 followed by 100 mg PO daily for 13 days based on clinical data comparing its efficacy and safety to FCZ [60]. Patients with persistent febrile neutropenia or refractory IFIs who have failed treatment with caspofungin and/or AMB, are recommended to receive PCZ PO 200 mg suspension four times daily for nine doses, followed by 400 mg PO twice daily up to 6 months or until recovery of neutropenia [51]. PCZ should be given as 200 mg PO three times daily for prophylactic use in immunocompromised adults, including patients with prolonged neutropenia from chemotherapy for acute myelogenous leukemia or myelodysplastic syndrome, acute or chronic extensive graft-*versus*-host disease (GVHD), and/or patients being treated with intensive immunosuppressive therapy. PCZ therapy is continued until recovery from neutropenia and complete remission, occurrence of invasive fungal infection or for up to 12 weeks (febrile neutropenia) or 112 days (GVHD) [47,55]. Since PCZ is primarily metabolised in the liver and has minimal renal elimination, there is no renal dosing adjustment in chronic kidney disease and end-stage renal disease patients on hemodialysis [42,43]. Currently there is no data on PCZ dosing adjustment in hepatic impaired, obese and bariatric surgery patients. PCZ dose should remain the same regardless of age, gender and race [45]. There is still limited data to support PCZ use in pediatrics [2]. During pregnancy and lactation this drug should not be used [2].

Table 3. Dosing and Administration of PCZ [2]

Conditions	Dosing and Administration
Oropharyngeal candidiasis in HIV/AIDS	200 mg on day 1 followed by 100 mg daily
Persistent febrile neutropenia	200 mg QID for 2 days followed by 400 mg BID
Refractory invasive fungal infection	200 mg QID for 2 days followed by 400 mg BID
Prophylaxis for prolong neutropenia from chemotherapy	200 mg TID
Prophylaxis for severe graft-*versus*-host disease	200 mg TID

BID = twice daily; TID = three times daily; QID = four times daily.

36. Special Populations—Age and Gender

Sansone-Parsons *et al.* conducted a randomized, placebo controlled, blinded study in healthy volunteers evaluating the effect of gender and age on the PK of PCZ suspension (400 mg PO twice daily) [45]. Subjects were stratified into four groups including males or females of 18 to 45 years, and males or females of 65 years or older. After an overnight fast, subjects were randomly assigned to a PCZ or placebo group (drug: placebo ratio = 3:1). The administration of the study drug or placebo occurred 10 min after a high fat meal. Blood samples were collected from the day before drug intake and up to 12 h after the morning doses on day 1 and up to 96 h on day 8. Plasma concentrations of PCZ were determined using LC-MS and PK of PCZ were characterized by model independent methods.

The majority of races in both groups were Caucasians (89% and 94%, respectively). The mean ± SD ages (years) in the non-obese young male and female groups were 30 ± 7.6 and 29.8 ± 10.5, respectively [45]. Contrastingly, the mean ± SD ages (years) in the non-obese elderly male and female groups were 71.3 ± 5.6 and 71.4 (6.1), respectively. The races of the elderly groups were similar to the young adult groups [46]. Pooled elderly subjects ($n = 24$) had a higher, but not clinically significant, PCZ exposure than pooled young subjects ($n = 24$) at steady state (day 8). The mean (CV) log-transformed C_{max} (ng/mL) and AUC_{0-12} (ng • h/mL) values between the two groups were 3374 (38) *vs.* 2607 (40) and 35,444 (39) *vs.* 26,740 (40), respectively [45]. The median T_{max} values ranged from 4 to 6 h, and the mean (CV) $t½$ and

CL/F values were similar between the two groups. The results of this study did not show a difference in the relative bioavailability of PCZ between genders of the same age groups. Adverse effects such as headache (18%) and abdominal pain (10%) were reported to be PCZ-related. Incidences of mild to moderate elevated hepatic enzymes were similar among the study groups. The authors concluded that dose adjustment for PCZ was not necessary in adults and elderly and in male and female patients. This conclusion was based on interpatient variability that could have influenced the results of this study, significant overlap of AUC_{0-24} parameters, as well as small CV values between young and elderly, and male and female subjects.

The most common PCZ adverse effects reported were headache (18%), musculoskeletal pain (12%), abdominal pain (10%), fever (8%), and pharyngitis (8%) [45]. There was no relationship between the occurrence of adverse effects among PCZ groups and age or gender [45].

37. Special Populations – Race

Sansone-Parsons *et al.* conducted an open-label and parallel study in healthy volunteers evaluating the effect of race/ethnicity on the PK parameters of PCZ [45]. Subjects who met the study criteria were divided into black and white race groups. After an overnight fast, patients were randomly assigned to receive PCZ or placebo. The administration of study drug or placebo occurred 10 min after a high fat meal. Blood samples were collected before and up to 12 h after the morning doses on day 1 and up to 96 h. Plasma concentrations of PCZ were determined using LC-MS and PK of PCZ were characterized by model independent methods.

The mean ± SD ages (years) in the black and white groups were 36.7 ± 6.7 and 32.6 ± 8.8, respectively, and both groups had similar mean ± SD weights (76.9 ± 7.4 and 75.6 ± 8.8, respectively) [45]. Pharmacokinetic parameters of PCZ were similar between white and black subjects during the initial dosing (day 1) and at steady state periods (day 3). The relative bioavailability values of PCZ were 84.4% (90% CI: 70% to 101% and 84.2% (90% CI: 70% to 101%), respectively [45]. There were no significant differences in the incidence of treatment-emergent adverse events between white and black subjects (71% *vs.* 80%, respectively). The most common adverse events were dry mouth (38%), headache (30%), dry skin (21%), increased frequency of micturition (20%), and insomnia (13%) [45]. No reports of elevated hepatic enzymes were mentioned in this study. The authors concluded that no dosage adjustment of PCZ was needed in different races.

38. Chronic Kidney Disease and Hemodialysis

Courtney *et al.* conducted an open-label and parallel group study to compare the PK, safety and tolerability of PCZ 400 mg PO suspension administered as a single dose in healthy volunteers and renal insufficient subjects after a high fat breakfast [43]. The sample size of this study was twenty four with six subjects assigned to each group. Renal insufficiency subjects were further divided into groups based on their creatinine clearance (CL_{Cr}, mL/min/1.73 m^2) as determined by a 24-h urine collection. Groups 1, 2, 3 and 4 consisted of subjects with normal renal function (CL_{Cr} >80), mild renal failure (CL_{Cr} 50–80), moderate renal failure (CL_{Cr} 20–49) and severe renal failure (CL_{Cr} <20 and/or on hemodialysis), respectively [43]. In addition, subjects, who were on hemodialysis, participated in two phases of PCZ dosing (*i.e.*, interdialytic and intradialytic). Each phase was separated by a washout period of at least 3 weeks. Sampling of blood was collected up to 120 h post PCZ dose for all groups, with the exception of Group 4 (interdialytic phase), 96 and 120 h samples were not performed if hemodialysis occurred before these designated time points. During the intradialytic phase (defined as the period after the administration of PCZ and 6 h prior to the initiation of the hemodialysis session) Group 4 blood samples were collected before the PCZ dose and up to 120 h post dose. Pre- and post- dialyzer blood samples were also collected during the dialysis period (~2.5 h). Total urine output was also collected up to 72 h post dosing. Plasma and urine PCZ concentrations were measured by LC-MS and PK of PCZ were determined by model independent methods [43].

In this study, the mean ± SD age (years) and weight (kg) were 52.5 ± 15.5 and 82.1 ± 14.5, respectively, and about 71% of subjects were male, 54% were white, 37% were black and 8% were classified as others [43]. The results demonstrated that the PK parameters were similar among the subjects with normal renal function when compared to those with renal insufficiency but not on hemodialysis [43]. Patients who were on hemodialysis showed a wide variability in PCZ exposure (AUC_{tf}, ng·h/mL) compared to subjects with normal to moderate renal function. These mean (%CV) values were 14238 (89) to 20826 (96) *vs.* 18425 (42), 16328 (27) and 18613 (34), respectively [43]. This phenomenon was suggested by drug-drug interactions between PCZ and concurrent medications in patients with severe renal insufficiency. The pre-dialysis and post-dialysis total plasma PCZ concentrations measured by AUC_{tf} were similar, suggesting PCZ was not dialyzable. The PK profiles of PCZ during the interdialytic and intradialytic phases were similar. The protein binding of PCZ was > 98% and was not affected by the various degrees of renal insufficiency, including subjects who were on hemodialysis. Adverse effects included somnolence, diarrhea and elevated liver function tests [43].

39. Hepatic Impairment, Obesity and Bariatric Surg ery

The PK parameters, safety and tolerability of PCZ in various degrees of hepatic impairment, obesity and bariatric surgery have not been evaluated [2].

40. Compromised Gastrointestinal Function

In a study by Cornely *et al.*, different dosing strategies that might lead to higher bioavailability of PCZ in patients with compromised gastrointestinal function were evaluated [62]. A secondary objective of this investigation was to determine whether measuring plasma levels of PCZ at an earlier stage in therapy can help predict steady-state plasma levels so they can be used to guide treatment in order to reach the desired threshold level. It was a phase IV, randomized, open-label, comparative, multicenter study in the United States and Europe with a total of 75 patients. Study participants were administered PCZ 200 mg PO three times a day from days 1 through 8. Thereafter, they were randomized into three groups from days 9 through 15. Group 1 received PCZ 200 mg PO TID; Group 2 received PCZ 400 mg PO BID; and Group 3 received PCZ 400 mg PO TID [62]. PCZ was administered 10 min after finishing a meal or an oral nutritional supplement. The primary PK parameter was mean plasma concentration of PCZ, which was defined as the mean of the 0 h (trough, pre-morning dose) and 5 h (post-morning dose) on days 2, 8, and 15. Blood samples were collected on days 1, 2, 3, 8, and 15 in the morning before the dose and five hours post-dose. The mean concentrations of PCZ were measured using a validated LC-MS. The lower limit of detection was set to 5.00 ng/mL with a calibration range of 5.00 to 5000 ng/mL.

The target plasma concentrations were 500 and 700 ng/mL on days 8 and 15, respectively. Plasma concentrations of 250 ng/mL and 350 ng/mL on day 2 were selected as desired levels that could result in the steady-state concentrations of 500 and 700 ng/mL. These target PCZ plasma concentrations were chosen based on previous PK studies of PCZ [62].

Inclusion criteria consisted of patients of any sex, race, and age >18 years receiving chemotherapy for acute myelogenous leukemia [62]. Patients also had to be at high risk of poor enteral absorption based on the effects of cytotoxic chemotherapy, such as nausea, vomiting, mucositis, and diarrhea. They also had to be at high risk of invasive IFIs, which was defined as an absolute neutrophil count <500/mm^3, but free from other significant diseases other than the acute myelogenous leukemia which was confirmed by normal clinical tests. Additionally, female participants had to have a negative pregnancy test at baseline and within 72 h before the start of the study, and be on an accepted method of contraception. Exclusion criteria included moderate-severe liver dysfunction, pregnancy, breastfeeding, and systemic antifungal therapy for proven or provable IFIs. Patients receiving treatment with omeprazole, cimetidine, vinca alkaloids, sirolimus, efavirenz, and anthracyclines, or any drugs that cause QT prolongation were also excluded from the study [62].

Results were provided for 49 out the 75 patients that were enrolled in the study (36 women and 39 men) [62]. The 75 study participants were mostly white (91%) and with a mean age of 53.5 years. Only 49 were included in the final analysis as it was desired to include only those who had no missing PK data on days 3, 8 and 15 (per-protocol analysis); reasons for study withdrawals and missing data were not stated. After evaluating the data, it was decided to use the plasma concentrations from day 3, rather than day 2, as they were found to better predict the concentrations for day 8. Even though there was a risk of compromised absorption due to the pre-existing conditions of the patients, the resulting PCZ plasma concentrations on days 3 and 8 reached the desired levels of 250 and 500 ng/mL, respectively. The mean plasma concentrations of PCZ on days 2, 3, and 8 were 230 ng/mL, 346 ng/mL, and 637 ng/mL, respectively. On day 15 of the study, the levels for the 200 mg TID, 400 mg BID, and 400 mg TID doses were 660 ng/mL, 930 ng/mL, and 671 ng/mL, respectively. By day 8, 37 out of 49 participants (76%) had reached the target level of 250 ng/mL for all dosing regimens of PCZ. Thirty out of 49 patients (61%) reached the target mean plasma concentration of 250 ng/mL on day 3, and 73% of these 30 patients reached the target of 500 ng/mL on day 8. Interestingly, out of the patients who did not achieve this target on day 8, 75% also failed to reach the target level of 500 ng/mL on day 15 of the investigation, demonstrating that administering higher doses of PCZ did not have a significant benefit. Moreover, food intake and fat intake during the study was not enough to provide a significant benefit on increasing PCZ absorption; therefore, no conclusions could be drawn regarding its impact on these poor absorbers. In terms of safety, a total of 74 patients (99%) experienced an adverse event during the study. The most common treatment-related adverse events were nausea [13/75 (17%)], diarrhea [10/75 (13%)], and rash [8/75 (11%)]. Elevated liver enzymes were also reported in five patients, but only considered to be related to treatment in two of these patients. A total of 15 patients did not complete the study due to an adverse event [62].

After analyzing these results, the authors concluded that even with compromised gastrointestinal absorption, a desired plasma concentration of PCZ can be expected in most patients [62]. However, those who were not able to reach the target concentration on day 3, tended to remain poor absorbers through the remainder of the study. Although only hypothesis-generating, the secondary aim of this study revealed that day 3 concentrations are better predictive of day 8 plasma concentrations of PCZ when compared to day 2 levels [62]. Limitations of this study include the use of descriptive statistics which do not provide the ability to see the statistical significance of the data. Also, compliance was not addressed and could have been a potential confounder in the study. Furthermore, restricting the concomitant use of several medications limits the ability to extrapolate the results to patients that have compromised gastrointestinal absorption, but that also need to be in some of these medications for the treatment of other conditions. Future studies could focus on introducing differential statistics that could provide additional valuable information, as well as allowing the use of concomitant medications to determine their impact on PCZ concentrations on patients with compromised gastrointestinal function.

41. Pediatrics

The PK data of PCZ in pediatric patients is limited [2]. Daily administration of PCZ 800 mg daily administered in divided doses represents salvage therapy in pediatric patients (n = 12) of 8 to 17 years of age with IFIs. Mean (median, range) steady-state concentrations (ng/mL) with this dose were 776 (580, 85.3–2891). These values were similar to those in adult patients who received the same dosing regimen [817 (626, 0–3710)] [63]. These results show that there is a large intersubject variability within each population. However, the study did not state whether PCZ was administered with or without a meal [63]. Furthermore, the efficacy and safety of the drug against invasive fungal infection were investigated in the same study groups. Despite the small sample size, the overall success rate in the pediatric group (45%, n = 11) was similar to the adult group (50%, n = 319) [2,63]. Adverse effects of PCZ in the pediatric population were primarily gastrointestinal related, fever and headache, which were comparable to the events in the adult group [2,63]. The authors concluded that PCZ was an effective salvage therapy in children with refractory IFIs. The clinical data on the use of PCZ in pediatric population is still limited [2].

42. Mechanism of Resistance

One major cause of resistance to azole antifungals is decreased binding via alteration of the CYP51A gene that encodes the enzyme lanosterol 14α-demethylase. This explains why the susceptibility of *C. albicans* isolates to azole antifungals (*i.e.* FCZ, ketoconazole, and ICZ) has decreased [64]. Another cause of resistance to these drugs is the reduced intracellular azole accumulation due to the expression of a membrane bound efflux pump [64].

Resistance to azole antifungal agents developed *in vitro* when amino acid substitutions occurred at specific positions in the binding site of CYP51A from *A. fumigatus* (AF-CYP51A) and *C. albicans* (CA-CYP51A) [65]. MIC values increased 100 fold with both PCZ and ICZ (MICs ranged from 0.5 to >16 mcg/mL) when Gly54 position was replaced with either Arg, Glu or Trp. This was seen in mutant forms of AF-CYP51A compared to the wild type isolates (MICs ranged from 0.03 to 0.12 mcg/mL) [65]. However, there was no change in the MIC values with VCZ. The long side chains of PCZ and ICZ (the triazole-3-one five membered ring) fit securely within the helix A′, the FG loop and β turn of CYP51A [65]. The replacement of Gly54 with amino acids that have side chains, such as Arg, Glu or Trp, created Van der Waals forces with the side chains of PCZ and ICZ. This resulted in alteration of receptor binding and increased MIC values. A 64 fold increase in MIC (mcg/mL) values was noted with VCZ when

Gly138 and Gly448 were located near the heme binding vicinity, or were replaced with Arg and Ser, respectively [65]. An eight-fold increase in MIC (2 mcg/mL) was reported with ICZ when Gly138 was substituted for Arg compared to the wild type isolate (MIC = 0.25 mcg/mL). However, when that same amino acid substitution occurred, it did not alter AF-CYP51A and the MIC values with PCZ.

Two clinically FCZ-resistant strains of *C. albicans* revealed amino acid substitutions in CYP51. The first strain revealed substitutions at Tyr257His and Gly464Ser and the second strain revealed substitutions at Lys128Thr, Typ132His, Asp278Asn, and Gly464Ser [65]. Both strains exhibited increased resistance in ascending order to PCZ, ICZ, VCZ and FCZ. The corresponding MICs (mcg/mL) values ranged from 0.5 to 128 in the first strain and 0.25 to 32 in the second, whereas the resulting MIC (mcg/mL) values for the wild type strains ranged from 0.03 to 0.125. Two additional amino acid substitutions (*i.e.*, Gly30Ser and Ala61Val) in the CA-CYP51 of the first strain resulted in less of an increase in MIC values with PCZ (1 and 4 mcg/mL) and ICZ (4 and 8 mcg/mL) as compared to the values with FCZ and VCZ (both >16 mcg/mL) [65]. Similarly, the amino acid substitution (Pro230Leu) in CA-CYP51 of the second strain displayed a significant increase in MIC values with FCZ and ICZ. The same amino acid substitution lead to an eight fold increase in MIC values with PCZ; however, there was no change in the MIC values with VCZ.

43. Safety and Tolerance

Based on the clinical data, PCZ is considered safe and well tolerated. The most commonly reported side effects (>10%) in the small, single and/or multiple dosing PK studies of PCZ, included headache, fatigue, nausea, and dry mouth [36,37,40,,42,43,45,51,52,57,66]. Table 4 shows the frequency of any adverse events that occurred in 1% or more of patients treated with either PCZ or FCZ [47,55,60]. These events seen in the larger efficacy and safety clinical trials, were similar between the two antifungals [47,55,60].

Table 4. Any adverse effects (≥1% of PCZ) in large, randomized, double-blind, parallel clinical trial evaluating PCZ *versus* fluconazole (FCZ) in Prophylaxis in patients with neutropenia, severe graft-*versus*-host disease and treatment of oropharyngeal candidiasis in patients with HIV/AIDS [47,55,60].

	PCZ	**FCZ**
Adverse Event	***n*** **= 783**	***n*** **= 711**
Nausea	5.0	6.0
Diarrhea	3.1	4.5
Neutropenia	2.8	2.5
Headache	2.0	3.1
Bilirubinemia	1.9	1.0
Increased hepatic enzymes	1.4	1.1
Vomiting	1.4	1.5
Fever	1.3	2.0
Hypotension	1.3	2.4
Abdominal pain	1.0	1.1
GI hemorrhage	1.0	0.3

44. Pregnancy

PCZ is a pregnancy category C drug [2]. In rats, it is excreted in breast milk and skeletal malformations were observed at doses ≥27 mg/kg [2]. These doses produced a 1.4 fold increase in PCZ steady state plasma concentrations as compared to 400 mg twice daily. In rabbits, teratogenic effects (*i.e.*, bone resorptions) were observed at PCZ doses ≥40 to 80 mg/kg. These doses produced a 2.9 to 5.2 fold increase in PCZ plasma concentrations [2]. Clinical trials have not been conducted in women because of the teratogenic effects in laboratory animals. Therefore, PCZ is recommended during pregnancy only if the potential benefits outweigh the risks to the fetus.

45. Drug Interactions

Antacids

Courtney *et al.* conducted a randomized, open label and four way crossover PK study in healthy volunteers ($n = 12$) to evaluate the effect of antacids on PCZ PO bioavailability [67]. Maximum strength Mylanta, containing aluminum hydroxide and magnesium hydroxide, was used. The antacid dose was 20 mL, providing a total of 102 mEq of acid neutralizing capacity. After 10-h of overnight fasting, all subjects were randomized to receive a single 200 mg PCZ tablet and 200 mL of regular water under four different conditions (either alone, immediately after a standardised high fat meal, antacid alone, or antacid and a standardised high fat meal) [67]. The meal contained 52% fat and provided a total of 841 calories. All meals were consumed within a 20-min period and the assigned treatments were initiated 5 min after meals were completed. Each subject was required to complete all four regimens with a 7-day washout period from the end of the study phase. Subjects were not released from the research center until 72 h after the PCZ dose. Plasma PCZ concentrations were measured by HPLC and the PK of PCZ were determined by model-independent methods. Safety and tolerance were monitored throughout the study.

The study population consisted of non-obese males with a mean age of 34 years. The proportion of black to white patients was a 2:1 ratio [67]. The results confirmed that the antacid did not significantly alter the relative bioavailability of PCZ under all the treatment conditions. In the presence of food and antacid, the mean (%CV) C_{max} (ng/mL) and AUC_{tf} (ng·h/mL) values were similar to those in the presence of food only [326 (47) *vs.* 366 (28) and 9513 (45) *vs.* 10220 (31), respectively] [67]. The relative PO bioavailability of PCZ was reported to be 88% [90% confidence interval (CI): 71%–110%]. The same effects were observed in the absence of food with or without antacid. The mean (%CV) C_{max} (ng/mL) and AUC_{tf} (ng·h/mL) values were 94.6 (36) *vs.* 92.5 (46) and 2930 (29) *vs.* 2718 (41), respectively [66]. The mean (%CV) T_{max} (h) and t½s (h) were similar among all conditions ranging from 8.5 (41) to 9.0 (47) and 18.3 (14) to 20.4 (18), respectively [67].

The mean (%CV) apparent volumes of distribution (liters) of PCZ were similar in the presence of food with or without the antacid [623 (55) *vs.* 526 (34)] [67]. Similar results were observed in the fasting state, but the values were three times higher than those in the non-fasting state. In addition, the mean (%CV) total body clearances (mL/min) of PCZ were three times higher in the fasting state with or without the antacid than in the non-fasting state with or without the antacid [1072 (18) and 1062 (35) *vs.* 345 (40) and 323 926), respectively] [67]. The authors explained that these observations were due to decreased absorption of PCZ under fasting conditions since the elimination rate constants did not change among all four treatment phases.

The authors concluded that, regardless of the presence or absence of food, PCZ PO absorption was independent of pH. However, the effects on PCZ bioavailability from a more potent acid suppressant, either a H2 receptor antagonist or a proton pump inhibitor, remain to be determined. Furthermore, PCZ PO absorption was enhanced (up to four fold) when PCZ was administered with a meal. Although the number of African Americans in this study was double compared to Caucasians ($n = 8$ *vs.* $n = 4$, respectively), the PK parameters were similar to those from previous published data, despite a moderate intrasubject variability (29% to 45%) [45,67]. It may be difficult to extrapolate this data to females, other age groups (especially children and elderly), races (including Hispanics and Asians), and to patients with other disease states (obesity, diabetes mellitus, HIV) and other factors (H2 receptor antagonist and proton pump inhibitor). Pharmacokinetic parameters of PCZ from multiple dosing studies are needed.

46. Proton Pump Inhibitors

Cojutti *et al.* investigated the influence that dose frequency and concomitant use of proton pump inhibitors (PPIs) have on the time to the PCZ target C_{min} of >700 ng/mL [68]. The study was performed on hematological patients who were administered PCZ prophylaxis after induction chemotherapy for acute myeloid leukemia. It consisted of a retrospective, observational study that was from August 2009 to November 2010 [68]. Inclusion criteria included subjects who had a minimum of three subsequent C_{min} levels during the initial 8 days of treatment. Blood samples were taken before the morning dose and analyzed LC-MS; the lower limit of detection was set to 15 ng/mL. The study had a total of 42 patients that were divided into four cohorts. Group 1 ($n = 10$) received PCZ 200 mg every 8 h without a PPI; Group 2 ($n = 11$) received PCZ 200 mg every 8 h with a PPI; Group 3 ($n = 10$) received PCZ 200 mg every 6 h without a PPI; and Group 4 ($n = 11$) received PCZ 200 mg every 6 h with a PPI [68]. The type of oral formulation administered was not stated.

The results of this investigation reported patients to have similar demographic and clinical characteristics with all p values > 0.05 [68]. A therapeutic median C_{min} was achieved by day 4 in Group 3 only, which reported a level of 935.5 ng/mL as compared to 567.0 ng/mL, 420.0 ng/mL, and 514.0 ng/mL in Groups 1, 2, and 4, respectively ($p < 0.01$). On day 8, the differences between the groups were more obvious, with a median C_{min} of 1550.0 ng/mL, 884.5 ng/mL, 716.0 ng/mL, and 589.0 ng/mL in Groups 3, 1, 2, and 4, respectively ($p = 0.006$). These results revealed that increasing the dosing frequency of PCZ, while avoiding the concomitant use of PPIs, can be an efficient approach to achieve a target C_{min} in acute myeloid leukemia patients being administered antifungal therapy for the prevention of breakthrough infections [68]. This was observed when analyzing the results in Group 4, where the expected benefit of increasing the dose of PCZ was counteracted by the concomitant use of a PPI and a subtherapeutic C_{min} level was observed. The authors concluded that avoidance of a PPI with a daily regimen of 200 mg q 6 h can achieve a therapeutic concentration of PCZ and serve as an effective strategy [68].

However, this study was limited in that it included a small sample size that restricts the ability to extrapolate the data to a wider population. Additionally, both increasing the dose frequency and coadministration of a PPI was left to the physician's discretion, which could have led to an increase in variability. Although not statistically significant, more patients in Group 4 had mucositis; this could have also contributed to the lower concentration of PCZ when compared to Group 2 on day 8 of the study. Nevertheless, this investigation served to demonstrate a potential impact of concomitant use of PPIs on PCZ serum concentrations and warrants future research in the area.

47. Cytochrome P450 System Cocktails

The effects of PCZ on the activity of several drug metabolizing CYP450 enzymes were investigated [68]. This study used 13 non-obese adult subjects (age range 18 to 45) who were randomly assigned to receive PCZ (200 mg tablet PO daily) or no drug for 10 days [69]. After a washout period of 14 days, subjects crossed over to the alternate study group. The standardised CYP450 cocktail with corresponding surrogate substrates included caffeine (CYP1A2) 200 mg, tobutamide (CYP2C8/9) 500 mg, dextromethorphan (CYP2D6 and total CYP3A4) 30 mg and chlorzoxazone (CYP2E1) 250 mg. This cocktail was given to both study groups 2 h after the administration of PCZ under fasting conditions on day 9. In addition, midazolam (0.05 mg/kg in 100 mL of 0.9% saline), a hepatic CYP3A4 substrate, was given as a 30 min infusion in place of the CYP450 cocktail on day 10 [69]. Blood samples were collected before and up to 24 h, and urine collection started 2 h and up to 48 h post-PCZ administration according to the research protocol [69]. Plasma PCZ concentrations were measured by HPLC and PK of PCZ were described by model independent methods. Concentrations of the CYP450 substrates and their metabolites were measured by HPLC and LC-MS based upon the specific enzyme isoforms [69]. Safety and tolerance were monitored throughout the study.

Steady state of PCZ was reached after 8 days with a reported mean (%CV) C_{max} (ng/mL), T_{max} (hours), AUC_{0-24} (ng·h/mL) and CL/F (mL/min) of PCZ of 1073 (31), 6.9 (21), 19,465 (32), and 188 (34), respectively [69]. Based on the information previously discussed, under fasting conditions, the systemic exposure of PCZ 200 mg PO tablets showed an accumulation index of 1.9, which was less than that reported with the PCZ PO suspension [36]. Plasma- or urine ratios of CYP450 substrates and their metabolites were evaluated to determine the effects of PCZ on the CYP450 isoenzymes. Plasma ratios of 1,7-dimethylxanthine to caffeine and 6-hydroxychlorzoxazone to chlorzoxazone were measured in order to assess the activities of CYP1A2 and CYP2E1, respectively. The urinary ratios of combined 4-hydroxytolbutamide + carboxytobutamide and tolbutamide, dextromethorphan and dextrorphan and dextromethorphan and 3-methoxymorphinan were calculated in order to evaluate the effects of CYP2C8/9, CYP2D6 and total CYP3A4, respectively [69]. Moreover, the hepatic activity of CYP3A4 was measured when midazolam was administered with PCZ. Overall, PCZ did not interact with CYP450 isoenzymes 1A2, 2C8/9, 2D6, 2E1 and total CYP3A4 with the exception of hepatic CYP3A4. The inhibitory effect of PCZ on hepatic CYP3A4 was confirmed by a significant increased mean AUC_{0-24} (%CV) (ng·h/mL) of midazolam in the presence of PCZ when compared with the absence of PCZ (93.4 (29) *vs.* 51.4 (29), respectively, $p < 0.01$). This leads to a relative 1.8 (90% confidence interval: 1.57 to 2.14) fold increase in midazolam exposure [69]. Based on the results of this study, the authors concluded that unlike other azole antifungal agents, PCZ has less potential for drug interactions due to its sole inhibition of hepatic CYP3A4.

Although this study suggested that PCZ was a CYP3A4 inhibitor, the magnitude of this effect could not be fully observed since the midazolam was administered as a single dose and PCZ was not given at its optimal dose, absorption state (*i.e.*, with food or nutritional supplement) or in the suspension formulation. In addition, the duration of urine collection may not have been long enough to allow for complete bladder emptying. This may have reduced urine metabolite concentrations. Lastly, the counter effect of midazolam on the PK of PCZ was not examined in this study.

48. Cyclosporine and Tacrolimus

Previous studies have shown that PCZ undergoes extensive hepatic metabolism to glucuronide metabolites [42]. PCZ is also a hepatic CYP3A4 enzyme inhibitor [2,69]. Sansone-Parsons *et al.* evaluated the effects of PO PCZ on the systemic exposures of cyclosporine (CSA) and tacrolimus (FK506) in two separate, open label, and single center, drug interaction studies [66]. The CSA-PCZ study was conducted in the United States on heart transplant recipients (n = 4) who had normal cardiac function; whereas the FK506-PCZ study was performed in England on healthy volunteers (n = 36). Subjects were excluded from the studies if they tested positive for hepatitis B surface antigen, hepatitis C antibody and human immunodeficiency virus antibodies. Additional exclusion criteria included subjects with a history of mental illness, vegetarian diet, current smoking, use of alcohol, or other medications. All study drug concentrations were analyzed by LC-MS [66,70].

Table 5a. Pharmacokinetics of PCZ in Different Single Dose Clinical Studies.

Ref	Sample Size	Subjects	Study Design	PCZ Dose (mg)	Dosage Form	With Breakfast (HF)	Cmax (ng/mL)	Tmax (h)	AUCtf (ng.h/mL)	AUCX-Y (ng.h/mL)	t½ (h)	CL/F (mL/min)	V/F (Liters)
							Mean (% CV)	Mean (%CV)	Mean (%CV)	Mean (%CV)	Mean (%CV)	Mean (%CV)	Mean (%CV)
[6]	20	Healthy	O, R, C	200	Susp	No	132 (50)	5.0 (149)		3553 (36) [b]	23.5 (25)		
				200	Susp	Yes (NF)	378 (43)	4.1 (21)		9511 (38) b	22.2 (18)		
				200	Susp	Yes	512 (34)	4.8 (9)		13885 (41) [b]	23 (19)		
				200	Tab	Yes	413 (33)	5.5 (32)		10304 (41) [b]	21 (15)		
[36]	54	Healthy	O, PL, P, DB, R	50	Tab	Yes	113 (46)	6.3 (51)	2317 (50)	2501 (45) [a]	15.9 (18)	389 (40)	511 (32)
				100	Tab	Yes	235 (26)	7.3 (36)	6101 (28)	6357 (27) [a]	18.3 (13)	275 (21)	431 (20)
				200	Tab	Yes	332 (21)	5.8 (35)	10354 (30)	10896 (31) [a]	24.5 (22)	341 (40)	674 (18)
				400	Tab	Yes	611 (31)	6.3 (44)	19401 (33)	20264 (33) [a]	24.1 (24)	363 (35)	781 (49)
				800	Tab	Yes	1320 (26)	6.2 (46)	46984 (40)	49841 (43) [a]	24.4 (33)	320 (48)	594 (19)
				1200	Tab	Yes	933 (28)	8.8 (85)	41755 (42)	45260 (44) [a]	28.5 (26)	585 (73)	1341 (58)
[38]	12	Healthy	O, R, C	200	Susp	Yes	354.29 [f]	7.38 [f]		12612.35 [a,f]	21.39 [g]		
						No	128 [f]	3.38 [f]		3196.18 [a,f]	22.11 [g]		
[39]	16	Healthy	R,C	400	Susp	Yes	608.38 [h]	4.88 [i]		21626.08[a]	22.0		
				400	Susp	No	279.00 [h]	3.15 [i]		7304.72[a]	22.0		
[40]	23	Healthy	O, R, C	400	Susp	Yes (Boost)	355 (43)	5 (4–8) *		11295 (40) [a]	26 (19)	710 (56)	1574 (51)
				400	Susp	No	121 (75)	4 (2–12) *		5258 (48) [a]	27.3 (26)	1520 (40)	3674 (51)
[43]	8	Healthy	O	400	Susp	Yes	654 (19)	9.25 (26)		26100 (26) [a]	20 (19)	271.7 (30)	465 (31)

Table 5a. *Cont.*

Ref	Sample Size	Subjects	Study Design	PCZ Dose (mg)	Dosage Form	With Breakfast (HF)	Cmax (ng/mL)	Tmax (h)	AUCtf (ng.h/mL)	AUCX-Y (ng.h/mL)	t½ (h)	CL/F (mL/min)	V/F (Liters)
							Mean (% CV)	**Mean (%CV)**	**Mean (%CV)**	**Mean (%CV)**	**Mean (%CV)**	**Mean (%CV)**	**Mean (%CV)**
		CLCR > 80		400 mg	Susp	Yes	555 (40	5.5 (5–8) *		18425 (42) [a]	24.1 (22)	421.7 (42)	834 (34)
		CLCR 50–79		400 mg	Susp	Yes	631 (47)	5 (5–6) *		16328 (27) [a]	28.1 (22)	436.7 (30)	1073 (37)
[42]	24	CLCR 20–49	O, P	400 mg	Susp	Yes	486 (37)	8 (5–12) *		18613 (34) [a]	29.6 (17)	406.7 (45)	1034 (49)
		Interdialytic HD period		400 mg	Susp	Yes	809 (93)	5.33 (15)	20826 (96)	14751 (140) [a]	68 (14)	1415 (81)	2893 (96)
		Intradialytic HD period		400mg	Susp	Yes	548 (84)	5.42 (17)	14238 (89)	14656 (115) [a]	76 (13)	1638.3 (105)	3061 (99)
[45]	10	Healthy	R, PL	200	Tab	No	778 (29)	4.0 (3–8) [d]	23000 (23)	23000 (23) [c]	25.1 (20)	8.80 (26) [e]	
	9			400	Tab	No	1290 (29)	5.0 (3–8) [d]	42800 (35)	42800 (35) [c]	26.1 (22)	9.55 (34) [e]	

PL = Placebo, O = open label, P = parallel, R = Randomized, C = Crossover, DB = double blind, B = Blind, NF = Non-fat, HF = High-fat, IF = If possible, Tab = Tablet, Susp = Suspension; HD = Hemodialysis, mg = milligrams, ng/mL = nanogram per milliliter, ng·h/mL = nanograms x hour per milliliter, mL/min = milliliter per min, %CV = percent coefficient of variation, * Median (range), CLCR = Creatinine clearance (mL/min); Cmax = Maximum concentration, Tmax = Time to reach Cmax; t½ = half-life, CL/F = Apparent total clearance, V/F = Apparent volume of distribution, AUCtf = Area under the concentration time curve from time zero to the time of recovery of the final sample with a quantifiable concentration, AUCx-y = Area under the concentration time curve from time X to a specific time Y, [a]: X-Y is from 0 to infinity; [b]: X-Y is from 0 to 72 h; c: X-Y is from 0 to 24 h; [d]: median (range); [e]: results reported in L/h; [f]: $p < 0.05$; [g]: $p > 0.05$; [h]: $p < 0.0001$; $p = 0.0176$.

Table 5b. Pharmacokinetics of PCZ in different multiple dosing clinical studies.

Ref	Sample Size	Subjects	Study Design	PCZ Dose (mg)	Doseage Form	With Breakfast (HF)	Cmax1 (ng/ mL)	Cmin (ng/ mL)	Cav (ng/ mL)	Tmax1 (h)	AUCX-Y (ng.h/ mL)	t½ (h)	CL/F (mL/min)	V/F (Liters)
							Mean (%CV)	**Mean (%CV)**	**Mean (%CV)**	**Mean (%CV)**	**Mean (%CV)**	**Mean (%CV)**	**Mean (%CV)**	**Mean (%CV)**
[36]	48	Healthy	O, PL, P, DB, R	50 BID	Tab	**Yes**	457 (38)			5 (12)	8295 (36) [a]	19.2 (16)	225 (34)	365 (29)
				100 BID	Tab	**Yes**	1141 (37)			6 (40)	21,778 (40) [a]	24.1 (20)	171.7 (24)	343 (24)
				200 BID	Tab	**Yes**	1753 (27)			4 (12)	31,106 (26) [a]	23.9 (26)	231.7 (34)	467 (32)
				400 BID	Tab	**Yes**	4150 (20)			5 (12)	73,105 (20) [a]	31 (46)	191.7 (25)	486 (34)
							Mean (SD)	**Mean (SD)**		**Mean (SD)**	**Mean (SD)**			
[37]	18	Healthy	O, R, C	800 QD	Susp	No	137 (90)	50 (26)		7.8 (4.7)	3900 [a]			
				400 BID	Susp	No	225 (115)	96 (46)		16.6 (3.9)	770 [a]			
				200 QID	Susp	No	405 (280)	189 (135)		24.2 (3.2)	12,400 [a]			
[45]	24	Healthy adults	B, R, PL	400 BID	Susp	Yes	2607 (40)			5 (4–8) *	26,740 (40) [b]	31.6 (18)	551.7 (29)	
	24	Healthy elderly		400 BID	Susp	Yes	3374 (38)			5 (0–12) *	35,444 (39) [b]	41.8 (27)	445 (45)	
[45]	13	Young male	B, R, PL	400 BID	Susp	Yes	2682 (51)			4 (4–8) *	27,784 (51) [b]	31.3 (21)	558.3 (22)	
	11	Young female		400 BID	Susp	Yes	2517 (18)			5 (4–8) *	25,507 (20) [b]	31.9 (14)	543.3 (22)	

Table 5b. *Cont.*

Ref	Sample Size	Subjects	Study Design	PCZ Dose (mg)	Doseage Form	With Breakfast (HF)	Cmax1 (ng/ mL)	Cmin (ng/ mL)	Cav (ng/ mL)	Tmax1 (h)	AUCX-Y (ng.h/ mL)	t½ (h)	CL/F (mL/min)	V/F (Liters)
	12	Elderly Male		400 BID	Susp	Yes	3250 (36)			5 (0–6) *	32,924 (35) [b]	37.1 (21)	468.3 (45)	
	12	Elderly female		400 BID	Susp	Yes	3498 (40)			6 (0–12) *	37,924 (43) [b]	42.4 (NC)	423.3 (46)	
[45]	28	Blacks	O, R, P	400 BID	Susp	Yes	2857 (36)			5 (4–8) *	30,091 (37) [b]	37.3 (24)	528.3 (50)	
	28	Whites		400 BID	Susp	Yes	2399 (36)			5 (2–12) *	25,107 (36) [b]	32.2 (24)	616.7 (44)	
							Mean (%CV)	Mean (%CV)	Mean (%CV)	Mean (%CV)	Mean (%CV)	Mean (%CV)	Mean (%CV)	Mean (%CV)
				200 QD	Tab	No	1800 (31)		1310 (32)	5.0 (2–8) ♦	31,400 (32) [a]			
[46]	24	Healthy	R, PL	200 BID	Tab	No	2980 (38)		2550 (38)	4.0 (2–8) ♦	30,600 (38) [a]			
				400 QD	Tab	No	2940 (46)		2360 (54)	5.0 (0–12) ♦	56,600 (54) [a]			
							Mean (SD)	Mean (SD)		Mean (SD)	Mean (SD)			
		Persistent FN		200 QID	Susp	Yes, IP	539 (82)		447 (84)	2.65 (0–11.8) *	5314 (83) [b]			
[51]	69	Refractory IFI	O, R, P	400 QID	Susp	Yes, IP	531 (71)		423 (70)	5.78 (2–12.4) *	5075 (71) [b]			
				800 BID	Susp	Yes, IP	417 (60)		340 (63)	4.21 (0–11.9) *	4035 (63) [b]			
		Persistent FN		400 BID	Susp	Yes, IP	851 (82)	640 (98)	723 (86)	3 (0–12.5) *	8619 (86) [c]	11.9 (3)	4716.7 (354)	2447 (421)
[51]	61	Refractory IFI	O, R, P	600 BID	Susp	Yes, IP	579 (71)	388 (64)	490 (71)	3.83 (0–10) *	5823 (71) [c]	12 (3)	2983.3 (82)	4984 (919)
				800 QD	Susp	Yes, IP	361 (74)	252 (100)	259 (72)	4.04 (2.42–12.5) *	6199 (71) [c]	24 (2)	3583.3 (81)	5061 (903)
[66]	12	Healthy	O, C	200 QD	Tab	No	1073 (31)			6.9 (21)	19,465 (32) [a]		188 (34)	

PL = Placebo, O = open label, P = parallel, R = Randomized, C = Crossover, DB = double blind, B = Blind, HF = High fat, IF = If possible, Tab = Tablet, Susp = Suspension, M = Males, F = Females, FN = febrile neutropenia, IFI = Invasive fungal infection, mg = milligrams, ng/mL = nanogram per milliliter, ng·h/mL = nanograms × hour per milliliter, mL/min = milliliter per min, %CV = percent coefficient of variation, QD = Daily, BID = Twice daily, QID = Four times daily, t½ = half-life, SD = Standard deviation, * median (range), CL/F = Apparent total clearance, V/F = Apparent volume of distribution; ♦ median (range), Cmax1 = Maximum concentration after first dose, Cmax2 = Maximum concentration after second dose, Tmax1 = Time to reach Cmax1, Tmax2 = Time to reach Cmax2, AUCtf = Area under the concentration time curve from time zero to the time of recovery of the final sample with a quantifiable concentration, AUCx-y = Area under the concentration time curve from time X to a specific time Y, [a]: X-Y is from zero to 24 h, [b]: X-Y is from zero to 12 h, [c]: X-Y = dose normalized at steady state dosing interval.

In the CSA-PCZ study, heart transplant recipients, who received CSA for 6 weeks or longer, were given PO PCZ 200 mg tablet daily for 10 days [66]. PCZ was administered in the evening on day 1 and after a high fat content breakfast between days 2 to 10. The CSA dose was adjusted for each subject depending on corresponding trough (C_0) concentration. Blood samples of whole blood CSA (2 mL) concentrations were collected before and up to 12 h after CSA administration on days 1 and 10. Plasma PCZ (4 mL) concentrations were collected before PCZ dosing on days 7 and 8, and at 1 and up to 120 h after PCZ dosing on day 10. In addition, CSA C_0 concentrations were also measured on days 2, 3, 5, 8, 21 and 28 [66,70].

The subjects in the CSA-PCZ study were all Caucasian males with an average age of 54 years. The investigators reported that the steady state plasma PCZ concentrations increased CSA levels. Thus, CSA dose reductions (ranging from 14 to 29%) were necessary in three out of the four study subjects [66,70]. Consequently, the authors recommended a three-fourths reduction of the CSA dose when starting therapy with PCZ. However, this was based on results from only three study subjects [70]. Also, it was difficult to interpret the results of whole blood CSA concentrations in this study because no statistical analysis was performed and the sample size was small. Furthermore, it was unclear how CSA doses were adjusted since CSA C_0 concentrations were collected but not reported. Lastly, the PK profile of PCZ was similar to that previously reported in healthy adults [36]. Reported adverse events that were determined to be drug-related in this study included diarrhea, nonherpetic cold sores, dysuria, flank pain, hematuria, urinary tract infection, pain, rash and gastritis [66,70].

Sansone-Parsons *et al.* also examined the effects of PCZ on FK506. Healthy adult subjects received a single PO dose of FK506, 0.05 mg/kg on days 1 and 14 after a 10 h fasting period. PCZ was administered as a 400 mg PO suspension twice daily between days 7 to 14 after a high fat breakfast. [69]. This allowed for a 5 day washout period of FK506. Blood samples for whole blood FK506 were collected before dosing and from 1 to 72 h after FK506 administration on days 1 and 14. Blood samples for plasma FK506 concentrations were also collected on days 1 and 12, before PCZ administration and 12 h after the morning dose on days 13 and 14 [66,70].

The study population consisted of non-obese patients who were 50% male and 92% Caucasians with a mean age of 26 years. The PK profile of PCZ was similar to previous studies [36]. The results of this study showed that PCZ significantly increased the systemic exposure of FK506. The means (%CV) C_{max} (ng/mL) and $AUC_{0-\infty}$ (ng·h/mL) values of FK506 in the absence and presence of PCZ were 24.2 (31) *vs.* 51.7 (18) and 207 (52) *vs.* 875 (27), respectively [66]. The mean (%CV) $t_{½}$ and CL/F values of FK506 in the presence of PCZ were 35.9 (10) and 4.31 (30), respectively. The corresponding values of FK506 when given alone were 29 (15) and 21.4 (56), respectively [69]. The median (range) T_{max} (h) values were the same in both study phases [1.5 (1–3)]. The most common adverse events reported during co-administration of FK506 and PCZ were mild-moderate paresthesia (56%) and headache (39%) [66,70].

Despite the similarities in the PK properties of PCZ when given concomitantly with CSA or FK506, there was high intersubject variability of plasma PCZ that was reported (74%–141% and 30% in PCZ-CSA and PCZ-FK506 study, respectively). This limits the ability to draw solid conclusions from these results and creates a need for further research to evaluate this variation in PCZ PK profile. Furthermore, more information is needed on the interaction pathways between PCZ and both CSA and FK506, which are believed to be mediated by inhibition of CYP3A4 and P-gp transport.

In another investigation, Vaes *et al*. analyzed the impact of different factors on PCZ concentrations in myeloid leukemia or myelodysplastic syndrome patients that were being treated prophylactically with PCZ [71]. It was a prospective, bicentric study that was carried out between February 2009 and August 2010. Inclusion criteria included patients 16 and older being treated with PCZ for prophylaxis during their chemotherapy treatment [71]. Study participants were administered an oral suspension of PCZ 200 mg three times a day at the time of meals which were 50 g of fat when possible. The prophylaxis was continued until the neutropenia was resolved (neutrophil count >1000/mm^3), or until another antifungal medication was initiated for prophylaxis or treatment of IFIs. Blood samples were taken on day 7 of treatment, followed by twice a week thereafter. They were collected before the first dose (time zero [T0].) and 5 h after the first dose (time 5 [T5].) which was correlated with the C_{max}. The PCZ concentrations were measured by HPLC. Ongoing treatments with concomitant medications such as proton pump inhibitors (PPIs), histamine (H2)-receptor antagonists, cyclosporine, and tacrolimus were recorded and analyzed. Additionally, the effects of other factors such as age, sex, BMI, comorbidities, and allogenic transplant status were investigated [71].

Results were reported for a total of 40 patients who underwent 74 episodes of treatment with PCZ [71]. Treatment duration had a median of 22 days and ranged from 4 to 93 days. After analyzing the PCZ concentrations for 20 of the study participants, it was confirmed that there was no difference in the results from T0 to T5 ($p = 0.58$); therefore, PCZ concentrations at T0 were used from that point on in the study. Additionally, study subjects were not able to eat more than 30 g of fat in a meal; therefore, a high-fat meal was considered to be one with more than 20 g of fat. PCZ concentrations revealed that age, sex, and BMI do not affect serum plasma levels of the drug ($p = 0.44$, $p = 0.62$, $p = 0.12$, respectively). Allogenic transplant status also did not have an impact on PCZ concentrations when compared to other patients ($p = 0.33$). However, patients with mucositis of grade 1, 2, and 3 had lower PCZ concentrations at 270, 280, and 200 ng/mL, respectively, when compared to patients without mucositis who had PCZ levels with a median of 430 ng/mL ($p < 0.001$). Caloric intake was also shown to affect serum plasma levels of PCZ with study participants who had a caloric intake >1000 kcal/day having a level of 470 ng/mL compared to 300 ng/mL in patients with reduced caloric intake ($p = 0.02$) [71]. In regards to concomitant use of medications, patients taking PPIs had a lower PCZ concentration at 390 ng/mL compared to 510 ng/mL for patients who were not being administered a PPI ($p = 0.02$). Moreover, the concomitant use of ranitidine or cyclosporine did not affect PCZ concentrations ($p = 0.07$ for both). On the contrary, the use of tacrolimus led to an increased PCZ concentration ($p = 0.03$), with patients taking both medications having an average level of 160 ng/mL higher than patients not taking tracolimus ($p < 0.001$). Incidence of adverse events was not addressed [71].

Based on these results, the authors concluded that the main factors that have an impact on PCZ concentrations include the severity of mucositis, caloric intake, and concomitant use of PPIs or tacrolimus [71]. They recommended the use of H2-receptors antagonists instead of PPIs when possible, as well as further research to confirm the effect of tracolimus since the higher PCZ concentrations were observed in only two patients [71]. However, this study had some limitations, including a small sample size and lack of optimization of the PCZ dose which could have allowed for patients to reach higher serum plasma concentrations of the drug. Additionally, the different factors that were analyzed were not labeled as primary or secondary outcomes; therefore, it cannot be determined whether the study was actually powered to find a difference between any of them. Also, baseline characteristics were not presented with p values, limiting our ability to determine if the study participants were similar at the beginning of the study. Lastly, there were discrepancies in the amount of measurements that were compared for each of the factors. For example, when determining the effect of concomitant use of tracolimus, only nine PCZ measurements from patients taking the medication were compared to 266 PCZ measurements from patients not on the drug. These limitations warrant the need for further studies in order to define the need for drug monitoring in patients taking PCZ and the extent to which drug interactions with these medications affect PCZ concentrations.

49. Rifabutin

Krishna *et al.* performed a nonrandomized, open label, parallel, multiple dose PK study in healthy volunteers (n = 24) in order to study the interaction between PCZ and rifabutin at steady state [72]. Subjects were randomly assigned to receive either PCZ alone for 10 days (Group 1) or rifabutin coadministered with PCZ for 10 days (Group 2). Study participants received daily doses of PCZ (tablet, 200 mg) and rifabutin (capsule, 300 mg). Steady state levels of rifabutin were established 7 days (days −7 to 1) prior to the administration of PCZ (between days 1–10) in Group 2. Study drugs were ingested in the morning after the consumption of a high fat content breakfast. Plasma PCZ concentrations were determined by a series of time sensitive blood samples collected on day 10 and up to 120 h post PCZ dose in both groups. Steady state PCZ troughs were also done on days 8–10. Contrastingly, plasma rifabutin concentrations were determined from blood samples collected up to 24 h after administration and up to 120 h on days −1 and 10, respectively. All plasma drug concentrations were measured and analyzed using HPLC. Safety and adverse effects were monitored according to the study protocol [70,72].

Study population consisted of Caucasian males with a mean age (range) of 27 (20 to 40) years and with a mean weight of 73 kilograms [72]. In Group 2, four subjects did not complete the study due to adverse events (*i.e.*, leukopenia in 3 subjects and dizziness, headache and fever in 1). In Group 1, the PK of PCZ alone were comparable to previous studies. The mean (%CV) C_{max} (ng/mL), AUC_{τ} (ng·h/mL) and median (range) T_{max} (h) of PCZ were 766 (37), 12629 (43) and 5 (5–15), respectively [72]. The PK parameters of PCZ were significantly changed with rifabutin (Group 2). The mean (%CV) of C_{max} (ng/mL), AUC_{τ} (ng·h/mL), and median (range) T_{max} (h) were 438 (29), 6389 (38) and 7 (3–10), respectively [72]. According to the study, concomitant use of rifabutin reported a 43% and 49% reduction in C_{max} and AUC_{τ} of PCZ, respectively. This reduction in systemic exposure of PCZ was related to a 2-fold increase in PCZ clearance (CL/F, 307 *vs.* 594 mL/min) and a 42% decrease in PCZ $t_{1/2}$ (27.4 *vs.* 15.9 h) [72]. In Group 2, the two consecutive mean rifabutin trough concentrations (ng/mL) on day −1 and day 1 of PCZ coadministration were similar (64.1 *versus* 72.1) [70,72].

It is interesting to note that the PK of rifabutin were changed with coadministration of PCZ. The mean (%CV) of C_{max} (ng/mL) and AUC (ng·h/mL) of rifabutin were 438 (23) and 3975 (20) respectively, on day −1 and 569 (20) and 6833 (21), respectively, on day 10. The results demonstrated that co-administration of PCZ with rifabutin resulted in a 31% and 72% increase in C_{max} and AUC_{τ} values, respectively. This increase in exposure of rifabutin was associated with a 42% decrease in total rifabutin clearance when compared to rifabutin administered alone (CL/F, 1300 *versus* 758 mL.min) [72].

The frequency of adverse events, which were mild in nature, was higher in Group 2 than in Group 1. In Group 1, the adverse events that were related to drug use included back pain (25%), cough (17%) and dry skin (17%); whereas headache (75%), back pain (67%), leukopenia (42%), eye abnormality (42%) and abdominal pain (42%) were observed in Group 2 [72]. Leukopenia was the only abnormal laboratory finding in both study groups. The investigators concluded that concomitant use of PCZ and rifabutin should be avoided and should only be given together when the benefits outweigh the risks [72]. Close monitoring for adverse events is necessary if PCZ and rifabutin are used together [72].

Some of the limitations of this study were that only healthy Caucasian male subjects were included, sample size was small, and the parallel study design did not account for intersubject variability [72]. Previous PK studies showed that PCZ had a large intersubject variability in the systemic exposure of PCZ. The fact that this study was not conducted in a cross-over manner would not minimize the intersubject variability issue.

50. Phenytoin and Cimetidine

Two individual drug interaction studies published in abstract form evaluated the effects of phenytoin and cimetidine on the PK of PCZ in healthy volunteers [73,74]. Due to the limited information provided in these studies, a summary of the results were discussed. The first study by Courtney *et al.* was a randomized, open label, parallel, and multiple dose study in which healthy subjects ($n = 36$) were randomly assigned to three 10 day treatment arms. Group 1 received PCZ 200 mg tablet PO daily, Group 2 received phenytoin 200 mg PO daily, and Group 3 was given the same doses of PCZ and phenytoin [73]. Blood samples measuring plasma concentrations of PCZ and phenytoin and data analysis were performed following study protocol. On day 10, the mean C_{max} (ng/mL) and AUC_{0-24} (ng·h/mL) were decreased by 41% and 50%, respectively, after the co-administration of PCZ (200 mg tablet PO daily) and phenytoin (200 mg PO daily) [73]. This was attributed to the increase in clearance of PCZ by 90% when coadministered with phenytoin. On the other hand, the systemic exposure of phenytoin was increased by 16% with concomitant use of PCZ [73]. Based on these results, the authors recommended avoiding the use of phenytoin in patients who are taking PCZ [73].

The second study was a randomized, open label, two-way crossover, multiple dose drug interaction study in which healthy subjects ($n = 12$) were randomly assigned to 10 days of either PCZ 200 mg tablet PO daily in phase 1 or the same dose of PCZ and cimetidine 400 mg PO twice daily in phase 2 [74]. The two phases were separated by a washout period of 7 days. Blood samples measuring plasma concentrations of PCZ and cimetidine and data analysis were performed. The mean C_{max} and AUC_t values of PCZ were both decreased by 39% in phase 2 when compared to phase 1 [74]. The relative systemic exposure of PCZ in the presence of cimetidine was estimated to be 61% [90% CI: 54%–59%]. In both treatment phases, the average T_{max} and t ½ was 7 h and 35 h, respectively. The authors concluded that PCZ is safe and well-tolerated as a multiple-dosing regimen, and that absorption is not affected by changes in gastric pH. Nevertheless, concomitant use should be avoided due to the decrease in PCZ relative bioavailability when the pH is 3 or higher [74].

51. Glipizide

Courtney *et al.* conducted an open-label, crossover study in order to analyze the effect of glipizide on the relative bioavailability of PCZ [75]. The study was performed on 12 healthy volunteers. Glipizide was administered at a dose of 10 mg on days 1 and 11, and PCZ was given at a dose of 400 mg daily between days 2 to 11 [75]. The results of the study demonstrated that glipizide had no significant effect on the relative bioavailability of PCZ and *vice versa* [70,75]. Consequently, the co-administration of PCZ and glipizide was determined to be safe, even though a non-clinical significant decrease in blood glucose was seen [70,75].

52. Caspofungin and Micafungin

Krishna *et al.* investigated the effects of PCZ on the PK of caspofungin or micafungin in a phase I, randomized, parallel study [76]. A total of 67 healthy subjects were randomized into one of two groups. Group 1 was administered caspofungin 70 mg on day 1, followed by 50 mg on days 2–14 as a 1-h IV infusion. Group 2 received micafungin 150 mg once daily on days 1–7 as a 1-h IV infusion [76]. PCZ 400 mg twice a day was administered as an oral suspension on days 1–14 in Group 1, and on days 1–7 in Group 2. The PK parameters that were assessed included C_{max}, steady-state AUC over the dosing interval (AUC(t)), and the time to C_{max} (T_{max}). Safety was addressed with clinical laboratory tests, vital signs, electrocardiograms, and recording of incidence of adverse events [76].

The results of this investigation revealed that coadministration of PCZ did not lead to affected PK of caspofungin or micafungin [76]. Caspofungin with concomitant use of PCZ reported log-transformed ratio estimates of C_{max} and AUC(t) that were 90% and 98%, respectively, of those with caspofungin alone on day 14 of the study [76]. Similarly, ratio estimates of micafungin coadministered with PCZ were 104% (C_{max}) and 109% (AUC (t)) of those with micafungin alone on day 7. There was no change in the median T_{max}. The authors concluded that concomitant use of PCZ with caspofungin or micafungin does not affect the PK of either echinocandin, and that it is mostly well-tolerated [76]. This study was limited in that PCZ concentrations were not reported. Future studies could address the effects that both echinocandins have on the PK of PCZ and determine if it has an impact on its efficacy.

53. Simvastatin and Midazolam

In a study by Krishna *et al.*, the effect of PCZ on the PK of simvastatin and midazolam was investigated [77]. It was a randomized, fixed-sequence, parallel, single-center study performed on 35 healthy subjects. Study participants were randomized to receive oral PCZ 50, 100, or 200 mg [77]. All participants were administered single doses of the reference drug midazolam 2 mg PO alone on day 9; simvastatin 40 mg PO alone on day 6; PCZ 50, 100, or 200 mg PO once daily on days 1–7; PCZ with midazolam on day 8; PCZ alone on days 9–10; PCZ with simvastatin on day 11; and PCZ alone on days 12–13 [77]. The results of this investigation showed that concomitant use of PCZ (at all doses) with simvastatin leads to increased C_{max} and AUC of simvastatin and simvastatin acid when compared to the use of simvastatin alone [77]. The increase was by 5- to 11-fold and by 5- to 8-fold for simvastatin and simvastatin acid, respectively. When compared to the administration of midazolam alone, PCZ (at all doses) inhibits the CYP3A4 metabolism of midazolam, leading to a 3- to 6-fold increase in AUC. The investigators of this study stated in their conclusions that these results confirm the classification of PCZ as a strong CYP3A4 inhibitor [77]. They recommended that the concomitant use of PCZ with simvastatin, and other statins that are mostly metabolised by CYP3A4, should be avoided, and that other statins that are not affected by CYP3A4 inhibition be used instead [77]. However, this study did not report any p values in order to determine the statistical significance of the results. Also, it would be important to translate these results into the clinical relevance that an increase of this magnitude in the AUC of simvastatin and midazolam would have in terms of efficacy and safety for patients.

54. Benzodiazepines

Heinz *et al.* explored the concentration of PCZ at steady-state when given concomitantly with benzodiazepines in a retrospective study [78]. Blood samples were collected from patients with different indications for antifungal therapy in several clinical settings [78]. Similar plasma concentrations of PCZ were reported from patients receiving both PCZ and temazepam compared to patients who were administered PCZ alone. However, a significant reduction in the concentration of PCZ was observed when coadministered with lorazepam compared to PCZ alone with median values of 336 ng/mL *vs.* 585 ng/mL, respectively ($p = 0.001$) [78]. Patients who received a total daily dose of PCZ of 800 mg also showed a similar trend with a concentration of 292 ng/mL with PCZ and lorazepam compared to 537 ng/mL when PCZ was given alone ($p = 0.003$). However, at a lower dose of 200 mg three times a day, the difference in plasma concentrations of PCZ was not statistically significant, even though the same pattern was observed (512 ng/mL *versus* 689 ng/mL; $p = 0.186$) [78]. Based on these results, the authors claimed that concomitant use of lorazepam with PCZ is associated with reduced concentrations of PCZ. They suggested that this could be due to induction of PCZ clearance by glucuronidation [78]. However, the data was not consistent with different doses of PCZ; therefore, further studies would be needed to confirm these results and determine the role of different PCZ strengths and glucuronidation in this potential drug interaction.

55. Posaconazole with HIV Antiretroviral Agents

55.1. Atazanavir +/− Ritonavir or Efavirenz

In a study by Krishna *et al.*, the PK interaction between PCZ and atazanavir, with and without ritonavir, as well as the interaction between PCZ and efavirenz was investigated [79]. It was a phase I, open label, randomized, crossover study that was divided in two parts. In part 1, 12 healthy Caucasian volunteers with an average age of 45 years old were randomized into two groups. Group 1 was administered atazanavir 300 mg and ritonavir 100 mg daily for 7 days, followed by atazanavir/ritonavir with PCZ 400 mg twice a day for 7 days. Afterwards, there was a 28-day washout period after which patients received atazanavir alone daily for 7 days, followed by atazanavir with PCZ daily for 7 days. Patients in Group 2 were administered the same medications in the opposite order. Part 1 of the study was carried out for a total of 59 days [79].

In part 2, 17 healthy Caucasian volunteers with an average age of 43 years old were also randomized into two groups. In Group 1, subjects were administered efavirenz 400 mg daily for 10 days, followed by efavirenz 400 mg daily with PCZ 400 mg twice a day for 10 days [79]. Subsequently, subjects were in a 28-day washout period, which was followed by the administration of PCZ alone 400 mg twice a day for 10 days. In Group 2, patients were administered the same medications in the opposite order. This second part of the study had a duration of 60 days. In both parts of this investigation, PCZ was given after a standardised high fat meal. Assessment of compliance to treatment was not addressed [79].

A one-way analysis of variance model was used to determine the differences in time to reach C_{max} and AUC, which was the primary endpoint of the study [79]. Safety was addressed by incidence of adverse effects and by monitoring of hematology parameters, ECG and vital signs. The power of the study was set to 80% to detect a difference of 22% in AUC in 12 subjects [79].

In part 1 of the study, the results showed that concomitant use of PCZ 400 mg twice a day and atazanavir 300 mg daily for 7 days lead to an increase in mean AUC and mean C_{max} of atazanavir by 3.7 and 2.6-fold, respectively, when compared to atazanavir alone [79]. There was also a delayed systemic absorption by 1.5–2 h, increased half-life (from 5.85 to 11.1 h), and a decreased clearance (from 49.7 L/h to 9.61 L/h) of atazanavir when used in combination with PCZ; this suggested that there is possible CYP3A4 enzyme inhibition by PCZ in the metabolism of atazanavir. Moreover, the addition of ritonavir to both atazanavir and PCZ reported similar results; C_{max} and AUC increased by 1.5 and 2.5-fold, respectively. Also, coadministration of atazanavir, ritonavir and PCZ resulted in 1.5 and 1.8-fold increase in mean C_{max} and AUC of ritonavir, respectively, when compared to atazanavir and ritonavir alone. The investigators attributed these results to a potential UGT1A1 enzyme inhibition by atazanavir in addition to CYP3A4 inhibition by PCZ [79]. Nevertheless, atazanavir and ritonavir did not affect the PK parameters of PCZ. Safety data reported that 92% of the participants experienced ocular icterus, which is possibly related to benign hyperbilirubinemia, an established side effect of atazanavir. An increase in bilirubin that was determined to be clinically significant was reported in a total of 11 subjects [48–156 mmoL/L (baseline bilirubin concentrations were not provided)]. This may have been due to the increase in atazanavir AUC. Other adverse events reported included pollakiuria and abdominal pain (50% and 25%, respectively) [79].

Part 2 of the study showed a 45% and 50% decrease in mean C_{max} and AUC of PCZ, respectively, when coadministered with efavirenz. The authors suggested that this can be due to UGT induction by efavirenz affecting the metabolism of PCZ. On the other hand, PCZ did not have a significant effect on the systemic absorption of efavirenz; it was delayed from 2–4 h when coadministered with PCZ. Commonly reported adverse events included dizziness (47%), fatigue (41%), and headache (41%) [79].

The investigators of this study concluded that there can be a potential increase in plasma concentrations of protease inhibitors and NNRTIs when used concomitantly with PCZ [79]. Their recommendation was to monitor for toxicity and adverse events regularly if coadministration was necessary [79]. Additionally, they did not support the use of efavirenz and PCZ together as their results reported a decreased exposure of PCZ [79]. This study was limited in that it had a small sample size and a short duration. Also, confidence intervals were limited and no p values were provided to show clinical and statistical significance. However, the package insert for posaconazole includes ritonavir, atazanavir, and efavirenz as interacting agents based on the results of this study [2].

55.2. Fosamprenavir +/− Ritonavir

Bruggeman *et al.* evaluated the effects of fosamprenavir alone *versus* fosamprenavir boosted with ritonavir on the PK of PCZ and *vice versa* [79]. It was an open-label, three period, cross-over, multiple-dosing study on 24 healthy volunteers with a mean age of 36 years old. The participants received PCZ suspension 200 mg daily on day 1, PCZ 200 mg twice a day on day 2, and PCZ 400 mg twice a day from day 3 forward combined with fosamprenavir 700 mg twice a day or fosamprenavir/ritonavir 700 mg/100 mg twice a day. The treatment regimen was given for a total of 10 days, followed by a washout period of 17 days after which the regimens were switched between the two groups. The power was set to 80% to find a 20% difference in PCZ AUC [79].

The results reported a statistically significant decrease in exposure to PCZ when administered concomitantly with fosamprenavir. The geometric mean ratio (GMR) for PCZ combined with fosamprenavir when compared to administration of PCZ alone was 0.77 (90% CI, 0.68–0.87) and 0.79 (90% CI, 0.71–0.89) for the AUC_{0-12} and C_{max}, respectively [79]. No statistical significance was found in the GMR free fraction of PCZ when compared to the combination group (1.10%; $p = 0.177$). The GMR for the AUC_{0-12} and C_{max} were 0.35 (90% CI, 0.23–0.39) and 0.64 (90% CI, 0.55–0.76), respectively, when comparing fosamprenavir with PCZ to fosamprenavir/ritonavir with PCZ [79]. There were a total of 141 adverse events; however, none were reported as serious. Details on these adverse events were not provided. Based on these results, the authors concluded that there is a significant bidirectional PK interaction between PCZ and fosamprenavir. They suggested that this could be due to a reduced exposure of PCZ by fosamprenavir because of UGT1A4 or p-glycoprotein induction, decreased PCZ absorption, or protein displacement of PCZ [79]. Nevertheless, small sample size and short duration of this study limit the ability to determine the long-term effects of concomitant use of PCZ and fosamprenavir. Also, with a study population composed of only healthy volunteers, extrapolating the results to patients with HIV is more challenging. After analyzing these results, it may be concluded that fosamprenavir boosted with ritonavir could be used concomitantly with PCZ; however, therapeutic drug monitoring is recommended. At the present moment, a target plasma concentration of PCZ has not been established due to significant interpatient variability in PK. Consequently, the coadministration should be avoided when possible.

56. Posaconazole in HIV-infected Patients

There are a few studies that have analyzed the use of PCZ in the treatment of oropharyngeal/esophageal candidiasis in patients with HIV. Two of these studies investigated the treatment of oropharyngeal candidiasis concentrating on patients who were azole-refractory [80,81]. Exclusion criteria for all trials included patients that had started on a protease inhibitor for the past 30 days. Skiest *et al.* reported that approximately 72% of the participants were receiving antiretroviral therapy [80]. This was a multicenter, international, phase III, open-label study [80]. It was noted that 38% of these patients were taking NNRTIs, 63% were taking NRTIs, and 53% were taking PIs. Study subjects were given a PCZ suspension for 28 days. The primary safety outcome was the incidence of adverse events. QT prolongation was reported as a reason for study withdrawal for at least one patient in the investigation, but the most common adverse events included diarrhea and neutropenia [80]. However, it is important to note that the authors did not discuss how the correlation between study drug use and adverse events was determined, especially with the antiretrovirals. The investigators did mention that the incidence of diarrhea and neutropenia could also be related to the underlying HIV disease, opportunistic infections, or the administration of concomitant medications. Another confounder of this study is related to these concomitant medications that were not listed in detail, even though the percentage of patients taking them was reported. This makes it challenging to determine if there is a direct correlation between the adverse events that were observed to a drug interaction with PCZ.

Another study by Vazquez *et al.* investigated the efficacy of PCZ compared to FCZ for the treatment of oropharyngeal candidiasis [60]. It was a multicenter, randomized, evaluator-blinded clinical study in 350 patients infected with HIV. The participants were administered PCZ or FCZ oral suspension for a total of 14 days. A total of 132 (66%) of these patients were receiving no antiretroviral therapy, 29 (8%) were taking a NNRTI, 117 (32%) were receiving a NRTI, and 85 (24%) were on a PI. Adverse events that were observed and determined to be serious included fever, asthenia, abdominal pain, respiratory insufficiency, and lymphadenopathy [60]. However, the investigators did not consider any of these serious adverse events to be related to the administration of the study drug [60]. As with the first study previously discussed, how the relationship between adverse events and potential drug interactions was determined, particularly with antiretrovirals, was not addressed.

Vazquez *et al.* evaluated the safety and efficacy of PCZ in another study that focused on the long-term treatment of patients infected with HIV and oropharyngeal/esophageal candidiasis who were azole-refractory [81]. The study was a multicenter, international, non-comparative, open-label investigation on a total of 100 patients [81]. Study subjects were administered PCZ oral suspension for a total of 3 months, and the option to continue treatment for up to 12 months for patients who were considered to be clinical responders was offered. At baseline, 70% of the participants were receiving antiretroviral therapy. Out of the patients taking antiretrovirals at baseline, 38% were taking NNRTIs, 64% were on NRTIs, and 48% were receiving PIs [81]. Adverse events reported included neutropenia, urticarial, and cardiac failure/sudden death, and they occurred after 3 months of treatment on a total of three patients. The investigators suggested that these adverse events could have been due to the HIV infection itself, opportunistic infections, or the use of concomitant medications [81]. As with the other two studies, the correlation between study drug use, potential drug interaction, mainly with the antiretrovirals, and the incidence of adverse events was not addressed. The possibility of elevated antiretroviral serum concentrations due to the concomitant use of PCZ remains an area that warrants further research as this increased antiretroviral exposure could have led to the laboratory abnormalities and other adverse events observed in the study.

57. Formulary Considerations

Although PCZ has a chemical structure similar to ICZ, it has a wider spectrum of antifungal activity. This drug covers not only selected *Candida* and *Aspergillus* species, but other breakthrough fungal infections including *fusarium*, *scedosporium* and *zygomycosis*. Posaconazole has a unique PK profile that does not require renal dose adjustment. Thus, the drug is considered safe and well tolerated. Posaconazole has been approved by the FDA for the prophylaxis of invasive *Aspergillus* and *Candida* infections in severely immunocompromised patients 13 years and older. However, the efficacy of PCZ in the treatment of IFIs has yet to be determined. The average wholesaler price (AWP) of a 105 mL PCZ oral suspension (40 mg/mL) bottle is $576.00 and the unit cost is $5.49 per 40 mg/mL [82]. Depending on the usage, the AWP cost of a week therapy of PCZ can range from $110 to $770.

Differences in formulation of PCZ have a significant impact on drug interactions, PK properties, and safety and tolerance of the antifungal. Currently, there are three FDA approved formulations that include the oral suspension, delayed-release tablets and injection for IV infusion. The oral suspension is indicated for the prophylaxis of invasive *Aspergillus* infections in patients who are immunocompromised. It is also approved for the treatment of oropharyngeal candidiasis, including cases that are refractory to ICZ and FCZ. The delayed-release tablets and injection, which became available on 2014, are indicated for the prophylaxis of invasive *Aspergillus* and *Candida* infections in severely immunocompromised patients. The FDA-approved indication for the delayed-release tablets and injection is based on PK and safety trials [2, 83–86]. On the other hand, more supporting data on the oral suspension formulation of PCZ, including PK, safety and efficacy trials, have allowed for the recommendations per IDSA guidelines for additional indications, such as treatment of invasive infections of aspergillosis, allergic bronchopulmonary aspergillosis, salvage consolidation therapy in meningeal cryptococcosis relapse, and pulmonary cryptococcosis in patients who are not immunocompromised [87–89].

The extent to which drug interactions can occur is also dependent on the different formulations of PCZ. While the bioavailability of the oral suspension is highly affected by the concomitant use of medications that affect gastric pH and motility, such as H2RA antagonists, PPIs, and metoclopramide, the delayed-release tablets were not significantly impacted by the concomitant use of these drugs [90]. This also applies to the IV injection which is unaffected by drug interactions by default since it bypasses first-pass metabolism. In terms of PK properties, the delayed-release tablets have more predictable bioavailability and higher serum concentrations [91]. However, they cannot be crushed or chewed, removing them as an option for critically-ill patients, or those unable to swallow; this is where the IV injection formulation plays a major role [91]. In general, the tablet formulation has less inter-patient variability, better bioavailability which allows for once-daily administration (*versus* four times daily administration with the oral suspension), and absorption that is not affected by changes in gastric pH or motility, as previously mentioned [92]. Additionally, the tablets can be taken without regards to meals, and they have higher and more consistent mean serum concentrations compared to the oral suspension. Consequently, using the tablet formulation can potentially optimize treatment efficacy in IFIs. [92]. The tablet and injection formulations have shown a slightly similar safety profile to that of the oral suspension and are generally well tolerated. The delayed-released tablets have shown to cause diarrhea, pyrexia, nausea and hypoglycemia; while the IV injection has shown to cause diarrhea, hypokalemia, pyrexia, and nausea [2]. In clinical trials, the IV injection has also shown to cause thrombophlebitis when multiple peripheral infusions are given through the same vein [2].

58. Summary

PCZ is an extended-spectrum antifungal agent with antifungal activity against yeasts, filamentous fungi and azole resistant *Candida* species. PCZ exerts its antifungal activity by inhibiting fungal cell wall synthesis. It is orally bioavailable and is absorbed through the GI tract independent of pH. The systemic exposure of PCZ is optimized when it is taken with food or a nutritional supplement. Nevertheless, this only applies to the suspension formulation since the bioavailability of PCZ tablet and injection formulations is unaffected by the presence of food. PCZ has a large volume of distribution and is highly protein bound. The antifungal agent is metabolsed in the liver to several inactive glucuronide metabolites through the UGT enzyme pathway. The major elimination route of PCZ and its metabolites is fecal (~77%) and only small fractions are detected in the urine (~14%). The half-life of PCZ is long (>24 h) which allows this drug to be administered once daily. However, due to its unique oral absorption profile, PCZ is best administered as divided doses with a maximum daily dose of 800 mg. Age, gender, race and diseases, such as persistent febrile neutropenia and refractory IFIs, do not appear to alter the PK of PCZ. Dose adjustments are not needed in patients with renal failure and patients who are on hemodialysis. Furthermore, anecdotal PK, efficacy and safety data support the use of PCZ as salvage therapy in pediatric patients with IFIs. The use of PCZ is contraindicated in pregnancy and lactation. In adults, PCZ is efficacious, safe and well tolerated in the area of oropharyngeal candidiasis associated with HIV/AIDS infection, prophylaxis in neutropenia secondary to chemotherapy or in severe graft-*versus*-host disease associated with hematopoietic stem-cell transplantation. The most common adverse effects of PCZ include headache, fatigue, nausea and dry mouth. Potential drug-drug interactions exist between PCZ and other therapeutic agents including cimetidine, proton pump inhibitors, cyclosporine, tacrolimus, phenytoin, and rifabutin through either hepatic enzyme inhibition (CYP3A4) or induction. However, the potential for drug interactions is highly dependent on the formulation of PCZ, especially when coadministered with medications that affect gastric pH and motility, as the tablet and injection formulations have shown to be unaffected. Drug interactions also exist between PCZ and antiretrovirals used for the treatment of HIV, such as atazanavir, ritonavir, efavirenz, and fosamprenavir. Further research is needed in order to establish drug interactions between PCZ and other NRTIs, NNRTIs and PIs. Formulary limitation warrants PCZ oral administration in immunocompromised patients with functional GI tracts who fail conventional antifungal therapies or who are suspected to have a breakthrough fungal infection. Although a comparative study demonstrated that most patients with compromised gastrointestinal function can still achieve a therapeutic serum concentration of PCZ, future studies are warranted in order to confirm these results. Nevertheless, the new IV injection formulation is an attractive option for this patient population and will play a significant role when patients are unable to receive oral formulations of PCZ. Published studies present with several limitations in their study designs, including their retrospective nature, small sample sizes, descriptive analysis of the data, and lack of assessment of compliance of concomitant medications. This provides ample room for future research with better-controlled clinical trials in order to establish the role of PCZ in the treatment and prevention of several fungal infections, and potentially expand its FDA indications and role in clinical practice.

Conflicts of Interest

The authors declare no conflict of interest.

References

1. FDA website. Available online: http://www.fda.gov/safety/medwatch/safetyinformation/ucm228417.htm (accessed on 7 September 2015).
2. *Noxafil [package insert]*; Schering Corp: Kenilworth, NJ, USA, March 2014.
3. Keating, G.M. Posaconazole. *Drugs* **2005**, *65*, 1553–1567.
4. Pfaller, M.A.; Diekema, D.J.; Jones, R.N.; Messer, S.A.; Hollis, R.J.; SENTRY Participants Group. Trends in antifungal susceptibility of *Candida* spp. isolated from pediatric and adult patients with bloodstream infections: SENTRY Antimicrobial Surveillance Program, 1997 to 2000. *J. Clin. Microbiol.* **2002**, *40*, 852–856.

5. Pfaller, M.A.; Diekema, D.J. Rare and emerging opportunistic fungal pathogens: Concerns for resistance beyoud Candida albicans and Aspergillus fumigatus. *J. Clin. Microbiol.* **2004**, *42*, 4419–4431.
6. Courtney, R.; Wexler, D.; Radwanski, E.; Lim, J.; Laughlin, M. Effect of food on the relative bioavailability of two oral formulations of posaconazole in healthy adults. *Br. J. Clin. Pharmacol.* **2004**, *57*, 218–222.
7. Xiao, L.; Madison, V.; Chau, A.S.; Loebenberg, D.; Palermo, R.E.; McNicholas, P.M. Three-dimensional models of wild-type and mutated forms of cytochrome P450 14α-sterol demethylases from aspergillus fumigatus and candida albicans provide insights into posaconazole binding. *Antimicrob. Agents Chemother.* **2004**, *48*, 568–574.
8. Ghannoum, M.A.; Rice, L.B. Antifungal agents: Mode of action, mechanisms of resistance, and correlation of these mechanisms with bacterial resistance. *Clin. Microbiol*. **1999**, *12*, 501–517.
9. Heimark, L.; Shipkova, P.; Greene, J.; Munayyer, H.; Yarosh-Tomaine, T.; DiDomenico, B.; Hare, R.; Pramanik, B.N. Mechanism of azole antifungal activity as determined by liquid chromatographic/mass spectrometric monitoring of ergosterol biosynthesis. *J Mass Spectrom.* **2002**, *37*, 265–269.
10. Munayyer, H.K.; Mann, P.A.; Chau, A.S.; Yarosh-Tomaine, T.; Greene, J.R.; Hare, R.S.; Heimark, L.; Palermo, R.E.; Loebenberg, D.; McNicholas, P.M. Posaconazole is a potent inhibitor of sterol 14α-demethylation in yeasts and molds. *Antimicrob. Agents Chemother.* **2004**, *48*, 3690–3696.
11. Sabatelli, F.; Patel, R.; Mann, P.A.; Mendrick, C.A.; Norris, C.C.; Hare, R.; Loebenberg, D.; Black, T.A.; McNicholas, P.M. *In vitro* activities of posaconazole, fluconazole, itraconazole, voriconazole, and amphotericin B against a large collection of clinically important molds and yeasts. *Antimicrob. Agents Chemother*. **2006**, *50*, 2009–2015.
12. Espinel-Ingroff, A. Comparison of *in vitro* activities of the new triazole SCH56592 and the echinocandins MK-0991 (L-743,872) and LY303366 against opportunistic filamentous and dimorphic fungi and yeasts. *J. Clin. Microbiol.* **1998**, *36*, 2950–2956.
13. Perfect, J.R.; Cox, G.M.; Dodge, R.K.; Schell, W.A. *In vitro* and *in vivo* efficacies of the azole SCH56592 against Cryptococcus neoformans. *Antimicrob. Agents Chemother*. **1996**, *40*, 1910–1913.
14. Barchiesi, F.; Schimizzi, A.M.; Caselli, F.; Giannini, D.; Camiletti, V.; Fileni, B.; Giacometti, A.; Di Francesco, L.F.; Scalise, G. Activity of the new antifungal triazole, posaconazole, against Cryptococcus neoformans. *J. Antimicrob. Chemother.* **2001**, *48*, 769–773.
15. Pfaller, M.A.; Messer, S.A.; Boyken, L.; Hollis, R.J.; Rice, C.; Tendolkar, S.; Diekema, D.J. *In vitro* activities of voriconazole, posaconazole, and fluconazole against 4169 clinical isolates of *Candida* spp. and Cryptococcus neoformans collected during 2001 and 2002 in the ARTEMIS global antifungal surveillance program. *Diagn. Microbiol. Infect. Dis.* **2004**, *48*, 201–205.
16. Pfaller, M.A.; Messer, S.A.; Hollis, R.J.; Jones, R.N. *In vitro* activities of posaconazole (Sch 56592) compared with those of itraconazole and fluconazole against 3685 clinical isolates of *Candida* spp. and Cryptococcus neoformans. *Antimicrob. Agents Chemother*. **2001**, *45*, 2862–2864.
17. Barchiesi, F.; Caggiano, G.; Maracci, M.; Arzeni, D.; Scalise, G.; Montagna, M.T. Antifungal susceptibility patterns of yeast isolates causing bloodstream infections. *J. Antimicrob. Chemother.* **2003**, *51*, 431–433.

18. Barchiesi, F.; Schimizzi, A.M.; Najvar, L.K.; Bocanegra, R.; Caselli, F.; Di Cesare, S.; Giannini, D.; Di Francesco, L.F.; Giacometti, A.; Carle, F.; *et al*. Interactions of posaconazole and flucytosine against cryptococcus neoformans. *Antimicrob Agents Chemother.* **2001**, *45*, 1355–1359.
19. Barchiesi, F.; Schimizzi, A.M.; Caselli, F.; Novelli, A.; Fallani, S.; Giannini, D.; Arzeni, D.; Di Cesare, S.; Di Francesco, L.F.; Fortuna, M.; *et al*. Interactions between triazoles and amphotericin B against Cryptococcus neoformans. *Antimicrob Agents Chemother.* **2000**, *44*, 2435–2441.
20. Perea, S.; Gonzalez, G.; Fothergill, A.W.; Sutton, D.A.; Rinaldi, M.G. *In vitro* activities of terbinafine in combination with fluconazole, itraconazole, voriconazole, and posaconazole against clinical isolates of candida glabrata with decreased susceptibility to azoles. *J. Clin. Microbiol.* **2002**, *40*, 1831–1833.
21. Oliveira, E.R.; Fothergill, A.W.; Kirkpatrick, W.R.; Coco, B.J.; Patterson, T.F.; Redding, S.W. *In vitro* interaction of posaconazole and caspofungin against clinical isolates of candida glabrata. *Antimicrob Agents Chemother.* **2005**, *49*, 3544–3545.
22. Cacciapuoti, A.; Loebenberg, D.; Corcoran, E.; Menzel, F., Jr.; Moss, E.L., Jr.; Norris, C.; Michalski, M.; Raynor, K.; Halpern, J.; Mendrick, C.; *et al*. *In vitro* and *in vivo* activities of SCH 56592 (posaconazole), a new triazole antifungal agent, against Aspergillus and Candida. *Antimicrob. Agents Chemother.* **2000**, *44*, 2017–2022.
23. Pfaller, M.A.; Messer, S.A.; Hollis, R.J.; Jones, R.N.; SENTRY Participants Group. Antifungal activities of posaconazole, ravuconazole, and voriconazole compared to those of itraconazole and amphotericin B against 239 clinical isolates of *Aspergillus* spp. and other filamentous fungi: Report from SENTRY Antimicrobial Surveillance Program, 2000. *Antimicrob. Agents Chemother.* **2002**, *46*, 1032–1037.
24. Manavathu, E.K.; Cutright, J.L.; Loebenberg, D.; Chandrasekar, P.H. A comparative study of the *in vitro* susceptibilities of clinical and laboratory-selected resistant isolates of *Aspergillus* spp. to amphotericin, B.; itraconazole, voriconazole and posaconazole (SCH 56592). *J. Antimicrob. Chemother.* **2000**, *46*, 229–234.
25. Sugar, A.M.; Liu, X.P. *In vitro* and *in vivo* activities of SCH 56592 against Blastomyces dermatitidis. *Antimicrob. Agents Chemother*. **1996**, *40*, 1314–1316.
26. Paphitou, N.I.; Ostrosky-Zeichner, L.; Paetznick, V.L.; Rodriguez, J.R.; Chen, E.; Rex, J.H. *In vitro* antifungal susceptibilities of Trichosporon species. *Antimicrob Agents Chemother.* **2002**, *46*, 1144–1146.
27. Meletiadis, J.; Meis FGM, Mouton, J.W.; Rodriquez-Tudela, J.L.; Donnelly, J.P.; Verweij, P.E.; EUROFUNG Network. *In vitro* activities of new and conventional antifungals agents against clinical *scedosporium* isolates. *Antimicrob. Agents Chemother.* **2002**, *46*, 62–68.
28. Carrillo, A.J.; Guarro, J. *In vitro* activities of four novel triazoles against *Scedosporium* spp. *Antimicrob. Agents Chemother.* **2001**, *45*, 2151–2153.
29. Gonzalez, G.M.; Tijerina, R.; Najvar, L.K.; Bocanegra, R.; Rinaldi, M.; Loebenberg, D.; Graybill, J.R. *In vitro* and *in vivo* activities of posaconazole against coccidioides immitis. *Antimicrob. Agents Chemother.* **2002**, *46*, 1352–1356.
30. Sun, Q.N.; Najvar, L.K.; Bocanegra, R.; Loebenberg, D.; Graybill, J.R. *In vivo* activity of posaconazole against *Mucor* spp. in an immunosuppressed-mouse model. *Antimicrob Agents Chemother.* **2002**, *46*, 2310–2312.

31. Gonzalez, G.M.; Tijerina, R.; Najvar, L.K.; Bocanegra, R.; Rinaldi, M.G.; Loebenberg, D.; Graybill, J.R. Activity of posaconazole against pseudallescheria boydii: *In vitro* and *in vivo* assays. *Antimicrob Agents Chemother.* **2003**, *47*, 1436–1438.
32. Barchiesi, F.; Arzeni, D.; Camiletti, V.; Simonetti, O.; Cellini, A.; Offidani, A.M.; Scalise, G. *In vitro* activity of posaconazole against clinical isolates of dermatophytes. *J. Clin. Microbiol.* **2001**, *39*, 4208–4209.
33. Manavathu, E.K.; Alangaden, G.J.; Chandrasekar, P.H. Differential activity of triazoles in two-drug combinations with the echinocandin caspofungin against Aspergillus fumigatus. *J. Antimicrob. Chemother.* **2003**, *51*, 1423–1425.
34. Manavathu, E.K.; Ramesh, M.S.; Baskaran, I.; Ganesan, L.T.; Chandrasekar, P.H. A comparative study of the post-antifungal effect (PAFE) of amphotericin, B, triazoles and echinocandins on aspergillus fumigatus and *Candida* albicans. *J. Antimicrob. Chemother.* **2004**, *53*, 386–389.
35. Nomeir, A.A.; Kumari, P.; Hilbert, M.J.; Gupta, S.; Loebenberg, D.; Cacciapuoti, A.; Hare, R.; Miller, G.H.; Lin, C.C.; Cayen, M.N. Pharmacokinetics of SCH 56592, a new azole broad-spectrum antifungal agent, in mice, rats, rabbits, dogs, and cynomolgus monkeys. *Antimicrob. Agents Chemother.* **2000**, *44*, 727–731.
36. Courtney, R.; Pai, S.; Laughlin, M.; Lim, J.; Batra, V. Pharmacokinetics, safety, and tolerability of oral posaconazole administered in single and multiple doses in healthy adults. *Antimicrob. Agents Chemother.* **2003**, *47*, 2788–2795.
37. Ezzet, F.; Wexler, D.; Courtney, R.; Krishna, G.; Lim, J.; Laudhlin, M. Oral bioavailability of posaconazole in fasted healthy subjects: Comparison between three regimens and basis for clinical dosage recommendations. *Clin. Pharmacokinet.* **2005**, *44*, 211–220.
38. Xu, H.R.; Chu, N.N.; Chen, W.L.; Wang, Z.D.; Li, X.N. Liquid chromatography-mass spectrometry method for the quantification of posaconazole in human plasma: Application to pharmacokinetics following single-dose administration in the fasted state and with a high-fat meal. *Pharmazie* **2013**, *68*, 173–177.
39. Lin, T.Y.; Yang, M.H.; Chang, F.Y. A randomized, phase, I, 3-way crossover study to examine the effects of food on the pharmacokinetics of single doses of 400 mg posaconazole oral suspension in healthy male Taiwanese subjects. *Ther. Drug Monit.* **2013**, *35*, 223–227.
40. Sansone-Parsons, A.; Krishna, G.; Calzetta, A.; Wexler, D.; Kantesaria, B.; Rosenberg, M.A.; Saltzman, M.A. Effect of a nutritional supplement on posaconazole pharmacokinetics following oral administration to healthy volunteers. *Antimicrob. Agents Chemother.* **2006**, *50*, 1881–1883.
41. Walravens, J.; Brouwers, J.; Spriet, I.; Tack, J.; Annaert, P.; Augustijns, P. Effect of pH and comedication on gastrointestinal absorption of posaconazole: Monitoring of intraluminal and plasma drug concentrations. *Clin. Pharmacokinet.* **2011**, *50*, 725–734.
42. Courtney, R.; Sansone, A.; Smith, W.; Marbury, T.; Statkevich, P.; Martinho, M.; Laughlin, M.; Swan, S. Posaconazole pharmacokinetics, safety and tolerability in subjects with varying degrees of chronic renal disease. *J. Clin. Pharmacol.* **2005**, *45*, 185–192.
43. Krieter, P.; Flannery, B.; Musick, T.; Gohdes, M.; Martinho, M.; Courtney, R. Disposition of posaconazole following single dose oral administration in healthy subjects. *Antimicrob. Agents Chemother.* **2004**, *48*, 3543–3451.

44. Ghosal, A.; Hapangama, N.; Yuan, Y.; Achanfuo-Yeboah, J.; Lannucci, R.; Chowdhury, S.; Alton, K.; Pateick, J.E.; Zbaida, S.; *et al.* Identification of human UDP-glucuronosyltransferase enzyme(s) responsable for th eglucuronidation of posaconazole (Noxafil). *Drug Metab. Dispos.* **2004**, *32*, 267–271.
45. Sansone-Parsons, A.; Krishna, G.; Simon, J.; Soni, P.; Kantesaria, B.; Herron, J.; Stoltz, R. Effects of age, gender, and race/ethnicity on the pharmacokinetics of posaconazole in healthy volunteers. *Antimicrob. Agents Chemother.* **2007**, *51*, 495–502.
46. Krishna, G.; Ma, L.; Martinho, M.; Preston, R.A.; O'Mara, E. A new solid oral tablet formulation of posaconazole: A randomized clinical trial to investigate rising single- and multiple-dose pharmacokinetics and safety in healthy volunteers. *J. Antimicrob. Chemother.* **2012**, *67*, 2725–2730.
47. Cornely, O.A.; Maertens, J.; Winston, D.J.; Perfect, J.; Ullmann, A.J.; Walsh, T.J.; Helfgott, D.; Holowiecki, J.; Stockelberg, D.; Goh, Y.T.; *et al.* Posaconazole *vs.* fluconazole or itraconazole prophylaxis in patients with neutropenia. *N. Engl. J. Med.* **2007**, *356*, 348–359.
48. De Pauw, B.E.; Donnelly, J.P. Prophylaxis and aspergillosis—Has the principle been proven? *N. Engl. J. Med.* **2007**, *356*, 409–411.
49. Kontoyiannis, D.P.; Lewis, R.E. Posaconazole prophylaxis in hematologic cancer. *N. Engl. J. Med.* **2007**, *356*, 2214–2215.
50. Van Nieuwkoop, C.; van Dissel, J.T. Posaconazole prophylaxis in hematologic cancer. *N. Engl. J. Med.* **2007**, *356*, 2215–2218.
51. Ullmann, A.J.; Cornely, O.A.; Hachem, B.R.; Burchardt, A.; Kontoyiannis, D.P.; Töpelt, K.; Courtney, R.; Wexler, D.; Krishna, G.; Martinho, M.; *et al.* Pharmacokinetics, safety and efficacy of posaconazole in patients with persistent febrile neutropenia or refractory invasive fungal infection. *Antimicrob. Agents Chemother.* **2006**, *50*, 658–666.
52. Huang, X.; Wang, F.; Chen, Y.; Liu, T.; Wang, J.; Hu, J.; Jie, J.; Chen, F.; Wang, S.; Shen, Z.; *et al.* A multicenter, open-label study of posaconazole oral suspension in the treatment of invasive fungal infections in patients refractory to or intolerant of first-line therapy. *Future Microbiol.* **2012**, *7*, 201–209.
53. Shen, Y.; Huang, X.J.; Wang, J.X.; Jin, J.; Hu, J.D.; Yu, K.; Wu, D.P.; Wang, S.J.; Yu, L.; Chen, X.Q.; Liu, T.; *et al.* Posaconazole *vs.* fluconazole as invasive fungal infection prophylaxis in China: A multicenter, randomized, open-label study. *Int. J. Clin. Pharmacol. Ther.* **2013**, *51*, 738–745.
54. Kaya, S.; Sonmez, M.; Koksal, I.; Gencalioglu, E.; Yilmaz, M.; Yilmaz, G. Comparison of fluconazole and posaconazole for fungal prophylaxis in high-risk patients with hematological malignity. *J. Microbiol. Infect.* **2014**, *4*, 1–6.
55. Ullmann, A.J.; Lipton, J.H.; Vesole, D.H.; Chandrasekar, P.; Langston, A.; Tarantolo, S.R.; Greinix, H.; Morais de Azevedo, W.; Reddy, V.; Boparai, N.; *et al.* Posaconazole or fluconazole for prophylaxis in severe graft-*versus*-host disease. *N. Engl. J. Med.* **2007**, *356*, 335–347.
56. Winston, D.J.; Bartoni, K.; Territo, M.C.; Schiller, G.J. Efficacy, safety, and breakthrough infections associated with standard long-term posaconazole antifungal prophylaxis in allogeneic stem cell transplantation recipients. *Biol. Blood Marrow Transplant.* **2011**, *17*, 507–515.
57. Raad, I.I.; Hachem, R.Y.; Herbrecht, R.; Graybill, J.R.; Hare, R.; Corcoran, G.; Kontoyiannis, D.P. Posaconazole as salvage treatment for invasive fusariosis in patients with underlying hematologic malignancy and other conditions. *Clin. Infect. Dis.* **2006**, *42*, 1398–1403.

58. Sponsel, W.E.; Graybill, J.R.; Nevarez, H.L.; Dang, D. Ocular and systemic posaconazole (SCH-56592) treatment of invasive *fusarium* solani keratitis and endophthalmitis. *Br. J. Ophthalmol.* **2002**, *86*, 829–830.
59. Lozano-Chiu, M.; Arikan, S.; Paetznick, V.L.; Anaissie, E.J.; Loebenberg, D.; Rex, J.H. Treatment of murine fusariosis with SCH 56592. *Antimicrob. Agents Chemother.* **1999**, *43*, 589–591.
60. Vazquez, J.A.; Skiest, D.J.; Nieto, L.; Northland, R.; Sanne, I.; Gogate, J.; Greaves, W.; Isaacs, R. A multicenter randomized trial evaluating posaconazole *versus* fluconazole for the treatment of oropharyngeal candidiasis in subjects with HIV/AIDS. *Clin. Infect. Dis.* **2006**, *42*, 1179–1186.
61. Heinz, W.J.; Egerer, G.; Lellek, H.; Boehme, A.; Greiner, J. Posaconazole after previous antifungal therapy with voriconazole for therapy of invasive aspergillus disease, a retrospective analysis. *Mycoses* **2013**, *56*, 304–310.
62. Cornely OA1, Helfgott, D.; Langston, A.; Heinz, W.; Vehreschild, J.J.; Vehreschild, M.J.; Krishna, G.; Ma, L.; Huyck, S.; McCarthy, M.C. Pharmacokinetics of different dosing strategies of oral posaconazole in patients with compromised gastrointestinal function and who are at high risk for invasive fungal infection. *Antimicrob. Agents Chemother.* **2012**, *56*, 2652–2658.
63. Krishna, G.; Sansone-Parsons, A.; Martinho, M; Kantesaria, B; Pedicone, L. Posaconazole plasma concentrations in juvenile patients with invasive fungal infection. *Antimicrob Agents Chemother* **2007**, *51*, 812–818.
64. Ghannoum, M.A.; Rice, L.B. Antifungal agents: Mode of action, mechanism of resistance and correlation of these mechanisms with bacterial resistance. *Clin. Microbiol. Rev.* **1999**, *12*, 501–517.
65. Sanglard, D.; Ischer, F.; Koymans, L.; Bille, J. Amino acid substitutions in the cytochrome P-450 lanosterol 14α-demethylase (CYP51A1) from azole-resistant Candida albicans clinical isolates contribute to resistance to azole antifungal agents. *Antimicrob. Agents Chemother.* **1998**, *42*, 241–253.
66. Sansone-Parsons, A.; Krishna, G.; Martinho, M.; Kantesaria, B.; Gelone, S.; Mant, T.G. Effect of oral posaconazole on the pharmacokinetics of cyclosporine and tacrolimus. Pharmacotherapy. **2007**, *27*, 825–834.
67. Courtney, R.; Radwanski, E.; Lim, J.; Laughlin, M. Pharmacokinetics of posaconazole coadministered with antacid in fasting or nonfasting healthy men. *Antimicrob. Agents Chemother.* **2004**, *48*, 804–808.
68. Cojutti, P.; Candoni, A.; Simeone, E.; Franceschi, L.; Fanin, R.; Pea, F. Antifungal prophylaxis with posaconazole in patients with acute myeloid leukemia: Dose intensification coupled with avoidance of proton pump inhibitors is beneficial in shortening time to effective concentrations. *Antimicrob. Agents Chemother.* **2013**, *57*, 6081–6084.
69. Wexler, D.; Courtney, R.; Richards, W.; Banfield, C.; Lim, J.; Laughlin, M. Effect of posaconazole on cytochrome P450 enzymes: A randomized open-label, two-way crossover study. *Eur. J. Pharm. Sci.* **2004**, *21*, 645–653.
70. Leung, S.; Poulakos, M. Drug interaction profile of posaconazole. *Internet J. Allied Health Sci. Pract.* **2008**, *8*, 1–8.
71. Vaes, M.; Hites, M.; Cotton, F. Therapeutic drug monitoring of posaconazole in patients with acute myeloid leukemia or myelodysplastic syndrome. *Antimicrob. Agents Chemother.* **2012**, *56*, 6298–6303.
72. Krishna, G.; Persons, A.; Kantesaria, B.; Mant, T. Evaluation of the pharmacokinetics of posaconazole and rifabutin following co-administration to healthy men. *Curr. Med. Res. Opin.* **2007**, *23*, 545–552.

73. Courtney, R.D.; Statkevich, P.; Laughlin, M.; Pai, S.; Lim, J.; Clement, R.P.; Batra, V.K. Potential for a drug interaction between posaconazole and phenytoin. In Proceedings of the 41st Interscience Conference on Antimicrobial Agents Chemotherapy, Chicago, IL, USA, 16–19 December 2001; Volume 4, p. 22.
74. Courtney, R.; Wexler, D.; Statkevich, P.; Lim, J.; Batra, V.; Laughlin, M. Effect of cimetidine on the pharmacokinetics of posaconazole in healthy volunteers. In Proceedings of the 42nd Interscience Conference on Antimicrobial Agents Chemotherapy, San Diego, CA, USA, 27–30 September 2002; pp. 24–30.
75. Courtney, R.; Sansone, A.; Statkevich, P.; Martinho, M.; Laughlin, M. Assessment of the Pharmacokinetic (PK), Pharmacodynamic (PD) interaction between posaconazole and glipizide in healthy volunteers. *Clin. Pharmacol. Ther.* **2003**, *73*, 45.
76. Krishna, G.; Vickery, D.; Ma, L.; Yu, X.; Noren, C.; Power, E.; Beresford, E.; Medlock, M. Lack of pharmacokinetic drug interaction between oral posaconazole and caspofungin or micafungin. *J. Clin. Pharmacol.* **2011**, *51*, 84–92.
77. Krishna, G.; Ma, L.; Prasad, P.; Moton, A.; Martinho, M.; O'Mara, E. Effect of posaconazole on the pharmacokinetics of simvastatin and midazolam in healthy volunteers. *Expert Opin. Drug Metab. Toxicol.* **2012**, *8*, 1–10.
78. Heinz, W.J.; Grau, A.; Ulrich, A.; Helle-Beyersdorf, A.; Zirkel, J.; Schirmer, D.; Lenker, U.; Einsele, H.; Klinker, H. Impact of benzodiazepines on posaconazole serum concentrations. A population-based pharmacokinetic study on drug interaction. *Curr. Med. Res. Opin.* **2012**, *28*, 551–557.
79. Poulakos, M.; Henneman, A.; Leung, S. Posaconazole: A Review of Drug Interactions with HIV Antiretroviral Agents. *Pharmacy* **2014**, *2*, 98–113.
80. Skiest, D.J; Vazquez, J.A.;Anstead, G.M.; Graybill, J.R.; Reynes, J.; Ward, D.; Hare, R.; Boparai, N.; Isaacs, R. Posaconazole for the treatment of azole-refractory oropharyngeal and esophageal candidiasis in subjects with HIV infection. *Clin Infect Dis.* **2007**, 15,607-614.
81. Vazquez, J.A.; Skiest, D.J.; Tissot-Dupont, H.; Lennox, J.L.; Boparai, N, Isaacs, R. Safety and efficacy of posaconazole in the long-term treatment of azole-refractory oropharyngeal and esophageal candidiasis in subjects with HIV infection. *HIV Clin. Trials* **2007**, *8*, 86–97.
82. American Academy of Pediatrics. *Red Book*; Thomson Healthcare, Inc.: Montvale, NJ, USA, 2007.
83. Duarte, R.; Lopez, J.; Cornely, O.; Ma, L.; van Iersel, M.; Waskin, H. Phase 1b study of the pharmacokinetics and safety of posaconazole solid oral tablet in patients at risk for invasive fungal infection. In Proceedings of the 52nd Intersceince Conference on Antimicrobial Agents and Chemotherapy (ICAAC), San Francisco, CA, USA, 9–12 September 2012.
84. Cornely, O.; Duarte, R.; Haider, S.; Chandrasekar, P.; Helfgott, D.; Lopez, J.; van Iersel, M.; Connelly, N.; Waskin, H. Phase 3 pharmacokinetics and safety study of posaconazole tablet in patients at risk for invasive fungal infection. In Proceedings of the 23rd European Congress of Clinical Microbiology and Infectious Diseases (ECCMID), Berlin, Germany, 27–30 April 2013.
85. Maertens, J.; Cornely, O.; Ullmann, A.; Heinz, W.J.; Krishna, G.; Patino, H.; Caceres, M.; Kartsonis, N.; Waskin, H.; Robertson, M.N. Pharmacokinetics and safety of posaconazole IV in patients at risk for invasive fungal infection: A phase 1B study. *Antimicrob. Agents Chemother.* **2014**, *58*, 3610–3617.

86. Cornely, O.; Haider, S.; Grigg, A.; van Iersel, M.; Caceres, M.; Hepler, D.; Waskin, H.; Kartsonis, N.; Robertson, M. Phase 3 Pharmacokinetics (PK) and safety study of posaconazole (POS) IV in patients (Pts) at risk for invasive fungal infection (IFI). In Proceedings of the 52nd Intersceince Conference on Antimicrobial Agents and Chemotherapy (ICAAC), Denver, CO, USA, 10–13 September 2013.
87. Walsh, T.J.; Anaissie, E.J.; Denning, D.W.; Herbrecht, R.; Kontoyiannis, D.P.; Marr, K.A.; Morrison, V.A.; Segal, B.H.; Steinbach, W.J.; Stevens, D.A.; *et al.* Treatment ofaspergillosis: clinical practice guidelines of the Infectious Diseases Society of America. *Clin. Infect. Dis.* **2008**, *46*, 327–360.
88. Pappas, P.G.; Kauffman, C,A.; Andes, D.; Benjamin, D.K.; Calandra, T.F.; Edwards, J.E.; Filler, S.G.; Fisher, J.F.; Kullberg, B.; Ostrosky-Zeichner, L.O.; *et al.* Clinical practice guidelines for management of candidiasis. 2009 update by the Infectious Diseases Society of America. *Clin. Infect. Dis.* **2009**, *49*, 1–45.
89. Perfect, J.R.; Dismukes, W.E.; Dromer, F.; Goldman, D.L.; Graybill, J.R.; Hamill, R.J.; Harrison, T.S.; Larsen, R.A.; Lortholary, O.; Nguyen, M.H.; *et al.* Clinical practice guidelines for the management of cryptococcal disease: 2010 update by the Infectious Diseases Society of America. *Clin. Infect. Dis.* **2010**, *50*, 291–322.
90. Kraft, W.K.; Chang, P.S.; van Iersel, M.L.; Waskin, H.; Krishna, G.; Kersemaekers, W.M. Posaconazole tablet pharmacokinetics: Lack of effect of concomitant medications altering gastric pH and gastric motility in healthy subjects. *Antimicrob. Agents Chemother.* **2014**, *58*, 4020–4025.
91. Percival, K.M.; Bergman, S.J. Update on posaconazole pharmacokinetics: Comparison of old and new formulations. *Curr. Fungal Infect. Rep.* **2014**, *8*, 139–145.
92. McKeage, K. Posaconazole: A review of the gastro-resistant tablet and intravenous solution in invasive fungal infections. *Drugs* **2015**, *75*, 397–406.

8

Analysis of Medications Returned During a Medication Take-Back Event

Christina H.J. Yang [1,*], Mitesh Doshi [2,†] and Nancy A. Mason [3,†]

[1] Nash Drugs, Inc., Hillsdale, MI 49242, USA

[2] Beaumont Health System, Royal Oak, MI 48073, USA; E-Mail: Mitesh.Doshi@beaumont.edu

[3] University of Michigan College of Pharmacy, 428 Church Street, Ann Arbor, MI 48109, USA; E-Mail: nmason@med.umich.edu

† These authors contributed equally to this work.

* Author to whom correspondence should be addressed; E-Mail: hyyang@umich.edu

Academic Editor: Maree Donna Simpson

Abstract: A medication take-back event was held in Lansing, MI, USA, for four hours in September 2013. The objective was to quantify medication waste by determining the ratio of medication units remaining *versus* dispensed and to identify therapeutic classes with greater ratios of remaining medication units. Drug name, strength, quantity remaining, quantity dispensed, dispensary source, and brand or generic were recorded from the label of each medication container returned. Out of the over 3600 medication containers collected, this study analyzed 2459 containers, which included 304 controlled substances. On average, 66 percent of the medications dispensed in these containers were unused, and therefore wasted. Immunologic medications had the lowest quantity of waste at 54%, while geriatrics/miscellaneous therapeutic class yielded the highest quantity of waste at 79%. The most common therapeutic classes collected were pain/spasm, cardiovascular, and mental health. Greater emphasis on patient education regarding medication adherence and health care professionals' judicious prescribing habits is warranted to reduce the frequency of unused medications. The increased accessibility to medication return sites may alleviate the prevalence of medication accumulation, environmental damage, and medication misuse.

Keywords: adherence; medication safety; unused medication; medication take-back; medication disposal

1. Introduction

Unused medications may accumulate in home medicine cabinets due to a variety of reasons including overprescribing, elimination of need for the medication, noncompliance to the regimen, or medication expiration. People with access to medicine cabinets can divert medications for use by someone other than the patient or use the medications for unintended purposes. Medications may also be disposed into the trash, toilet or sink, risking the safety of others and damaging the environment. Even when there is no intention for mishandling, patients may retain medications due to the high cost of the medication, lack of disposal method, or the possibility of needing these medications again in the future.

Accessible storage of these medications poses a particular threat to children and elders, who may not understand the dangers of medications and may inadvertently ingest these medications, with consequences ranging from stomachache to death. In 2011, more than 68,000 children in the US suffered from medication poisoning and were seen in emergency departments, with 86% of these cases involving children ingesting adult medicine [1]. The most common places children found medications included on the ground, in purses or bags, on counters or nightstands, in pillboxes, and in cabinets or drawers [1]. Out of the more than two million calls made annually to poison control centers regarding unintentional child poisonings, nine out of 10 involve poisonings at home [2].

More common than accidental ingestion is the misuse of medications by young adults and adolescents with 21.7% and 13.0% of 12th graders in the US admitting to medical misuse of prescription medications and narcotics, respectively, as surveyed by the National Institute of Drug Abuse in 2014 [3]. Nationally, 4.5 million people over the age of 11 reported being current nonmedical users of prescription pain relievers, tranquilizers, stimulants, and sedatives based on the 2013 National Survey on Drug Use and Health [4]. Fifty-three percent of these nonmedical users stated they received analgesics for free from a friend or relative [4]. The reported 6.5 million Americans abusing prescription drugs in 2013 is more than double the number of those who have admitted to using heroin, cocaine, and hallucinogens combined [4]. With this high prevalence of medication being used for unintended persons or purposes, it can be deduced that, for many patients, the quantity of medications prescribed must far exceed the quantity needed for intended treatment.

The public media and scientific community have also highlighted the environmental impact of disposed medications. Flushing medications down the toilet or sink, disposal in household trash, and normal human and animal excretions containing pharmaceutical ingredients can all lead to medications being released into the environment [5]. On a list of more than 100 active ingredients found in the environment, amoxicillin, acetaminophen, and metoprolol stand at the top [6]. Unfortunately, some of these drugs that have seeped into the sewage system have failed to be eliminated through conventional sewage treatment, rendering the public and the environment more susceptible to contaminated water and antibiotic resistance [6,7]. Studies examining the effects of medication-contaminated drinking water have not yet produced reliable results. Additionally, there is a lack of information regarding biodegradation of these chemicals in soil environments, further providing concern for public and environmental safety.

To help relieve these concerns, the Drug Enforcement Administration (DEA) sponsored a National Prescription Drug Take-Back Day biannually where the public can bring their unused medications to designated sites. This program collected 309 tons of unwanted medications at 5495 locations during the most recent Drug Take-Back Day in September 2014, with each year's collections reported greater than the previous year's [8]. While this event cleared out medicine cabinets of many patients across the country, the increasing utilization of these types of events shows that there are still homes with unused or expired medications and an ongoing accumulation through new prescriptions. In response to the Secure and Responsible Drug Disposal Act, enacted by Congress in 2010, the DEA implemented new disposal regulations that allow retail pharmacies to register to become authorized collectors of controlled medications, replacing the biannual take-back events [8].

Because of the growing concern of accumulating unused medications, this study was initiated with the purpose to assess the quantity of medications gathering in homes by determining the ratio of medication units remaining *versus* dispensed, and to identify the therapeutic classes with greater ratios of remaining medication units.

2. Methods

A medication take-back event, held for four hours on 10 September 2013, was the site for data collection. The event was part of the Michigan Pharmacists Association's (MPA) annual Pharmacy Day at the Capitol. Event volunteers consisted of student pharmacists and faculty of Ferris State University, Wayne State University, and the University of Michigan attending Pharmacy Day at the Capitol, as well as MPA staff. Because this operation included controlled medications, local police officers supervised all aspects of the event from medication collection to disposal and incineration.

All members of the public were welcome to drop-off their unused medications. These medications were then counted and the following information was recorded and transcribed onto Microsoft Excel spreadsheets: drug name, strength, amount remaining, amount prescribed, generic or brand, and source (local pharmacy, mail-order pharmacy, or sample). Collected medications were transported from the site for incineration upon the conclusion of the event.

In addition to collecting medications, event volunteers asked all donors to complete an optional nine-question anonymous web-based survey (Appendix) within the following week to further gather information about their medication disposal habits. The survey was not administered on-site to allow for donors to quickly donate their medications and to minimize the wait time to do so.

Statistical analysis was completed only for prescription medications in tablet or capsule formulations. Medications were categorized into the following therapeutic classes: allergy (antihistamines), cardiovascular, dietary (related to electrolyte or vitamin imbalances), endocrine (e.g., diabetes, hypothyroidism, reproductive hormone replacement), gastrointestinal, immunologic (e.g., cancer, rheumatoid arthritis, immunosuppression), infectious disease, mental health (e.g., depression, bipolar disorder, schizophrenia, anxiety, attention deficit disorder, insomnia, seizure disorder), nausea, pain/spasm, respiratory, and geriatric/miscellaneous (e.g., urinary incontinence, osteoporosis, dementia, Parkinson's disease, benign prostatic hyperplasia, erectile dysfunction). Exclusion criteria included medications never available in the US, pet medications, medications in containers without a legible label, and containers with remaining medication amounts larger than the amount dispensed as this may have been the result of patients combining medications into the same container. Medications not in tablet or capsule formulations were also excluded as limited package sizes may intend for patients to have more than needed. For example, amoxicillin suspension is manufactured in 100 and 150 mL formulations, but a patient may require only 120 mL of the 150 mL formulation to complete therapy.

Medications analyzed in this study were grouped by therapeutic classes except the grouping called geriatric/miscellaneous. Medications were quantified by the average ratio of the quantity of units remaining out of the quantity dispensed. The averages were compared using a one-way analysis of variance (ANOVA), and a two-sample unpaired Student's *t*-test with Bonferonni adjustment evaluated the statistical difference between the averages of each therapeutic class to each other. A *p*-value less than 0.05 was considered statistically significant. To avoid confusion, the term "container" will be used to describe the box, bottle, or other packaging the medications were enclosed in.

3. Results

The event gathered 3633 containers of medications, including over-the-counter, prescription, and pet medications. Out of 2,830,094 units (tablets or capsules) originally dispensed in these containers, 1,824,854 units of medications were collected. The top 15 most commonly returned out of the 348 different prescription drugs collected are listed in Table 1. The majority of the medications were generic products, composing 69.0% of all medications collected. Most were obtained at local pharmacies (89.4%), compared to mail order (5.7%), or samples from physician offices (4.8%).

Table 1. Quantities of most commonly returned medications.

	Medication	Quantity of Containers	Percentage of All Containers Returned
1	Acetaminophen/hydrocodone	110	4.4
2	Ibuprofen	73	2.9
3	Tramadol	44	1.8
4	Acetaminophen/codeine	42	1.7
5	Naproxen	42	1.7
6	Prednisone	41	1.7
7	Amoxicillin	37	1.5
8	Omeprazole	37	1.5
9	Levothyroxine	35	1.4
10	Aspirin	32	1.3
11	Acetaminophen/propoxyphene	27	1.1
12	Cyclobenzaprine	27	1.1
13	Cephalexin	26	1.1
14	Lisinopril	26	1.1
15	Warfarin	26	1.1

For this study 2459 containers were analyzed, with 304 of them holding controlled medications (excluding tramadol as it was not a controlled substance in the state of Michigan at the time of the event).

Figure 1 displays the quantity of containers collected at the event and the respective average ratio of remaining units of medications per container, grouped by therapeutic drug class. The pain/spasm therapeutic class accounted for the largest number of containers collected with 615 containers, followed by 431 containers of cardiovascular medications, and 341 containers of mental health medications.

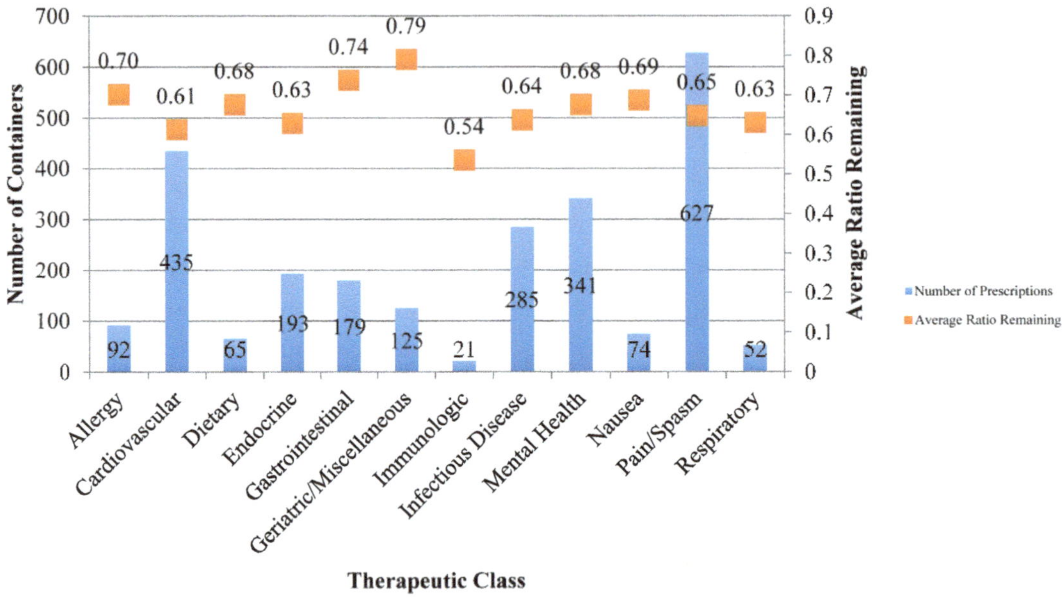

Figure 1. Quantities of containers collected and average ratios remaining categorized by therapeutic class.

The overall ratio of remaining medication units to units dispensed was 0.66 for all medications included in this study. A one-way ANOVA was calculated on the average ratios, grouped by therapeutic class. The analysis revealed a significant difference among the therapeutic groups' ratios of remaining units, $F(11, 2447) = 3.37$, $p < 0.001$. The average ratio remaining for each therapeutic drug class was compared to that of the other therapeutic classes utilizing Student's *t*-tests with Bonferonni adjustment. Six pairs showed a significant difference, five of which included the geriatric/miscellaneous therapeutic class: geriatric/miscellaneous > cardiovascular ($p < 0.001$), geriatric/miscellaneous > endocrine ($p < 0.001$), geriatric/miscellaneous > infectious diseases ($p < 0.001$), geriatric/miscellaneous > mental health ($p = 0.027$), geriatric/miscellaneous > pain ($p < 0.001$), and gastrointestinal > cardiovascular ($p = 0.001$).

Seventy participants responded to the online survey. Fifty of the seventy respondents were female, and nearly 60% were adults above the age of 50. Over 75% of respondents reported returning a family member's medication(s), and 67% reported returning their own. Medication expiration was the most common reason for medication disposal at the event, while discontinuation of the medications due to side effects or lack of necessity without professional recommendation were the least common reasons (Figure 2). Nearly 59% of respondents cited drug take-back events as their usual method for disposing unused medications, while over 25% stated they disposed of them in the garbage and 14% flushed medications down the toilet or sink.

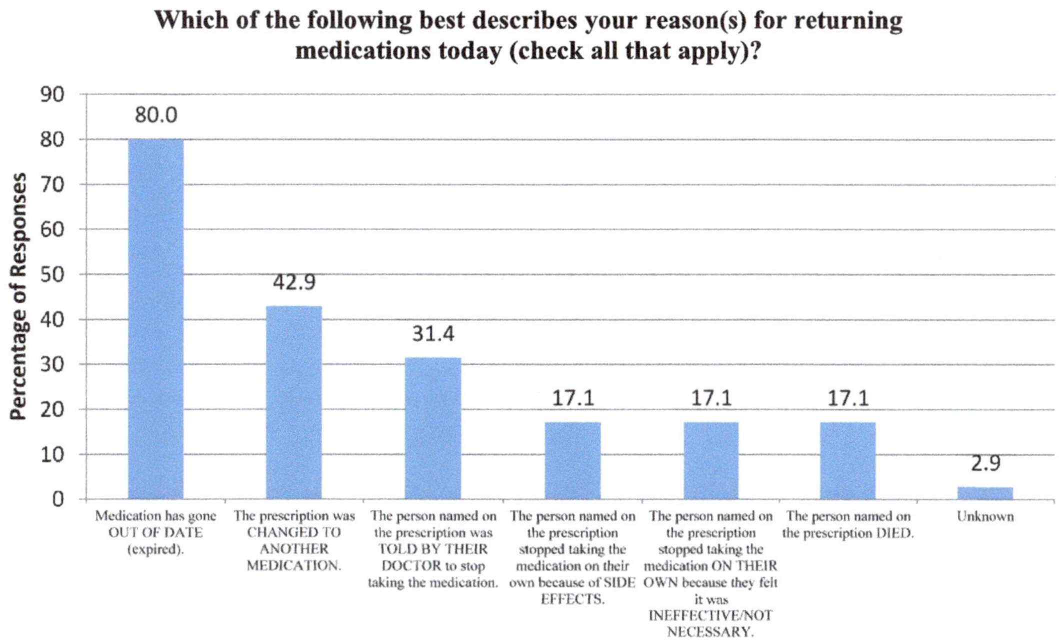

Figure 2. Participant Survey Question.

4. Discussion

While this event gathered 345 different prescription medications, the top five most common were pain relievers. The pain/spasm therapeutic class had the greatest number of containers collected, with more than a quarter of all containers analyzed falling into this category. Likewise, similar medication take-back events in rural Appalachia and Findlay, Ohio gathered high rates of pain medications, with hydrocodone-, propoxyphene-, and codeine-containing medications being three of the most common medications collected [9,10]. A survey of Cook County, Illinois, residents by researchers at the University of Illinois revealed the first and the fifth most common type of medication in homes were over-the-counter pain (82.5% of respondents) and prescription pain (39.2%) medications, respectively [11]. The similarity of these studies justifies the widespread concern that patients are accumulating analgesics in the home, which provides opportunity for abuse, diversion, and accidental ingestion.

The high rate of having unused pain relievers in the home not only raises the concern of potential misuse, but the concern that pain relievers may be overprescribed. Thirty-seven percent of the Cook County survey participants stated they had leftover unexpired medications from a previous illness [11]. The most common reasons for this were that they felt better or the directions stated take as needed and the drug was no longer necessary. As patients prescribed analgesics for short-term use are directed to take as needed, a portion of the quantity returned during the event was due to prescribing a greater amount of analgesics than the patients found necessary.

Across all therapeutic categories, the proportion of remaining medications was fairly consistent, with nine of the 12 categories falling between the range of 60% to 70%. This narrow range also yields great concern related to patient nonadherence. The data show remaining proportions are similar despite differences in acute or chronic use, such as between medications for nausea (0.69) *vs.* endocrine disorders (0.63).

While the medications included in the geriatric/miscellaneous class are not exclusive to the elderly population, this class interestingly had a relatively high ratio of remaining medications and was included in five of the six comparison groups that noted a statistically significant difference in average ratios. The high use of these medications by the elderly population may be the result of having greater time to accumulate unused medications, potentially due to dose adjustments or therapy modifications, or to caretakers or family members disposing of medications after the patient's death.

Eighty percent of survey respondents cited medication expiry as a reason for disposing medications. This high number may be because the survey allowed for donors to indicate multiple reasons. For example, a patient may have selected two answers if he was told to discontinue a medication by his physician and kept it at home for several years before disposing of it at this event. The fact that the majority of respondents cited drug take-back events as their usual method for medication disposal is alarming because these events are only offered to local residents a few days of the year, if any, for some areas of the country. As medication accumulation is ongoing, the DEA's intention of allowing pharmacies to register to take back controlled and noncontrolled medications would allow avenues for greater access to environmentally safe medication disposal.

There were several limitations in this study. Numerous reasons aside from non-adherence and overprescribing contribute to medications being unused. Patient allergies or intolerances, ineffective therapeutic effect, or diagnosis changes may have restricted patients from taking the full amount of medication dispensed. Data gathered during a medication take-back day are only reflective of a small percentage of the population in Lansing, MI and the surrounding areas who willingly disposed of their unused medications. The participants were primarily older adults, which is expected as this demographic tends to have more diseases and disorders for which medications are needed. The total number of participants was not recorded due to the operational logistics of this medication take-back event, but the number of survey respondents reflects a small percentage of this total.

5. Conclusion

Among all medications collected at the medication take-back event, approximately two-thirds of the quantity dispensed was remaining. Only 17% of survey respondents admit to discontinuing use on their own accord as they felt the medication was unnecessary, while the most common reason for donating medications to the event was medication expiration.

Currently, there are limited works published regarding what medications are collected at take-back events. Our study broadly matches the data gathered by groups in Findlay, Ohio, and rural Appalachia, with the high quantities of analgesics and cardiovascular agents collected during the event [9,10]. However, more studies are needed to further assess the incidence of drug accumulation and patients' reasons for disposal.

The popularity of medication take-back events has primarily focused on disposing of unused medications rather than addressing the sources of this accumulation, namely overprescribing and the patient's failure to complete full courses of therapy. While health care professionals should continue to stress the importance of patient adherence, prescribers can help reduce medication accumulation by prescribing more conservative quantities for medications. Local pharmacies can also aid in reducing accumulation by registering as authorized medication return sites with the DEA, which would offer patients an environmentally friendly method of medication disposal nearly every day of the year.

Author Contributions

Christina H.J. Yang, Mitesh Doshi, and Nancy A. Mason were all involved in the planning and development of the project, collection, analysis of data and writing of the manuscript.

Conflicts of Interest

The authors declare no conflicts of interest.

Appendix. Medication Donor Survey.

Q1. Which of the following best describes your age?

- ☐ Less than 20
- ☐ 21 to 30
- ☐ 31 to 40
- ☐ 41 to 50
- ☐ 51 to 60
- ☐ 61 to 70
- ☐ 71 or greater

Q2. Gender?

- ☐ Male
- ☐ Female

Q3. Are you an employee of the state, city, or local government?

- ☐ Yes
- ☐ No

Q4. The medications you returned today were prescribed for (you may check all that apply):

- ☐ You
- ☐ A Family member
- ☐ Friend(s) or acquaintance(s)
- ☐ Other (please specify) ______________________________

Q5. Which of the following best describes your reason(s) for returning medications today (check all that apply)?

- ☐ Medication has gone out of date (expired).
- ☐ The prescription was changed to another medication.
- ☐ The person named on the prescription stopped taking the medication on their own because of side effects.
- ☐ The person named on the prescription stopped taking the medication on their own because they felt it was ineffective/not necessary.
- ☐ The person named on the prescription was told by their doctor to stop taking the medication.
- ☐ The person named on the prescription died.
- ☐ Unknown
- ☐ Other (please specify) ______________________________

Q6. Where do you usually get your prescription medication filled?

- ▯ A local pharmacy (chain, supermarket, independent, etc.)
- ▯ I choose to get my prescription(s) filled by a mail order pharmacy (Medco, Caremark, Express Scripts, etc.)
- ▯ I am forced to get my prescription(s) filled by a mail order pharmacy (Medco, Caremark, Express Scripts, etc.)
- ▯ Doctor's office samples
- ▯ Other (please specify) ______________________

Q7. How do you normally dispose of your unused medications?

- ▯ Garbage
- ▯ Flush down toilet/sink
- ▯ Take to a pharmacy
- ▯ Drug take-back program (such as this program)
- ▯ Other (please specify) ______________________

Q8. Which of the following best describes the prescription insurance used to obtain the medication being returned? (Prescription insurance refers to the insurance plan that pays for part or all of your prescription drugs with or without copays.)

- ▯ Medicare Part D plan
- ▯ Medicaid insurance plan
- ▯ TRICARE or VA Health System
- ▯ Employer-based prescription insurance
- ▯ There was no prescription drug insurance in place
- ▯ Unknown
- ▯ Other (please specify) ______________________

Q9. Describe in percentages how many of your medications are prescribed by each of the following types of providers (Response options: 0, 25, 50, 75, 100 %):

_____% Primary care physician
_____% Specialist
_____% Nurse practitioner/physician's assistant
_____% Other health care professional (dentist, optometrist, etc.)

References

1. Ferguson, R.W.; Mickalide, A.D. An In-Depth Look at Keeping Young Children Safe Around Medicine. Available online: http://www.safekids.org/medsreport (accessed on 5 March 2015).
2. Consumer Product Safety Commission. CPSC warns that 9 out of 10 unintentional child poisonings occur in the home. News from CPSC, 18 March 2009. Available online: http://www.cpsc.gov/cpscpub/prerel/prhtml09/09159.html (accessed on 5 March 2015).
3. National Institutes of Health. Monitoring the future. January 2015. Available online: http://www.drugabuse.gov/related-topics/trends-statistics/monitoring-future (accessed on 7 March 2015).
4. Substance Abuse and Mental Health Services Administration. *Results from the 2013 National Survey on Drug Use and Health: Summary of National Findings*; NSDUH Series H-48; HHS Publication No. (SMA) 14-4863; Substance Abuse and Mental Health Services Administration: Rockville, MD, USA, 2014.

5. Wu, M.; Atchley, D.; Greer, L.; Janssen, S.; Rosenberg, D.; Sass, J. Dosed without prescription: Preventing pharmaceutical contamination of our nation's drinking water. December 2009. Available online: http://docs.nrdc.org/health/files/hea_10012001a.pdf (accessed on 10 July 2015).
6. Monteiro, S.C.; Boxall, A.B. Occurrence and fate of human pharmaceuticals in the environment. *Rev. Environ. Contam. Toxicol.* **2010**, *202*, 53–154.
7. Thach, A.V.; Brown, C.M.; Pope, N. Consumer perceptions about a community pharmacy-based medication take back program. *J. Environ. Manag.* **2013**, *127*, 23–27.
8. Drug Enforcement Administration. DEA and partners collect 309 tons of pills on ninth prescription drug take-back day. 5 November 2014. Available online: http://www.dea.gov/divisions/hq/2014/hq110514.shtml (accessed on 29 December 2014).
9. Gray, J.A.; Hagemeier, N.E. Prescription drug abuse and DEA-sanctioned drug take-back events: Characteristics and outcomes in rural Appalachia. *Arch. Intern. Med.* **2012**, *172*, 1186–1187.
10. Perry, L.A.; Shinn, B.W.; Stanovich, J. Quantification of ongoing community-based medication take-back program. *J. Am. Pharm. Assoc.* **2014**, *54*, 275–279.
11. Wieczorkiewicz, S.M.; Kassamali, Z.; Danziger, L.H. Behind closed doors: Medication storage and disposal in the home. *Ann. Pharmacother.* **2013**, *47*, 482–489.

9

Education Intervention on Chronotherapy for Final-Year Pharmacy Students

Gagandeep Kaur [1,*], Maya Saba [1], Craig L. Phillips [2], Keith Wong [2] and Bandana Saini [1]

1 Faculty of Pharmacy, The University of Sydney, Camperdown, NSW 2006, Australia; E-Mails: maya.saba@sydney.edu.au (M.S.); bandana.saini@sydney.edu.au (B.S.)

2 Woolcock Institute of Medical Research, Glebe, NSW 2037, Australia; E-Mails: craig.phillips@sydney.edu.au (C.P.); keith.wong@sydney.edu.au (K.W.)

* Author to whom correspondence should be addressed; E-Mail: gaga8947@uni.sydney.edu.au

Academic Editor: Janine M. Traulsen

Abstract: Chronotherapy involves altering the timing of medication administration in coordination with the body's circadian rhythms to improve the overall control of disease and to minimise treatment side effects. Training on chronotherapy requires students to map different topics learnt in earlier years of their professional degree and apply these concepts clinically. This requires strategic educational design. Therefore, the aim of the study was to develop, implement and evaluate an educational intervention focusing on the application of chronotherapy for final-year undergraduate pharmacy students. An educational intervention utilizing multiple learning strategies for enhancing chronotherapy related awareness was designed and implemented in the final year undergraduate pharmacy cohort at the University of Sydney Australia (2013). A custom-designed questionnaire measuring awareness about (13 items scored 0 or 1), and attitudes (12 items scored on a Likert scale of 1–5) towards chronotherapy was administered pre and post intervention to evaluate its impact. The pre-intervention mean total awareness and attitude scores were 6.5 ± 2.0 (score range 0–13) and 47.4 ± 6.9 (score range 12–60) respectively. The mean total post-intervention scores were significantly higher for total awareness (10.1 ± 1.9) and attitude (54.0 ± 6.0). Carefully designed educational interventions utilising pedagogic principles for pharmacy students can improve awareness of and enhance positive attitudes toward pharmacists' roles in optimizing drug therapy using chronotherapy.

Keywords: chronotherapy; circadian rhythms; intervention; pharmacy students; work shop; education

1. Introduction

Clinical knowledge about biological rhythms, the importance of the sleep-wake routine, and the effect of circadian timing on medicine administration is significant for the management of particular disease conditions and for potentiating the therapeutic effects and/or reducing the adverse effects of certain medications. Broadly referred to as chronotherapy, the administration of medications at optimal circadian times represents a multifaceted concept that exploits diverse mechanisms and principles such as formulation science, pharmacology, physiology, and pathophysiology [1,2]. Though not applicable in all cases, chronotherapy may be of significance in disease conditions that exhibit circadian variability such as asthma, gastroesophageal reflux, cardiovascular diseases, cancer, metabolic diseases, rheumatoid arthritis and sleep disorders [3–6]. Further, evidence from the various clinical effectiveness and drug disposition studies demonstrates improved outcomes when the administration of certain medications is timed in synchrony with circadian patterns [4,7,8]. A prime example is that of the statins, where short-acting statins are more effective when administered at night time, the circadian point when cholesterol synthesis is at its peak and HMG-CoA reductase enzyme exhibits maximal activity [9].

With recent advances in sleep and circadian medicine, awareness of chronotherapeutic principles has been growing, and clinicians have started to incorporate this research evidence into clinical practice [10]. As primary health professionals, community pharmacists can undoubtedly play a significant role in this area. This is particularly pertinent since community pharmacists often represent the last point of contact with patients prior to medication administration. Similarly, in hospital settings, pharmacists utilize their broad therapeutic expertise to optimize patient medication regimens [11]. Given that pharmacists are among the most accessible healthcare professionals who can provide medication and health-related advice without the need for appointment or consulting fees, patients are highly likely to seek pharmacists' advice on various health-related matters, including queries about the most appropriate time for administering a particular medication [12].

Although it may be one of several niche concepts in the pharmacists' armament, chronotherapy represents a novel way of optimizing the patient experience of medications and delivering individualized care. In Australia, the Pharmacy Guild, a national body representing community pharmacies, highlighted the importance of timing of drug administration to support patient adherence to their prescribed treatment over time [13,14]. The Accreditation Standards for Pharmacy Programs in Australia and New Zealand require pharmacy degree programs to establish a curriculum that equips students with the knowledge and skills to ensure the safe and effective use of medicines in consumers. [15]. Therefore, it is important that students, as future pharmacists are equipped with up-to-date knowledge about recent research in various clinical areas related to medication use including, for example, chronotherapy. As future pharmacists, they need to be well-positioned to educate their patients about the optimal timing of medication administration, chronotherapeutic technologies, and circadian and pathophysiological advantages of chronotherapy.

Although the fields of chronobiology and sleep and circadian rhythms have been around since the 1950s [16], until recently in clinical pharmacy circles it was believed that evidence for this concept was in equipoise. This concept was thus not usually covered in depth in clinical pharmacy courses [17], except at a very practical level [18]. Most pharmacists and pharmacy students may be aware, for example, that medications that interfere with sleep should be taken earlier in the daytime, *i.e.*, a single-dose diuretic might be better taken in the morning rather than at night. However, a deeper understanding of the concepts underpinning chronotherapy and exposure to newly emerging data is not included in most undergraduate pharmacy programs. This may be linked to the novelty of the sleep and circadian medicine field itself, which is only now being introduced in nursing and medical education in a meaningful manner [19,20].

Given recent evidence, supporting chronotherapy, education and training to improve pharmacy professionals' understanding of this concept is essential. Since chronotherapy represents an advanced clinical concept requiring learners to cross-link and apply their previous basic understanding of several underlying concepts in pharmacology, physiology and therapeutics, educational experiences constructed to diffuse awareness about chronotherapy need to be carefully planned with attention to pedagogical principles. Further, given the novelty of the concept, it may be likely that for many drugs, specific chronotherapeutic information would not be available, hence future graduates would need the skills to apply training in chronotherapy to such drugs, so that drug administration times are circadianly optimised for enhanced safety or efficacy. The final year curriculum would be the best place to situate such training, as learners at this stage would have the required pre-requisite learning, and with imminent entry to the profession, they would be keen to learn knowledge application skills. Therefore, the aim of the study was to develop, implement, and evaluate an education intervention focusing on principles of chronotherapy for final year undergraduate pharmacy students.

2. Experimental Section

2.1. Design of Education Intervention

The main purpose of the educational intervention was to provide students with evidence-based knowledge of principles on which chronotherapy is based and to enhance their awareness of the application of these principles in pharmacy practice. The study was approved by the Human Research Ethics Committee at the University of Sydney (HREC number 2012/2885).

The research design used to evaluate this experiment was a pre-post evaluation, where the evaluation instrument comprised a custom devised questionnaire. The questionnaire was used to assess participants' knowledge of circadian rhythms and chronotherapy and their attitudes and willingness to apply principles of chronotherapy throughout their professional life. The construction of the questionnaire was based on a review of the literature [2], a previous survey (1996 Gallup survey of medical chronobiology and chronotherapeutics) [21] and practical considerations in the clinical application of chronotherapy. It comprised three sections as highlighted in Table 1. Experienced practicing pharmacists, pharmacy academics, sleep and circadian specialists reviewed the questionnaire for face and content validity. The questionnaire was pilot tested with five practicing pharmacists. Prior to the questionnaire administration, all final-year pharmacy students ($n = 216$) enrolled in the "Pharmacy Management" (PHAR 4814) course during 1 Semester 2013 (Faculty of Pharmacy, University of Sydney, Australia) were offered a verbal invitation to participate in the study and requested to complete this questionnaire. For an implementation plan timed for the 2nd Semester 2013 (July–October), the questionnaire administration in Semester 1 allowed researchers to map knowledge deficits and construct an intervention that addressed existing needs. The same questionnaire was then administered after the intervention was delivered in the 2nd Semester 2013 as well.

Table 1. The content of the utilized questionnaire.

Section	Questionnaire Section	Description
1	General Demographics and Information Section	9 items that included statements with Yes/No answers and short questions covering demographic and general data about the students' work experience and information on the chronotherapy.
2	Awareness Section	13 items that included brief statements or clinical case studies with multiple-choice response options. The possible score for each item was either 0 or 1. The total possible score range for the section was 0–13.
3	Attitude Section	12 items that included statements with multiple options covering attitudes and willingness to use principles of chronotherapy. Each item was measured using the Likert scale of "Strongly Agree", "Somewhat Agree", "Neither Agree Nor Disagree", "Somewhat Disagree", and "Strongly Disagree". The possible score range for each item was 1 to 5. The total possible score range for the section was 12–60.

When developing a method to provide the education, it was hypothesized that the participation in a multi-component interactive educational intervention would increase students' knowledge about and attitudes towards the concept of circadian rhythms and principles of chronotherapy Compared to traditional directive teaching, interactive educational experiences enable students to become more active, independent and self-directed learners. Ultimately, this enhances their learning process by facilitating appropriate application of their knowledge in new contexts [22]. Thus, the educational intervention was designed based on the principles of active learning [23], and the learning outcomes were couched in accordance with Bloom's taxonomy of cognitive constructs [24]. The learning objectives, teaching activities and assessment tasks were aligned carefully (Table 2).

The educational intervention protocols and educational artifacts were developed by the first author in consultation with academics and clinicians who have extensive expertise in pharmacy education research, and sleep/circadian medicine. The educational activity was embedded in an existing practice based course on Professional Pharmacy (PHAR 4821). This course, offered to final year students, focuses on knowledge consolidation, therapeutics, application of knowledge, continuing professional education practices, and disease-state management. It consists of lectures, hands-on workshop sessions, online learning, and problem-based tutorial classes [18]. A detailed description of the intervention is provided below.

Table 2. Learning objectives and alignment with instruction and assessment plans.

Learning Objectives	**Instructional Strategies**	**Type of Learning (*Bloom's taxonomy*)**	**Assessment Strategy**
Define the key terms used in the field of circadian rhythms and chronotherapy.	Knowledge transfer through the delivery of a didactic lecture. Provision of references to background articles in the workshop	Factual knowledge/ Remembering	Performance in post-workshop questionnaire and exam questions
Understand the significance of circadian rhythms in various disease conditions	Delivery of the lecture. Screening of a BBC documentary and a few research articles as background references in the workshop	Comprehension	Discussion towards the end of the lecture and workshop. Performance in post-workshop questionnaire and exam questions
Apply the scientific rationale behind the timing of administration of medicine	Delivery of a lecture. Screening of a BBC documentary and a few research articles as background references in the workshop. Discussion of case studies and role-play during the workshop	Comprehension	Assessing the quality of case discussion, *i.e.*, how learners provided convincing support or evidence for the basis of their proposed case solution throughout their presentation. Performance in post-workshop questionnaire and exam questions
Demonstrate an understanding of different aspects of chronotherapy in terms of pharmacokinetics, dynamics, formulation and effectiveness	Delivery of a lecture. Provision of in-depth information on various aspects of chronotherapy. Discussion of case studies during the workshop	Application, Analysis, and Synthesis	Assessing the quality of case discussion, *i.e.,* how learners provided convincing support or evidence for the basis of their proposed case solution throughout their presentation. Performance in post-workshop questionnaire and exam questions
Compare the limitations and benefits of chronotherapy applications in clinical practice	Delivery of a lecture. Provision of in-depth information on different aspects of chronotherapy. Discussion of case studies, poster-making and role-play during the workshop	Analysis	Observation and analysis of case studies, poster and role-play. Peer critique, followed by group discussion.
Justify the role of pharmacists in implementing principles of chronotherapy and optimize drug therapy.	Discussion of case studies, role-play and poster making	Analysis, Evaluation, and Skill Acquisition	Observation and analysis of case studies, poster and role-play. Peer critique, followed by group discussion

2.1.1. "Medications Around the Clock"—Lecture

A 1-h lecture entitled "Medications around the clock" was prepared following a thorough review of the literature. The main purpose of the lecture was to provide the students with an overview of circadian rhythms, key definitions, and concepts used in chronobiology and chronotherapy. A meta-cognitive approach was applied in the construction and presentation of the lecture. The lecture, thus, covered fundamental concepts ranging from linking chronotherapy terms and explaining mechanisms of how chronotherapy may work to highlighting the latter relationally with case examples in a laddered approach, *i.e.*, proceeding from simple to more complex matters [25,26]. In other words, during the lecture, the lecturer provided "knowledge" or "facts" based on chronotherapy—and then linked these in (1) a backward integration to knowledge/concepts learnt in previous years and (2) a forward integration to how the knowledge could be applied in a clinical case patient presenting to a pharmacy. This sequence was used to direct cognitive processes in learners in their learning effort. The lecture was delivered by an experienced clinical pharmacist (last author) to 216 final-year pharmacy students in the fourth week of studies during the 2nd Semester 2013. An open discussion addressing questions and stimulating feedback was encouraged at the end of the lecture. The lecture was recorded and posted online along with the corresponding presentation slides (Microsoft PowerPoint® format) for future study reference.

2.1.2. "Medications Around the Clock—Chronotherapy"—Workshop

A 3-h workshop entitled "Medications around the clock—Chronotherapy" was carefully designed to reinforce and "scaffold" the knowledge acquired from the lecture [27]. It consisted of multiple collaborative and group learning activities including a video screening, case studies, poster making, and role plays. Table 3 describes the content of the workshop. The workshop was delivered by the first and last authors during the final week (week 13) of studies in the 2nd Semester 2013. The workshop took place in an allocated room over a period of one week and was administered to 192 final-year pharmacy students in "Professional Pharmacy" course. The subject coordinator for PHAR 4821 had divided the students into six groups of 30–34 students each, and each group was allocated to a single workshop session in the last week of the semester. On the day of any particular workshop, the instructors gave an introduction, outlining the objectives and content of the workshop. Following this, screening of a short, publicly available, British Broadcasting Corporation (BBC) documentary video was carried out [28]. This was intended to stimulate a relaxed learning environment and allow audio-visual engagement with the topic. Following the screening, students were allocated to one of the four groups, referred to as "stations"; with each station comprising 7–9 students. Information packages containing group activity details, research articles on the subject, and relevant medical references were provided for each station. Each station received a different set of activities covering 1 of 4 themes: (1) Concepts in chronotherapy; (2) Chronotherapy of pain; (3) Chronotherapy of hypertension; and (4) Chronotherapeutic drug delivery systems. The workshop room was also equipped with computers/other resources to facilitate the students' research.

Table 3. The content of the workshop.

Activity (Time Allotted for the Activities) [a]	Objective	Description
Video screening of a BBC documentary (30 min)	Introducing the audio-visual support for scaffolding clinical learning	BBC documentary: "Horizon - The Secret life of your biological clock" was screened. The documentary explained how the human biological clock works and how it affects and controls routine life activities. The video helped grasp students' interest and engagement in the topic through the visualization of real-life scenarios.
Clinical case studies and poster making (100 min: 40 min for solving the cases and 60 min for class discussion)	Clinical concept learning-collaborative learning, critical thinking, and generating a new idea in a team environment.	Clinical case studies related to circadian rhythms and chronotherapy principles that could be encountered in future practice were provided to each group. During the first 40-min, each group was asked to read, discuss, and analyze their case. The key clinical query was to determine an appropriate time for administering the medication in question. Students in each station were then asked to design a single poster addressing awareness of chronotherapy with their patients. Then 60 min were allocated for class discussion of the case studies. The case studies were presented using multimedia screen and read out by corresponding students from each station. Discussions covered issues such as counseling patients about the right time of administration, explaining to patients about the circadian variability in symptoms of disease conditions in lay language, and differences between conventional drug delivery systems and chronotherapeutic drug delivery systems. Each station displayed their poster on a multimedia screen, and an instructor-led the discussion. This activity was engaging and collated various ideas whilst providing learners with a creative outlet. The instructor guided the discussion by asking questions and answering queries from the students. All groups were encouraged to take part in the debate and provide input.
Role Play (10 min)	Collaborative learning-Practicing acquired knowledge.	A group of students role-played the "patient", the "pharmacist" and observer from clinical case studies. In the role play, the "pharmacist" counsels the "patient" regarding the "right time" of administration of medicines and promoting chronotherapy application in pharmacy.
Debriefing (10 min)	Solidifying learning concepts, synthesizing new knowledge	The instructor initiated the discussion by summarizing key points covered in the lecture and throughout the workshop focusing on variability in circadian rhythms and timing of medication administration.

Note: ([a]) 10 min were allotted at the beginning for the introduction and a brief description of the workshop; 20 min at the end of the workshop was reserved for the assessment.

Each station had a set of clinical case studies allocated to their topic; these were designed to integrate scientific and collaborative learning by improving student's clinical knowledge and practice skills related to the timing of drug administration. Table 4 summarizes the content of clinical cases. Students at each station also presented their "solutions" to their set cases to the entire class. The question-answer session that followed the presentations stimulated collaborative learning with different groups learning from each other (as each station had different cases). Some clinical cases were role played out; a structured approach to role-playing was utilized by rotating students through the roles of the pharmacist, patient, and observer. Each role helped the students acquire new communication skills via adopting different perspectives. In one station, an activity requiring students to develop a poster (to explain chronotherapy in lay terms) provided an opportunity to generate new ideas in a creative manner and to practice and refine presentation skills. Every element of the workshop was designed to encourage a highly interactive learning environment. The instructors provided assistance by answering questions, facilitating task completion, and guiding the flow of the workshop activities. The overall instructional design followed an upward trajectory, *i.e.*, learning was commenced at lower levels of Bloom's taxonomy of cognitive constructs (didactic lecture) and proceeded to higher cognitive levels [29].

Table 4. Examples of clinical case studies in the workshop.

Case Studies	Clinical Expertise Tested
Chronotherapy of pain: A 40-year-old male presents with epigastric burning pain. His physician prescribed omeprazole 40 mg for 14 days and advised him to change his diet.	Counseling for administration (right time of administration), lifestyle modification, contraindications, precautions, and storage
Chronotherapy of pain: A 49-year-old male had been waking up during the night-time with heartburn and reflux. The physician advised Antacid and zantac 300 mg.	Counseling for administration (right time of administration), lifestyle modification, contraindications, precautions, and storage.
Chronotherapy of pain: A 33-year-old female gradually developed painful wrists and early morning stiffness. The physician prescribed her ketoprofen 200 mg.	Counseling for administration (right time of administration), lifestyle modification, contraindications, precautions, and storage.
Chronotherapy of hypertension: A 62-year-old male has a past medical history of hypertension. His 24h ambulatory blood pressure indicates that nighttime blood pressure is about 25% lower than his daytime blood pressure.	Addressing patients' concerns, therapy selection/counseling, lifestyle modifications.
Chronotherapy of hypertension: A 52-year-old female has a history which includes type-2 diabetes, hypertension, and obstructive sleep apnea. Her 24 ambulatory blood pressure monitoring indicates that her blood pressure declines less than 10% during the night compared with daytime.	Addressing patients' concerns, therapy selection/counseling, lifestyle modifications.
Chronotherapeutic drug delivery systems: A 50-year-old female who presents to the pharmacy with a new prescription for Covera-HSR (verapamil).	Counseling for administration (right time of administration, how to take the medication), lifestyle modification, contraindications, precautions, and storage.
Concepts in chronotherapy: After an acute asthma attack, a 32-year-old woman is prescribed 40 mg of prednisone daily.	Counseling for administration (right time of administration), lifestyle modification, contraindications, precautions, and storage.

3. Results and Discussion

3.1. Evaluation and Assessment of Education Intervention

Pedagogical procedures should be carefully planned and continuously examined [30]. During the course of workshop, students' performance was continuously examined by the instructors by means of observing their in-class progress which included completion of assigned tasks, their participation in group discussions, their queries, enthusiasm and attentiveness to the presentation.

To evaluate the impact of the educational activity on students' knowledge about and attitudes toward chronotherapy and its application, the pre-intervention questionnaire was administered after the implementation of the education activities, at the completion of the workshops. During the administration of both the pre and post intervention questionnaires, the students were requested to complete their questionnaires within 10–20 min without discussing or seeking help from each other nor checking any relevant resources for responses. The questionnaire was administrated by the first author.

Data from the questionnaires was collected and analyzed using the Statistical Package for Social Sciences (version 22.0, IBM, Armonk, NY, USA). A total of 212 students completed the pre-workshop questionnaire (response rate 98%) and 192 students completed the post-workshop questionnaire (response rate 100%). Complete paired data sets were available for 157 students as 35 students did not provide their allocated identification code correctly, which resulted in utilizing a sample size of 157 students for statistical analysis purposes. Out of 157 students, 98.7% were under the age of 30, and 62.4% were females. Seventy-nine percent of the students were employed at pharmacies, and only 12.7% had previous knowledge about chronotherapy. Mean total awareness (knowledge) and attitude scores were calculated for the 13-item awareness section and the 12-item attitude sections items of the questionnaire. The awareness questions were scored either 1 (correctly answered) or 0 (incorrectly answered). The attitude questions were scored on 5 point Likert scale from "strongly disagree" to "strongly agree". Item with strongly agree scored 5 at one end and strongly disagree scored a 1 at the other end of the Likert scale. Pre and post-intervention scores were compared using paired *t*-tests. The pre-intervention mean total awareness and attitude scores were 6.5 ± 2.0 (score range 0–13) and 47.4 ± 6.9 (score range 12–60) respectively. The post-intervention total awareness score was 10.1 ± 1.9, and the attitude score was 54.0 ± 6.0. Post-intervention scores were significantly higher than pre-intervention scores with a score difference of 3.6 (95% CI, 3.2–3.9) and 6.6 (95% CI, 5.6–7.7) respectively.

From an educational perspective, pre and post intervention item difficulty and discrimination indices of the awareness section of the questionnaire were calculated [31,32]. The mean item difficulty, which corresponds to the proportion of students who answered an item correctly, was calculated to be 0.50 for pre-intervention and 0.78 for post-intervention. Item discrimination indices were used to review the ability of the awareness items of the questionnaire to discriminate between respondents who scored at either end of the scoring spectrum. It was computed from equal-sized high and low scoring groups to measure the ability of a particular item to differentiate between students with high scores and those with low scores. Item discrimination index was calculated to be 0.37 for pre-intervention and 0.33 for post-intervention.

To further evaluate the content of the provided educational activity, students' feedback was sought anonymously using a feedback form at the end of the workshop. The form comprised open-ended questions and 5-point Likert scale responses evaluating four key criteria of the workshop: (1) quality of teaching; (2) content of supporting material; (3) learning objectives; and (4) relevance of the workshop to future pharmacy practice. Mean scores were calculated for the Likert scale responses while the open-ended questions were thematically analyzed.

A total of 160 students completed the provided feedback form. Table 5 summarizes the results of the Likert scale questions. The majority of students (95%) highlighted the significance of chronotherapy-related education and advocated its retention in the curriculum for final-year pharmacy students. Most of the students reported that the introduction of a video screening was unique and made the workshop activities more engaging.

> "Great introduction video to introduce the mood of the workshop."
>
> "The tutors were very helpful, the video was interesting, the workshop was fun and we could see the relevance of it for our careers as pharmacists."

Many students also reported that the workshop was comprehensive and relevant to future practice:

> "I found the workshop very informative. It helped settle down all the pieces of what I have learned in the last four years. It provided me with the practical advice that can be used in real practice. I totally enjoyed the workshop."
>
> "It really opened my eyes more on the reasoning of time in relation to dosing regimen."

Table 5. Result of the feedback evaluation.

Feedback	Mean (SD) *
The workshop meets the stated learning objective.	2.1 (1.4)
The supporting materials used in the workshop (video, reference materials, PowerPoint template) were useful, and they enhance my learning experience.	2.1 (1.4)
The instructors used appropriate teaching techniques to enhance my learning.	1.8 (1.4)
Overall, the workshop was relevant and useful for my future practice.	2.1 (1.5)

Note: * The score was based on a Likert scale from 1–5, where 1 is strongly agree, and 5 is strongly disagree.

As a follow-up to the provided educational intervention, the subject of chronotherapy was then included at the end of semester examinations of final-year pharmacy students. Four questions (3 multiple choice and 1 short-answer) on the subject were included in "Professional Pharmacy Final Exam" (PHAR 4821) that took place at the end of the 2nd Semester 2013.

The students' overall performance at the end of the semester examination was favorable. Most students handled the multiple choice question well and proposed optimal therapeutic plans for the short descriptive question. The mean item difficulty for the three multiple choice exam questions in the final exam was 0.73. This result indicated considerable improvement in knowledge about chronotherapy. Item discrimination for the three multiple choice questions using the point bi-serial correlation was 0.37, 0.39 and 0.31; this is within the acceptable range of 0.3–0.6 [31].

3.2. Discussion

This research study reports on the design of an educational intervention on chronotherapy for final-year undergraduate pharmacy students. The aim of the study was to assess students' awareness and understanding of circadian rhythms and principles of chronotherapy and provide them with up-to-date education on this advanced clinical concept. Given that not much is known about effective methods for teaching students about this advanced concept, the design of an educational intervention with careful attention to pedagogic principles was warranted. This was achieved by balancing a spectrum of educational components ranging from didactic lectures to interactive case discussions within a scaffolding structure of contextual support materials. A significant improvement in pharmacy students' awareness of principles of chronotherapy and their application was observed following the exposure to the 4-h educational intervention. The improvement was significant in terms of both general knowledge about circadian rhythms and clinical-based information on prinicples of chronotherapy which was evident from improvements in scores of awareness items of questionnaire, class performance in the workshop and scores at end semester examination. The intervention highlighted that complex clinical aspects can be successfully delivered using well-designed educational interventions.

While the pre-intervention attitude score was already high, a further improvement was observed after the implementation of the educational activity. This indicated that pharmacy students were enthusiastic and motivated to learn new skills that could assist them in optimizing pharmacotherapeutic outcomes throughout their professional career. The delivered intervention, thus, facilitated the students' learning and achieved the desired outcomes. With respect to knowledge gains, an increase in the mean item difficulty and a decrease in the discrimination index values post-intervention were also observed. This indicates that, after the education, the proportion of awareness questions answered correctly was higher, and the gap between high-scoring and low-scoring students was reduced. These results may be attributed to the pedagogic design of the intervention. This could also highlight the sensitivity of the utilized questionnaire to the established changes in knowledge. Additionally, students' feedback on teaching standards, course organization, and the interactive nature of the workshop were overwhelmingly positive and highlighted the careful attention paid to the construction of the intervention. This resulted in the inclusion of a chronotherapy module in the curriculum of undergraduate pharmacy students at the University of Sydney (e.g., 2014 onwards).

From an instructional perspective, several studies have demonstrated that educational interventions with teaching methods fostering students' participation and engagement could enhance knowledge and positive attitudes [22,32]. Various learning techniques were, thus, employed during the design of the educational intervention. For instance, the use of professionally-designed, audio-visual tools to scaffold student learning was an effective strategy, integral to the flow and design of the intervention. Most students reported that the use of a video documentary was interesting and highly engaging, and they recommended its future use in other academic courses. Videos have, in fact, been used in continuing education training for pharmacists and as educational tools for pharmacy students [33]. Studies have shown that videotapes are effective in teaching clinical methods to medical students [34,35]. For example, videos have been used to introduce particularly difficult subjects, such as psychological adaptation to terminal illnesses and to illustrate the progressive changes that may occur in chronic disease conditions within a limited course schedule [36]. Another learning strategy utilized in our intervention was the employment of small-group activities and discussions. Small group formats have been particularly useful in medical education [37]. Studies have shown that small group discussions allowed students to apply their knowledge in solving problem-based case studies and to develop clinical and professional skills and reflective discussions [38]. Moreover, the role-play technique that we utilized has been regularly used in several studies to build communication skills [39] and was found out to be useful in improving the confidence of pharmacy students and pharmacists when counseling patients about common diseases and medications [22]. The literature also indicates that artwork and drawing have been efficient in building stronger communication skills [40]. The results of a study, in which students collaborated in pairs to research a public health topic related to pharmacy practice, demonstrated that a poster creation activity was effective in increasing knowledge and awareness of public health issues [41]. Similarly, in our intervention, the poster-making activity helped students to improve their verbal presentation abilities, drug information skills, and the ability to collaborate with other team members. All in all, the use of these combined learning strategies stimulated the students' critical thinking, clinical decision-making, and communication and counseling skills, particularly about the timing of drug administration and circadian rhythms.

It should be noted this study had a number of limitations. The questionnaire utilized to assess students' knowledge and attitudes was developed by the authors for the purpose of this study and was not validated or previously psychometrically-tested. Since the workshop was conducted in the last week of semester, the post-intervention questionnaire had to be administered on the same day of the workshop; hence, the recency of learning may have elicited the positive responses obtained. A possible limitation also includes test-retest bias as the same survey instrument was used to assess students' awareness and attitudes both before and after the education. To add, a follow-up study to examine the degree of knowledge retention was not conducted. In future research, it would be wise to do further content validation through administrating the questionnaire to sleep and circadian experts and to follow up with the students after they become registered pharmacists, possibly through the use of questionnaires or simulated patient scenarios.

4. Conclusions

An educational intervention on chronotherapy for pharmacy students was successful in improving awareness of circadian rhythms and principles of chronotherapy and enhancing attitudes toward the application of these principles in pharmacy practice. After the conclusion of this study, a two-hour chronotherapy module has been adopted into the curriculum of final-year pharmacy students at the University of Sydney. While interactive teaching techniques have been found to be useful in training pharmacy students on chronotherapy, similar strategies should be employed in the design of an adapted chronotherapy-based educational intervention or training program for pharmacy practitioners, possibly as part of their continuing professional education program. Other healthcare professionals, such as general practitioners, physicians, and practice nurses may also benefit from a similar intervention.

Acknowledgments

We acknowledge the University of Sydney for facilitating the research and data collection process. The authors thank Ms. Jocelyn Bussing for her assistance with the pre-workshop questionnaire and workshop administration. The authors also thank all final-year undergraduate pharmacy students for completing the questionnaire and providing valuable feedback about the workshop. Ms. Gagandeep Kaur is the recipient of scholarships from the NHMRC Centre for Integrated Research and Understanding of Sleep (CIRUS) and gratefully acknowledges this support.

Author Contributions

Gagandeep Kaur designed questionnaire, content of the workshop and wrote the manuscript. Bandana Saini, Craig Phillips and Keith Wong critically reviewed the questionnaire, content of workshop and the manuscript. Maya Saba reviewed the manuscript.

Conflicts of Interest

The authors declare no conflict of interest.

References and Notes

1. Ohdo, S. Chronopharmacology focused on biological clock. *Drug Metab. Pharmacokinet.* **2007**, *22*, 3–14.
2. Kaur, G.; Phillips, C.; Wong, K.; Saini, B. Timing is important in medication administration: A timely review of chronotherapy research. *Int. J. Clin. Pharm.* **2013**, *35*, 344–358
3. Strohl, K.P.; Haponik, E.E.; Sateia, M.J.; Veasy, S.; Chervin, R.D.; Zee, P.; Papp, K. The need for a knowledge system in sleep and chronobiology. *Acad. Med.* **2000**, *75*, 819–821.
4. Hassan, A.; Haefeli, W.E. Appropriateness of timing of drug administration in electronic prescriptions. *Pharm. World Sci.* **2010**, *32*, 162–171.
5. Smolensky, M.H.; Portaluppi, F.; Manfredini, R.; Hermida, R.C.; Tiseo, R.; Sackett-Lundeen, L.L.; Haus, E.L. Diurnal and twenty-four hour patterning of human diseases: Cardiac, vascular, and respiratory diseases, conditions, and syndromes. *Sleep Med. Rev.* **2015**, *21*, 3–11.
6. Smolensky, M.H.; Portaluppi, F.; Manfredini, R.; Hermida, R.C.; Tiseo, R.; Sackett-Lundeen, L.L.; Haus, E.L. Diurnal and twenty-four hour patterning of human diseases: Acute and chronic common and uncommon medical conditions. *Sleep Med. Rev.* **2015**, *21*, 12–22.
7. Smolensky, M.H.; Peppas, N.A. Chronobiology, drug delivery, and chronotherapeutics. *Adv. Drug Deliv. Rev.* **2007**, *59*, 828–851.
8. Stranges, P.M.; Drew, A.M.; Rafferty, P.; Shuster, J.E.; Brooks, A.D. Treatment of hypertension with chronotherapy: Is it time of drug administration? *Ann. Pharmacother.* **2015**, *49*, 323–334.
9. Plakogiannis, R.; Cohen, H. Optimal low-density lipoprotein cholesterol lowering-morning *versus* evening statin administration. *Ann. Pharmacother.* **2007**, *41*, 106–110.
10. Zhu, L.L.; Zhou, Q.; Yan, X.F.; Zeng, S. Optimal time to take once-daily oral medications in clinical practice. *Int. J. Clin. Pract.* **2008**, *62*, 1560–1571.
11. Karin, W.; Rob, S.S.; Clare, M.; Gous Andries, G.S.; Marthe, E.; Dick, T.; World Health Organization; International Pharmaceutical Federation. *Developing Pharmacy Practice—A Focus on Patient Care*; World Health Organization: Geneva, Switzerland, 2006; Volume 97.
12. The Pharmacy Guild of Australia. "Pre-Budget Submission." Available online: http://www.guild.org.au/docs/default-source/public-documents/issues-and-resources/Pharmacy-Issues/pdf-nbsp-guild-pre-budget---submission.pdf?sfvrsn=0 (accessed on 2 November 2015).
13. The Pharmacy Guild of Australia. "Pharmacy innovations in ehealth." Avaliable online: http://www.guild.org.au/docs/default-source/public-documents/issues-and-resources/Fact-Sheets/pharmacy-innovations-in-ehealth.pdf?sfvrsn=0 (accessed on 31 March 2015).
14. Ortiz, M.; Cecere, R.; Gallagher, R. Impact of the mirixa program on patient compliance to therapy. *Aust. Pharm.* **2011**, *30*, 244–248.
15. Accreditation Council for Pharmacy Education. "Accreditation standards and guidelines for professional program in pharmacy leading to the doctor of pharmacy degree." Avaliable online: https://www.acpe-accredit.org/pdf/FinalS2007Guidelines2.0.pdf (accessed on 25 March 2015).

16. Duffy, J.F.; Czeisler, C.A. Effect of light on human circadian physiology. *Sleep Med. Clin.* **2009**, *4*, 165–177.
17. Purvis, C.C.; Lechnar, J.M.; Hagen, K.; Evans, C. Sleep medicine education benefits pharmacists. *Med. Sci. Educ.* **2003**, *13*, 51–59.
18. The University of Sydney. "Bachelor of pharmacy-unit of study descriptions." Avaliable online: http://sydney.edu.au/handbooks/pharmacy/undergraduate/b_pharmacy_descriptions.shtml (accessed on 31 March 2015).
19. Lee, K.A.; Landis, C.; Chasens, E.R.; Dowling, G.; Merritt, S.; Parker, K.P.; Redeker, N.; Richards, K.C.; Rogers, A.E.; Shaver, J.F.; *et al.* Sleep and chronobiology: Recommendations for nursing education. *Nurs. Outlook* **2004**, *52*, 126–133.
20. Penzel, T.; Pevernagie, D.; Dogas, Z.; Grote, L.; de Lacy, S.; Rodenbeck, A.; Bassetti, C.; Berg, S.; Cirignotta, F.; d'Ortho, M.P. Catalogue of knowledge and skills for sleep medicine. *J. Sleep Res.* **2014**, *23*, 222–238.
21. Smolensky, M.H. Knowledge and attitudes of american physicians and public about medical chronobiology and chronotherapeutics. Findings of two 1996 gallup surveys. *Chronobiol. Int.* **1998**, *15*, 377–394.
22. Katoue, M.G.; Al Haqan, A. Implementation and evaluation of a workshop on patient counseling about antidiabetic medications for final-year pharmacy students. *Med. Princ. Pract.* **2013**, *22*, 489–494.
23. Gleason, B.L.; Peeters, M.J.; Resman-Targoff, B.H.; Karr, S.; McBane, S.; Kelley, K.; Thomas, T.; Denetclaw, T.H. An active-learning strategies primer for achieving ability-based educational outcomes. *Am. J. Pharm. Educ.* **2011**, *75*, 186.
24. Bloom, B.S. *Taxonomy of Educational Objectives. Cognitive Domain*; Addison Wesley Publishing Company: New York, NY, USA, 1956; Volume 1.
25. Lovrich, D. A ladder of thinking. *Sci. Teach.* **2004**, *71*, 56–59.
26. Kamp, M.T.; Admiraal, W.; Drie, J.; Rijlaarsdam, G. Enhancing divergent thinking in visual arts education: Effects of explicit instruction of meta-cognition. *Br. J. Educ. Psychol.* **2015**, *85*, 47–58.
27. Tsai, F.-H.; Kinzer, C.; Hung, K.-H.; Chen, C.-L.A.; Hsu, I.Y. The importance and use of targeted content knowledge with scaffolding aid in educational simulation games. *Interact. Learn. Environ.* **2012**, *21*, 116–128.
28. Sussman, A. *The Secret Life of Your Body Clock*; BBC: London, UK, 2009.
29. Poirier, T.; Crouch, M.; MacKinnon, G.; Mehvar, R.; Monk-Tutor, M. Updated guidelines for manuscripts describing instructional design and assessment: The ideas format. *Am. J. Pharm. Educ.* **2009**, *73*, 55.
30. Boyer, E.L. *Scholarship Reconsidered: Priorities of the Professoriate*; Carnegie Foundation for the Advancement of Teaching: Princeton, NJ, USA, 1990.
31. Sateia, M.J.; Reed, V.A.; Christian Jernstedt, G. The dartmouth sleep knowledge and attitude survey: Development and validation. *Sleep Med.* **2005**, *6*, 47–54.
32. Saba, M.; Bittoun, R.; Saini, B. A workshop on smoking cessation for pharmacy students. *Am. J. Pharm. Educ.* **2013**, *77*, doi:10.5688/ajpe779198.

33. Felton, L.A.; Keesee, K.; Mattox, R.; McCloskey, R.; Medley, G. Comparison of video instruction and conventional learning methods on students' understanding of tablet manufacturing. *Am. J. Pharm. Educ.* **2001**, *65*, 53–55.
34. Mir, M.A.; Marshall, R.J.; Evans, R.W.; Dannatt, R.J.; Hall, R.; Duthie, H.L. Videotapes for teaching clinical methods: Medial students' response to a pilot project. *J. Audiov. Media Med.* **1985**, *8*, 90–93.
35. Kline, P.; Shesser, R.; Smith, M.; Turbiak, T.; Rosenthal, R.; Chen, H.; Walls, R. Comparison of a videotape instructional program with a traditional lecture series for medical student emergency medicine teaching. *Ann. Emerg. Med.* **1986**, *15*, 16–18.
36. LeGardeur, B.Y.; Fe-Bornstein, M.; Lopez-S, A. The use of video tape in teaching how psychological factors influence nutritional status in chronic/terminal illness. *J. Cancer Educ.* **1991**, *6*, 213–217.
37. Fryer-Edwards, K.; Arnold, R.M.; Baile, W.; Tulsky, J.A.; Petracca, F.; Back, A. Reflective teaching practices: An approach to teaching communication skills in a small-group setting. *Acad. Med.* **2006**, *81*, 638–644.
38. Jaques, D. Teaching small groups. *BMJ* **2003**, *326*, 492–494.
39. Nestel, D.; Tierney, T. Role-play for medical students learning about communication: Guidelines for maximising benefits. *BMC Med. Educ.* **2007**, *7*, 3.
40. Biggerstaff, D.E.; Schnitz, G.W.; Wingrove, M.S. Enhanced communication skills for medical students through drawing. *J. Biocommun.* **1984**, *11*, 2–4.
41. Kelsch, M.P.; Werremeyer, A.B. Poster project to emphasize public health in the pharmacy curriculum. *Am. J. Pharm. Educ.* **2011**, *75*, 2.

10

An Algorithm to Identify Compounded Non-Sterile Products that Can Be Formulated on a Commercial Scale or Imported to Promote Safer Medication Use in Children

Varsha Bhatt-Mehta [1,2,*], Robert B. MacArthur [3], Raimar Löbenberg [4,5], Jeffrey J. Cies [2,6,7], Ibolja Cernak [2,8] and Richard H. Parrish II [2]

1 Department of Clinical, Social and Administrative Sciences, College of Pharmacy and Department of Pediatrics, Medical School, University of Michigan, Ann Arbor, MI, 48109, USA

2 Med4Kids Research Collaborative, Ltd., Edmonton, AB, T6M 2J9, Canada; E-Mails: info@meds4keds.ca; Jeffrey.Cies@tenethealth.com; ibicernak@yahoo.com

3 Clinical Development, Pharmaceutics International, Inc., Hunt Valley, MD, 21031, USA; E-Mail: RMacarthur@pharm-int.com

4 Pharmaceutical Sciences Division, Faculty of Pharmacy and Pharmaceutical Sciences, Edmonton, AB, T6G 2R3, Canada; E-Mail: Raimar@ualberta.ca

5 Drug Discovery and Innovation Centre, University of Alberta, Edmonton, AB, T6G 2R3, Canada

6 Drexel University College of Medicine, Philadelphia, PA, 19129, USA

7 St. Christopher's Hospital for Children, Philadelphia, PA, 19140, USA

8 Military and Veterans' Clinical Rehabilitation Research, University of Alberta, Edmonton, AB, T6G 2G4, Canada

* Author to whom correspondence should be addressed; E-Mail: rxvarsha@gmail.com

Academic Editor: Sandra Benavides Caballero

Abstract: The lack of commercially-available pediatric drug products and dosage forms is well-known. A group of clinicians and scientists with a common interest in pediatric drug development and medicines-use systems developed a practical framework for identifying a list of active pharmaceutical ingredients (APIs) with the greatest market potential for development to use in pediatric patients. Reliable and reproducible evidence-based drug formulations designed for use in pediatric patients are needed vitally, otherwise safe and consistent clinical practices and outcomes assessments will continue to be difficult to ascertain. Identification of a prioritized list of candidate APIs for oral formulation using the described algorithm provides a broader integrated clinical, scientific, regulatory, and market basis to allow for more reliable dosage forms and safer, effective medicines use in children of all ages. Group members derived a list of candidate API molecules by factoring in a number of pharmacotherapeutic, scientific, manufacturing, and regulatory variables into the selection algorithm that were absent in other rubrics. These additions will assist in identifying and categorizing prime API candidates suitable for oral formulation development. Moreover, the developed algorithm aids in prioritizing useful APIs with finished oral liquid dosage forms available from other countries with direct importation opportunities to North America and beyond.

Keywords: compounded medications; formulation development; patient safety; pediatric

1. Introduction

Childhood illnesses often require the use of medications under the premise of "off-label" use. In February 2014, the American Academy of Pediatrics (AAP) released a policy statement from its Committee on Drugs regarding the off-label use of drugs (medications) in children [1]. For the purpose of the statement the Committee defined "off-label" use as that use which is not included in the package insert (US Food and Drug Administration (US-FDA)-approved labeling) for that drug and is "neither experimentation nor research" [1]. Such off-label use of drugs in children does not require any oversight by any institutional committee, Investigational Review Board, or federal regulatory agency. Use of drugs without appropriate research in children can put this population at significant risk for adverse events. Off-label use combined with use of medication management systems designed for adults and adapted for use in children can compound the risk of adverse events due to increased potential for medication errors. We have addressed the issue of medication management systems elsewhere in this Special Edition [2]. Here, we make an attempt to identify other issues related to off-label use of drugs and present potential solutions. That is, an algorithm that identifies compounded non-sterile products (CNPs) suitable for commercial scale pediatric formulation development, or importation, to address the medical needs of children.

2. Why Is off-Label Use of Drugs in Children Still a Problem?

The issue of "off-label" use of drugs in neonates, infants and children has prevailed for many decades. Federal legislation to address this issue was first proposed in 1998 and reauthorized in 2012. Since that time, various government agencies, including US-FDA and the National Institute of Child Health and Human Development (NICHD), have worked together to develop product labeling for pediatric patients for existing and new drug molecules coming to the market, if the drug has been or could be used in children.

According to a recent study published in JAMA-Pediatrics, the legislation has produced 406 pediatric labeling changes; out of those only 24 include data on neonatal drug dosing [3]. Identified factors responsible for the lack of appropriate drug dosing data in children go beyond the efforts of the US-FDA and NICHD, which formed partnership almost two decades ago to address this issue and formed collaborations with academia and a number of other entities to enhance this knowledge. Current dosing regimens for most drugs used in neonates, infants and children are extrapolated from adult pharmacokinetic (PK)/pharmacodynamics (PD) data rather than PK and PD data derived for pediatric populations. A major barrier to generation of appropriate dosing regimens based on sound PK/PD data is lack of commercial availability of uniform and stable drug formulations. Many drug dosage forms used in pediatric populations today within health care institutions in North America and elsewhere are extemporaneously compounded and lack validated product uniformity. This results in significant variability in drug disposition (ADME) estimates when these products are studied in children, as it is often unclear whether measured ADME variation originates from the patient or the product. Thus, research in pediatrics is not only necessary for new drug moieties, but also for existing active pharmaceutical ingredients APIs. Variations in dose preparation can significantly affect bioavailability, plasma concentrations and therapeutic effect.

Effective delivery and viable manufacturing are essential to improve the clinical and commercial value of a pharmaceutical product. A reliable formulation will not only ensure optimal clinical outcomes, but also assure reproducibility in manufacturing and increased stability. This gap between commercial availability and clinical utility is bridged daily primarily by the efforts of compounding pharmacists, especially in the hospital setting, where APIs are extemporaneously compounded from adult solid oral dosage forms to provide medications that otherwise are not available to vulnerable pediatric populations, such as children with cardiovascular disease, cancer, cystic fibrosis, organ transplants, and other life threatening conditions.

It has been noted that these compounding practices, despite best efforts and intentions, do not incorporate the necessary manufacturing controls to assure reproducible product potency, stability, and purity. Formal efforts to assist pharmacists and other practitioners to compound the best products possible include methods and guidelines found in the United States Pharmacopeia, US-FDA regulations and guidance documents, professional working groups, and elsewhere [4]. Working groups focusing on the topic date back to at least 1977, when the American Society of Hospital Pharmacists Special Interest Group on Pediatric Pharmacy Practice started working on the issue. This group continues to meet to the current day [5].

When compared to Good Manufacturing Practices (GMPs), the manufacturing standards required by FDA for commercial products, there are multiple recognized deficiencies inherent in extemporaneous formulation-compounding suitable for pediatric patients, which include the following:

- Lack of specifications required for component development by compounding pharmacies.
- No onsite testing of active ingredients and excipients for purity, potency, content and stability.
- No onsite specifications or testing of product containers and closures.
- Site-to-site variations in compounding procedures, equipment, and the degree of product handling/manipulation.
- Lack of environmental control, which might lead to unintentional contamination and generation of degradation products due to inconsistent exposure to light, temperature and processing controls.
- Lack of testing of finished products for purity, potency, content or stability.

- Stability data for establishing expiry dates of compounded products are derived from published data, where preparation methods likely vary from local methods, or are simply default expiry periods defined by regional pharmacy regulations and "best practices".
- Published preparation methods provide only a portion of the information needed to consistently prepare a stable potent final product.
- Limited options available to mask bad-tasting active ingredients.
- The dose administration technologies used such as droppers, syringes, scoops, spoons, *etc.*, vary between sites and between prescription fills.
- Weak regulatory oversight.

Unfortunately, there are a number of barriers to the development of pediatric drug formulations under GMPs, not the least of which are economic in nature [6]. The first barrier concerns the market size. The elderly population (65 years of age and older) spends, on average, about 10 times more than the pediatric population (0–17 years of age) on medications. With regard to production, development of a unique pediatric formulation can take up to two years or more, with a cost ranging from $8 million to $15 million [7]. The second barrier relates to the need for incorporating taste-masking methods suitable for children; whereas the third one is due to the need to develop dosage forms such as liquids, suspensions, small tablets, films and chewable tablets that can be easily administered to children.

In the following sections, we present an algorithm that incorporates clinical and market-oriented variables in relation to existing APIs commonly used in pediatric practice that lack mass-produced formulations suitable for younger patients. Further, we overlay an array of scientific factors that support the selection of these APIs for mass-production, including Biopharmaceutical Classification System (BCS) and hot-melt extrusion (HME) as a flexible production technique for low solubility APIs.

3. Development of the Algorithm for a Tiered Selection Model for Candidate APIs

3.1. Clinical and Market Considerations

Between September and December 2013, a North-American group of pharmacists, pediatricians, and pharmaceutical scientists formed Meds4Kids Research Collaborative, LTD (M4KRC). This group of clinicians and scientists with a common interest in pediatric drug development and medicines-use systems developed a framework for developing drugs in dosage forms suitable for use in pediatric patients (Figure 1). The group met in a series of six conference calls to create a list of candidate API molecules that possess the greatest clinical, scientific, and market potential for mass production. The proposed criteria for determining potential candidate API molecules were prioritized primarily based on Best Pharmaceuticals for Children Act (BPCA), which lists broad-based clinical developmental needs within pediatrics. Below are the first phase criteria that the group selected for the API molecules:

(1). Listed on BPCA priority document (clinical need—broad base);

(2). Available in an injection (API is stable in solution for at least 18–24 months);

(3). Not a federally controlled substance in Canada or the US (minimal paperwork for chain of custody);

(4). Potential applicability for oral adult market (for adult patients that cannot swallow tablets or capsules);

(5). Established indication for any age group in the official labeling of the API (immediate marketability through accelerated ANDA mechanism) and

(6). Off-patent in both Canada and the US, and available in a pharmaceutical grade powder from a reputable supplier.

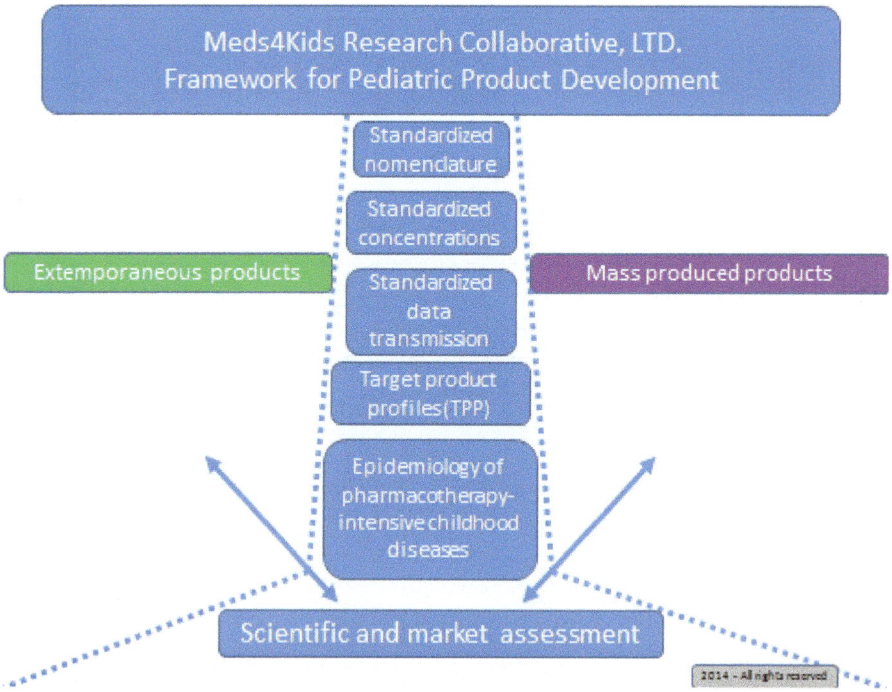

Figure 1. M4KRC framework for collaborative pediatric drug development.

The group reviewed the BPCA list and compared it to the list of 50 compounded non-sterile products (CNPs) prepared extemporaneously at St. Christopher's Hospital for Children, all of which had scientific evidence for stability in a standardized concentration [8]. The clinicians (VBM, RHP, and JJC) adjudicated the list using a scoring system that assigned a score for each API molecule's potential from a pharmacotherapy perspective. In the third meeting, a seventh factor was incorporated into the algorithm; the existence of a commercially-available oral liquid dosage form in the United Kingdom. Then, in the last two meetings, the scientists (RBM and RL) integrated the clinician-derived list with each API's biopharmaceutical and mass-manufacturing properties that complemented and validated the clinical rankings.

The original list was then segmented into four tiers:

- The first tier included API molecules that met at least five of the six criteria;
- The second tier fulfilled four criteria;
- The third tier included API molecules not listed by name in the BPCA list but met all others except availability in the United Kingdom; and
- The fourth tier included those available in the UK that could be imported readily for pharmacokinetic (PK), pharmacodynamics (PD), and/or pharmacogenomics (PG) studies in children.

Several API molecules were removed from the list because of new market entry (enalapril), availability of one oral liquid strength (levetiracetam), known pharmaco-chemical problems (acetylsalicylic acid), or low use potential in children (pravastatin). The final, fourth tier API molecules identified based on criteria of potential viability as candidates ready for PK/PD/PG studies, are listed in Table 1. Of note, while sildenafil is available in a mass-produced product in the UK, the 10 mg/mL formulation too concentrated for use in younger infants children, thereby necessitating an extemporaneous 2.5 mg/mL strength.

Table 1. M4KRC fourth tier candidate API molecules.

Generic Name	BCPA Listed?	Injection?	Non-Scheduled?	Oral Adult Market?	Established Adult Indication?	Off Patent?	Dose Form in UK?
Baclofen	1	1	1	1	1	1	Yes [a]
Warfarin	1	1	1	1	1	1	Yes [b]
Sildenafil	1	1	1	1	1	1	Yes [c]
L-thyroxine	1	1-lyo	1	1	1	1	Yes [d]

[a] Available as 5 mg/mL oral solution; [b] Available as 1 mg/mL oral suspension; [c] Available as 10 mg/mL suspension powder; [d] Available as 5 microgram/mL and 20 microgram/mL oral solution

3.2. Scientific and Production Considerations—Applying BCS and HME

The next step for the group was to apply scientific principles of drug delivery and formulation techniques to the clinically-derived list that would enhance the likelihood of the commercial availability of a mass-produced product.

The Biopharmaceutical Drug Classification System (BCS) was introduced by Amidon *et al.* in 1995 [9]. Today, this classification system is accepted by most regulatory agencies like the US FDA, Health Canada and European Medicines Agency (EMA). APIs are classified into one of four quadrants according to their potential bioavailability [10]. Solubility and permeability are the two parameters used for the classification. Only if a drug can dissolve in the gastrointestinal tract can it be absorbed, and only if it is absorbed it can have a systemic effect. BCS class I drugs have high solubility and high permeability; class II are poorly soluble but highly permeable; class III are highly soluble but poorly permeable and class IV are poorly soluble and poorly permeable. Wu and Benet linked metabolism to the BCS classification, and showed that classes I and II drugs can be highly metabolized and be subject to transporters, while classes III and IV drugs are poorly metabolized or transported [11]. If two pharmaceutically equivalent drug products have similar dissolution behavior at pH 1.2, 4.5 and 6.8, then they can be considered therapeutically equivalent and bioequivalence is assumed without the need of an *in vivo* bioequivalence study [12].

To be able to adopt the BCS classification to paediatric drugs, some consideration have to be made: (a) what are the differences in drug metabolism and transport in the GI tract between adults and children in different age groups; (b) age-relevant changes in the physiology of the GI tract which can change the permeability or solubility classification (c) changes in permeability due to transporters in children. Such data could be developed in paediatric physiologic and population-based pharmacokinetic databases. The volume of fluid the drug is taken and paediatric dose strength will also be different in a paediatric BCS classification compared to the current BCS [13].

If these considerations are included, a BCS approach can be used in the development of pediatric dosage forms if a suitable strength exists. The knowledge of the BCS class helps pharmaceutical companies in drug development. For example, a class I drug might need much less formulation work compared to a class II drug where solubility must be improved [14]. The BCS classes of APIs with the highest potential for pediatric formulation development are listed in Table 2, and could be applied to all WHO-listed essential medicines for children [15–18]. One of the manufacturing methods that can address many of these barriers is the hot-melt extrusion (HME) technology [19–21]. HME disperses the active ingredient(s) as a matrix at the molecular level, thus forming solid solutions without the use of excessive heat or solvents while preserving drug potency. The HME approach has been successful in improving the delivery and human absorption of poorly water-soluble compounds. Extruded solid solutions (*i.e.*, the end product of HME) offer greater thermodynamic stability compared to products prepared by alternative processes such as spray drying, solvent evaporation and other hot melt methods.

Table 2. BCS Class and potential APIs for pediatric drug development.

API Generic Name	BCS Class	Reference
Metoprolol	II	[15]
Clopidogrel	II	[16]
Lisinopril	III	[16]
Amlodipine	I	[17]
Ursodiol	Uncl.	n.d.
Bosentan	Uncl.	n.d.
Pantoprazole	Uncl.	n.d.
Acetazolamide	IV	[17]
Spironoloactone	II/IV	[16]
Valaciclovir	I/III	[17]
Captopril	III	[18]
Nifedipine	II	[16]
Baclofen	Uncl.	n.d.
Warfarin	I	[16]
Sildenafil	I	[15]
L-thyroxine	III	[16]

Uncl. = unclassified; n.d. = no data.

Concerning economics, HME can be used to produce small (on a GMP scale) lots of a formulated product. The final production sizes of these small lot sizes, denoted by contract manufacturers as research and development batches or Clinical Trial Manufacturing (CTM) batches, are within the range of 10,000 to 50,000 units. The flexibility to produce small batches using HME process may provide a sufficient commercial market for a given pediatric population for a year or more. Compared to commercial tableting or capsule manufacturing approaches, which incorporate processes such as milling, mixing, spray drying, pre-compression, compression, tableting/encapsulation, HME is a much more economical process with reduced production time, fewer processing steps, and is suitable for continuous operation [21].

With regards to formulation attributes and taste masking, HME can produce final drug products with sustained, modified, and targeted release properties, and can also coat poor tasting products. So, the finished product can then be milled in a single step to form powders suitable for incorporation into child-friendly dosage forms such as mini-tablets, orally disintegrating tabs, and liquid suspensions. The output of the extrusion process, known as an extrudate, can be optimized to protect the API against changing pH conditions, light, heat, and moisture levels, thus confer good stability properties to the final formulation.

While characterization of the pediatric gut awaits a more complete description, HME provides a useful tool for poorly soluble, highly permeable APIs [22–24].

An example of an API suitable for HME process is metoprolol succinate. Metoprolol is one of the most commonly used beta-blocking agents used in children from infancy through adolescence and into adulthood to treat a variety of cardiovascular conditions as an antihypertensive and heart rate modulator [25]. Metoprolol is a highly-soluble (~5 mg/mL) and permeable drug with no pH-dependent solubility. The required average pediatric dose ranges from 5 mg to 50 mg/day. Hence, a minimum concentration of about 2.5 mg/mL, with a maximum concentration of 10 mg/mL, is desired. When compounded in hospitals, a suspension with a concentration of 10 mg/mL is typically prepared. It is not possible to simply fill metoprolol succinate powder into a bottle to make a solution due to its poor solubility relative to dose volume and solution concentration as well as the formation of powder aggregates.

Metoprolol is an excellent candidate for HME as this process can increase in the dissolution rate of the drug for deriving clinically-appropriate concentrations, hence ease of reconstitution for a given strength. The process will also deliver good content uniformity of the drug and minimize risk for segregation. Overall, the manufacturing process is very simple, and involves only blending and processing using tight process controls. The HME process allows for in-process monitoring of the product quality using process analytical tools (e.g., Near Infra-Red (NIR) Spectroscopy). Moreover, there is no need for scaling up and down for different batch sizes.

In summary, the M4KRC-derived list of candidate API molecules has been derived from selection matrix that factored in a number of pharmacotherapy, scientific, production, and regulatory variables absent in other rubrics. These additions guided the group to identify the prime API candidates suitable for children in mass produced dosage forms. Further, the market-focused algorithm helped to prioritize useful APIs, and to facilitate clinical studies with finished oral liquid dosage forms available from other countries with direct importation potential to North America. Class II molecules are best suited for formulation using HME technologies Incorporating BCS classification and HME application into the final selection of candidate APIs, the following class II molecules are suggested for formulation and development: metoprolol, clopidogrel, spironolactone, and nifedipine. The assessment of these other variables, in addition to clinical and market parameters, is very important to increase the likelihood that a pharmaceutical manufacturer would successfully mass-produce and market these oral liquid dosage forms for children [26,27].

4. Conclusions

Successful public private partnerships have moved the science of pediatric clinical pharmacology forward. However, without reliable and reproducible evidence-based drug formulations designed for use in pediatric patients, safe and consistent clinical practices and outcomes assessments will continue to be difficult to ascertain. Identification and prioritization of prime candidate APIs with the algorithm has provided a broader integrated clinical, scientific, regulatory, and market basis, allowing for more reliable oral dosage forms for safe and effective medicines use in children of all ages.

The M4KRC group derived a list of candidate API molecules by factoring in a number of these pharmacotherapeutic, scientific, manufacturing, and regulatory variables into the selection algorithm that were absent in other rubrics. These additions have assisted in identifying and categorizing prime

API candidates suitable for oral formulation development. Finally, the developed algorithm aids in prioritizing useful APIs with finished oral liquid dosage forms available from other countries with direct importation opportunities to North America and beyond. These finished and standardized oral dosage forms await further clinical testing.

Author Contributions

Varsha Bhatt-Mehta, Richard Parrish, and Jeffrey Cies (the clinical practice group) created the molecule review criteria and algorithm; Robert MacArthur and Raimar Löbenberg (the production group) identified novel formulation methodologies and matched them to the BCS classification system to determine potential targets for mass production. Jeffrey Cies identified molecules available from the British National Formulary that may be suitable for clinical trials. Each group wrote the section of the paper pertaining to their respective expertise. Each author reviewed the final version of the paper. Varsha Bhatt-Mehta, Ibolja Cernak, and Richard Parrish finalized the manuscript in its present form.

The preparation of this manuscript received no financial subsidy from commercial, governmental, or other non-commercial sources.

The contents of this manuscript have not been presented previously at any scientific conference or published in any conference proceeding, and do not represent the positions of any of the author's respective organizations, commercial enterprises, governments, or employers.

Conflicts of Interest

The authors declare no conflict of interest.

References and Notes

1. Committee on Drugs. Off-label use of drugs in children. *Pediatrics* **2014**, *133*, 563–567.
2. Parrish, R.H., II; Cernak, I. Creating a distinct medicines-use system for children: The time is now. *Pharmacy* **2015**, *3*, 72–78.
3. Laughon, M.M.; Anat, D.; Tripathi, N.; Hornik, C.P.; Cohen-Wolkowiez, M.; Clark, R.H.; Smith, P.B.; Rodriguez, W. Drug labeling and exposure in neonates. *JAMA Pediatr.* **2014**, *168*, 130–136.
4. *Compounding Compendium*; The United States Pharmacopeial Convention: Rockville, MD, USA. Available online: http://www.usp.org/sites/default/files/usp_pdf/EN/products/2015_usp_compounding_compendium_feb_2015_toc.pdf (accessed on 21 August 2015).
5. Jew, R.K.; Soo-Hoo, W.; Erush, S.C. *Extemporaneous Formulations for Pediatric, Geriatric, and Special Needs Patients*, 2nd ed.; American Society of Health-System Pharmacists: Bethesda, MD, USA, 2010.
6. Vanchieri, C.; Stith Butler, A.; Knutsen, A. *Addressing the Barriers to Pediatric Drug, Development: Workshop Summary Forum on Drug Discovery, Development, and Translation*; The National Academies Press: Washington, DC, USA, 2008. Available online: http://www.nap.edu/catalog/11911.html (accessed on 31 March 2015).
7. Milne, C. Economic Issues for Making Available Adequate Drug Dosage Forms. In Proceedings of the Pediatric Formulations Initiative Workshop; NIHCD: Potomac, MD, USA, 2011.

Available online: http://bpca.nichd.nih.gov/collaborativeefforts/documents/pfi_workshop_11-1-2011.pdf (accessed on 31 March 2015).
8. Compounded Non-Sterile Product List. St. Christopher's Hospital for Children, 2013. (List is available upon request).
9. Amidon, G.L.; Lennernäs, H.; Shah, V.P.; Crison, J.R. A theoretical basis for a biopharmaceutic drug classification: The correlation of *in vitro* drug product dissolution and *in vivo* bioavailability. *Pharm. Res.* **1995**, *12*, 413–420.
10. Löbenberg, R.; Amidon, G.L. Modern bioavailability, bioequivalence and biopharmaceutics classification system. New scientific approaches to international regulatory standards. *Eur. J. Pharm. Biopharm.* **2000**, *5*, 3–12.
11. Wu, C.Y.; Benet, L.Z. Predicting drug disposition via application of BCS: Transport/absorption/ elimination interplay and development of a biopharmaceutics drug disposition classification system. *Pharm. Res.* **2005**, *22*, 11–23.
12. Löbenberg, R.; Chacra, N.B.; Stippler, E.S.; Shah, V.P.; DeStefano, A.J.; Hauck, W.W.; Williams, R.L. Toward global standards for comparator pharmaceutical products: Case studies of amoxicillin, metronidazole, and zidovudine in the Americas. *AAPS J.* **2012**, *14*, 462–472.
13. Abdel-Rahman, S.M.; Amidon, G.L.; Kaul, A.; Lukacova, V.; Vinks, A.; Knipp, G.T. Summary of the National Institute of Child Health and Human Development-Best Pharmaceuticals for Children Act Pediatric Formulation Initiatives Workshop—Pediatric Biopharmaceutics Classification System Working Group. *Clin. Ther.* **2012**, *34*, S11–S24.
14. Almukainzi, M.; Okumu, A.; Wei, H.; Löbenberg, R. Simulation of *in Vitro* Dissolution Behavior Using DDDPlus™. *AAPS PharmSciTech* **2014**, *16*, 217–221.
15. Takagi, T.; Ramachandran, C.; Bermejo, M.; Yamashita, S.; Yu, L.X.; Amidon, G.L. A provisional biopharmaceutical classification of the top 200 oral drug products in the United States, Great Britain, Spain, and Japan. *Mol. Pharm.* **2006**, *3*, 631–643.
16. Ramirez, E.; Laosa, O.; Guerra, P.; Duque, B.; Mosquera, B.; Borobia, A.M.; Lei, S.H.; Carcas, A.J.; Frias, J. Acceptability and characteristics of 124 human bioequivalence studies with active substances classified according to the Biopharmaceutic Classification System. *Br. J. Clin. Pharmacol.* **2010**, *70*, 694–702.
17. World Health Organization. *WHO Expert Committee on Specifications for Pharmaceutical Preparations*; WHO Technical Report Series; WHO Press: Geneva, CH, 2013. Available online: http://www.who.int/medicines/areas/quality_safety/quality_assurance/expert_committee/TRS981.pdf (accessed 05 November 2015).
18. Dahan, A.; Wolk, O.; Kim, Y.H.; Ramachandran, C.; Crippen, G.M.; Takagi, T.; Bermejo, M.; Amidon, G.L. Purely in silico BCS classification: Science based quality standards for the world's drugs. *Mol. Pharm.* **2013**, *10*, 4378–4390.
19. Crowley, M.M.; Zhang, F.; Repka, M.A.; Thumma, S.; Upadhye, S.B.; Battu, S.K.; McGinity, J.W.; Martin, C. Pharmaceutical applications of hot-melt extrusion—Part I. *Drug Dev. Ind. Pharm.* **2007**, *33*, 909–926.
20. Repka, M.A.; Battu, S.K.; Upadhye, S.B.; Thumma, S.; Crowley, M.M.; Zhang, F.; Martin, C.; McGinity, J.W. Pharmaceutical applications of hot-melt extrusion—Part II. *Drug Dev. Ind. Pharm.* **2007**, *33*, 1043–1057.

21. Maniruzzaman, M.; Boateng, J.S.; Snowden, M.J. A Review of Hot-Melt Extrusion: Process Technology to Pharmaceutical Products. *ISRN Pharm.* **2012**, 436763, doi:10.5402/2012/436763.
22. Batchelor, H.K.; Fotaki, N.; Klein, S. Paediatric Biopharmaceutics. *Adv. Drug Deliv. Rev.* **2014**, *73*, 102–126.
23. Batchelor, H.K.; European Paediatric Formulation Initiative (EUPFI). Paediatric Biopharmaceutics Classification System: Current status and future decisions. *Int. J. Pharm.* **2014**, *469*, 251–253.
24. Tannergren, C.; Bergendal, A.; Lennermas, H.; Abrahamsson, B. Toward an increased understanding of the barriers to colonic drug absorption in humans: Implications for early controlled release candidate assessment. *Mol. Pharm.* **2009**, *6*, 60–73.
25. Flynn, J.T.; Daniels, S.R.; Hayman, L.L. Maahs, D.M.; McCrindle, B.W.; Mitsnefes, M.; Zachariah, J.P.; Urbina, E.M.; American Heart Association Atherosclerosis, Hypertension and Obesity in Youth Committee of the Council on Cardiovascular Disease in the Young. Update: Ambulatory blood pressure monitoring in children and adolescents: A scientific statement from the American Heart Association. *Hypertension* **2014**, *63*, 1116–1135.
26. The Netherlands. Public Assessment Report for paediatric studies submitted in accordance with Article 45 of Regulation (EC) No1901/2006, as amended. Metoprolol succinate. Available online: www.sukl.cz/file/76992_1_1 (accessed 05 November 2015).
27. Allen, L.V.; Erickson, M.A. Stability of labetalol hydrochloride, metoprolol tartrate, verapamil hydrochloride, and spironolactone with hydrochlorothiazide in extemporaneously compounded oral liquids. *Am. J. Health Syst. Pharm.* **1996**, *53*, 2304–2309.

11

Medication Reconciliation at Discharge from Hospital: A Systematic Review of the Quantitative Literature

Maja H. Michaelsen [1,2], Paul McCague [1,2,3], Colin P. Bradley [4] and Laura J. Sahm [1,5],*

[1] Pharmaceutical Care Research Group, School of Pharmacy, University College Cork, College Road, Cork, Ireland; E-Mails: m.hoetoft@gmail.com (M.H.M.) ; pmccague01@qub.ac.uk (P.M.)

[2] Department of Drug Design and Pharmacology Faculty of Health and Medical Sciences, University of Copenhagen, Universitetsparken 2, DK-2100 Copenhagen, Denmark

[3] School of Pharmacy, Queen's University Belfast, Lisburn Road, Belfast, UK

[4] Department of General Practice, Department of General Practice,1st Floor, Brookfield Health Sciences Building, University College Cork, Cork; Ireland; C.Bradley@ucc.ie

[5] Department of Pharmacy, Mercy University Hospital, Grenville Place, Cork, Ireland

* Author to whom correspondence should be addressed; E-Mail: l.sahm@ucc.ie

Academic Editor: Keith A. Wilson

Abstract: Medicines reconciliation is a way to identify and act on discrepancies in patients' medical histories and it is found to play a key role in patient safety. This review focuses on discrepancies and medical errors that occurred at point of discharge from hospital. Studies were identified through the following electronic databases: PubMed, Sciences Direct, EMBASE, Google Scholar, Cochrane Reviews and CINAHL. Each of the six databases was screened from inception to end of January 2014. To determine eligibility of the studies; the title, abstract and full manuscript were screened to find 15 articles that meet the inclusion criteria. The median number of discrepancies across the articles was found to be 60%. In average patient had between 1.2–5.3 discrepancies when leaving the hospital. More studies also found a relation between the numbers of drugs a patient was on and the number of discrepancies. The variation in the number of discrepancies found in the 15 studies could be due to the fact that some studies excluded patient taking more than 5 drugs at admission. Medication reconciliation would be a way to avoid the high number of discrepancies that was found in this literature review and thereby increase patient safety.

Keywords: Medication reconciliation; medication errors; medication discrepancies; review

1. Introduction

Ensuring patient safety in the healthcare system is a complex challenge and involves many health care professionals across multiple institutions. One of the most common ways to prevent, manage and cure diseases and illnesses is by the use of medicines. This, however, does not come without its own set of risks. Medication errors (ME) are prevalent and costly; both in terms of patient injury and economics. Over half of these errors occur during transitions of care or at the interface of care [1–4]. According to Ferner and Aronson (2006), a medication error can be defined as "a failure in the treatment process that leads to, or has the potential to lead to, harm to the patient" [5]. This is in contrast to an adverse drug event (ADE), which is, "an actual unintended medication related event that occurs during treatment of the patient with pharmaceuticals". The difference therefore lies in the event having taken place (ADE) rather than the error (which may result in an event) being noted (ME). An example of a medication error is when a patient has not been prescribed one of their regular medicines on admission to hospital; this would be an error of omission and an ME. However, if the patient had been prescribed a medicine (even at the correct dose) that resulted in the patient experiencing an unintended side-effect (which could be anything from pruritus to anaphylaxis), this would be classed as an adverse drug event (ADE) [6,7]. It has been documented that there is a positive association between the number of medicines prescribed for a patient and the likelihood of experiencing an ME [8]. A structured handover between carers is one way in which MEs can be reduced [9]. Medication reconciliation has been acknowledged as one of the key elements to improve patient safety by decreasing MEs at discharge and transitions of care [1,10].

Medication reconciliation is defined as the process of "creating the most accurate list possible of all medications a patient is taking—including drug name, dosage, frequency and route—and comparing that list against the physician's admission, transfer and/or discharge orders, with the goal of providing correct medication to the patient at all transitions points within the hospital" [11]. Medication reconciliation consists of four steps that help to ensure patient safety across the healthcare system: (1) verification: the current medication list is obtained; (2) clarification: the medication and dosages are checked for adequacy; (3) reconciliation: newly-prescribed and previous medications are compared and documented; and (4) transmission: an updated and verified medication list is communicated to the next healthcare provider [11,12].

Two other terms that are commonly used when discussing medication reconciliation are: intentional and unintentional discrepancies. An unintentional discrepancy is one that occurs without the professional involved making a conscious decision to alter therapy. In contrast, those discrepancies that are made due to an underlying co-morbidity or change in drug metabolism (for example, a decline in renal function) are termed intentional. These intentional discrepancies will have been usually documented in a standard manner, in the medical notes, by the physician amending the prescription, as they are consciously making the decision to alter the therapy. Whilst only the unintended discrepancies can be classified as MEs, it is important to note that an intentional discrepancy may still lead to confusion and errors at discharge, if not documented clearly [7].

The aims of this literature review are to compile and analyse journal articles that focus on medication reconciliation at discharge. The objectives are to report the prevalence of ME and the mean number of discrepancies at discharge (expressed as the percentage of patients where available), as well as the most common types of errors and medications (or classes of medications) most frequently implicated.

2. Experimental Section

The following databases were used: PubMed, Sciences Direct, Excerpta Medica dataBASE (EMBASE), Google Scholar, Cochrane and, Cumulative Index to Nursing and Allied Health Literature (CINAHL). To ensure that all relevant articles were found, an advanced search strategy was undertaken. The search strategy is described in Table 1.

Articles had to meet the following inclusion/exclusion criteria.

Inclusion criteria:

- Published in English
- Quantitative studies, *i.e.*, studies that examine the prevalence of ME, or the mean number of discrepancies at discharge (expressed as the percentage of patients where available), or studies that quantify the most common types of errors and medications (or classes of medications) most frequently implicated in these errors.

Exclusion criteria:

- Duplicates
- Articles not published in English
- Review articles, meta-analysis and editorials
- Qualitative studies

The titles and abstracts of the articles found in the searches were screened for relevance before final inclusion.

Table 1. Results of the search strategy, including: search terms, limits, results, relevant studies and included studies.

Database	Search Terms	Limits	Results	Relevant Studies	Included Studies
PubMed	Medication reconciliation AND discharge AND error *	• English	105	12 (8 articles were duplicates from other databases)	4
Science Direct	Medication reconciliation AND discharge AND error *	Search in author, title and keywords	34	3	3
Cochrane	Medication reconciliation AND discharge AND error *	Search in author, title and keywords	14	2 (both duplicates from other databases)	0

Table 1. *Cont.*

Database	Search Terms	Limits	Results	Relevant Studies	Included Studies
Cumulative Index to Nursing and Allied Health Literature(CINAHL)	Medication reconciliation AND discharge AND error *	• English	25	5	5
Excerpta Medica dataBASE (EMBASE)	Medication reconciliation AND discharge AND error *	• Advanced search • English	51	10 (all duplicates from other databases)	0
Google Scholar	• With all words: error * • With the exact phrase: medication reconciliation • Where my words occur: in the title of the article		35	4 (1 was a duplicate from another database)	3
Total = 15					

The asterisk (*) is used to allow for terms that have error or errors.

Figure 1 shows a flow chart of the selection of relevant articles.

3. Results and Discussion

The key results from each article included in the literature review are summarised in Table 2.

This literature review was conducted to give an overview of the quantitative research on medicine reconciliation at hospital discharge. During the review, 270 articles were screened, after the advanced search strategy was conducted; see Figure 1. This resulted in the inclusion of 15 articles for this review (Table 2). The data from these 15 articles represent international data from over 6000 hospital discharges.

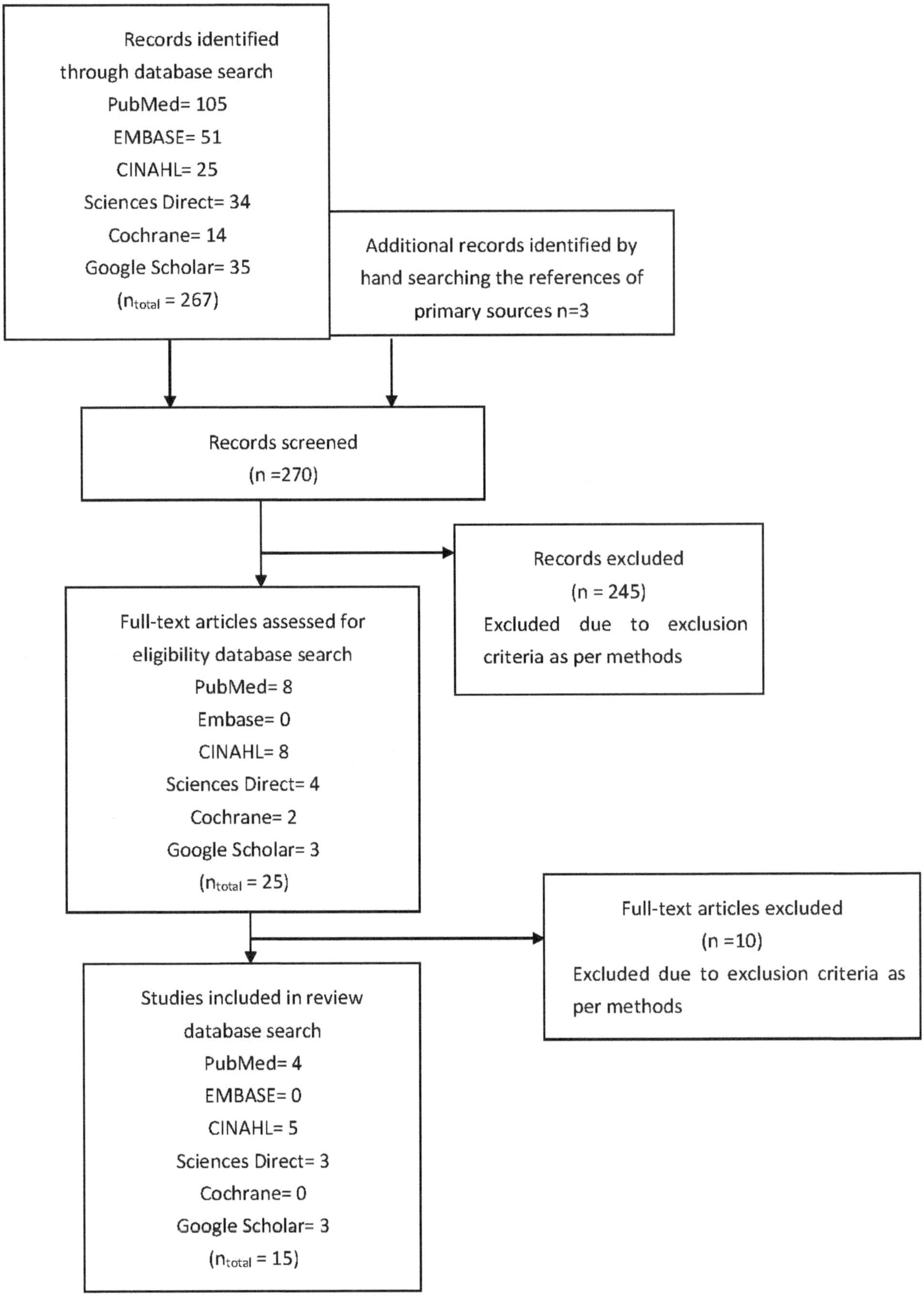

Figure 1. Flow diagram of studies assessed and included.

Table 2. Presentation of results. Key elements for each article are described.

Year	Study	Study Design	Study Population
Climente-Martí *et al.*, 2010 [13].	Potential Risk of Medication Discrepancies and Reconciliation Errors at Admission and Discharge from an Inpatient Medical Service [13]	Observational prospective study Preadmission treatment was compared with treatment prescribed on admission and discharge	Country: Spain 120 patients included Mean age: 76 years (SD 14.4) Mean number of preadmission drugs: 7.5
Key findings: 46 patients had a discrepancy at discharge corresponding to 38.3%. The most common therapeutic groups related to reconciliation errors were: blood/hematopoietic organ drugs (30%), cardiovascular (20%) and gastrointestinal agents (20%). **Limitations:** Medication list prior to admission was done through an interview with the patient or care giver; they might not always be able to give the correct information. Small sample size (n = 120) meant lack of power in the study. Clinical significance of the errors was decided in a group, which could lead to subjective bias.			
Cornu *et al.*, 2012 [14].	Effect of Medication Reconciliation at Hospital Admission on Medication Discrepancies During Hospitalization and at Discharge for Geriatric Patients [14]	Retrospective single-centre cohort study Medication reconciliation at admission, during hospitalization and at discharge was conducted by an independent pharmacist	Country: Belgium 199 patients were included Mean age: 83.7 years (SD 5.8) Mean number of preadmission drugs: 7.2
Key findings: 278 of the 682 discrepancies at admission resulted in discrepancies at discharge (40.8%). The reconciliation process at discharge revealed 554 discrepancies and a mean of 3 per patient. Omitted drugs were the cause in 47.7% of the errors at discharge. All types of discrepancy except for "drugs prescribed even though discontinued" occurred more often at discharge than during hospitalization. For every additional drug in the medication history, the likelihood of a discrepancy increased by 47%, but for every additional source used to make the medication history, the likelihood of a discrepancy decreases by 78%. **Limitations:** Recall bias; the doctor made a medication history prior to the pharmacist.			

Table 2. *Cont.*

Year	Study	Study Design	Study Population
Vira *et al.*, 2006 [15].	Reconcilable Differences: Correcting Medication Errors at Hospital Admission and Discharge [15]	Prospective study At discharge, pre-admission and in-patient medications were compared with discharge orders and written instruction	Country: Canada 60 patients included in the study only 56 at discharge Mean age: 56 years (SD 24)
Key findings: 41% had at least one unintended discrepancy at discharge, and the mean per patient was found to be 1.2. Types of unintended discrepancies: omitted medication/prescription (45%), lack of discharge instructions (51%) and incorrect details of frequency/dose/route (4%). **Limitations:** Clinical importance of the interventions was judged by a single review. Results are not generalizable due to the small sample size.			
Kripalani *et al.*, 2012 [16].	Effect of a Pharmacist Intervention on Clinically Important Medication Errors after Hospital Discharge [16]	Randomized, controlled trial Pharmacist-assisted medication reconciliation	Country: United States of America (USA) 851 patients included Mean age: 60 years (SD 14.4)
Key findings: Between 0.87 and 0.95 clinically-important errors were found per patient; 50.8% had at least one clinically-import error after discharge. 30.3% of the patients experienced a preventable adverse drug event after discharge; 13% of these resulted in a visit to the emergency department. 424 (29.7%) potential adverse drug events (ADEs) were found, half of which were related to medication discrepancies and half of which were related to non-adherence. The most common medication discrepancies were found to be: omission (34.5%), incorrect dose (32.9%), incorrect frequency (15.9%) and additional medicine that should not be on the list (11.9%). **Limitations:** The patient population had acute cardiovascular problems. The types of interventions may differ from other wards and make generalization difficult. Not all patients received the full intervention as intended			

Table 2. *Cont.*

Year	Study	Study Design	Study Population
Karapinar-Carkit *et al.*, 2009 [10].	Effect of Medication Reconciliation with and without Patient Counselling on the Number of Pharmaceutical Interventions among Patients Discharged from the Hospital [10]	Prospective observational study To examine the effect of medication reconciliation with and without patient counselling	Country: Netherlands Including 262 patients Mean age: 65 years (SD 17.3) Mean number of drugs preadmission: 6.6 Mean number of drugs at discharge: 9.1
Key findings: For patients without counselling, the number of intervention after medication reconciliation at discharge was 2.7 per patient, compared to 5.3 interventions per patient whom received counselling. 72.5% of the study population had discrepancies at discharge; the most common were that the physician forgot to restart medication, which had been temporarily discontinued during hospitalization. Interventions for stopping a drug were made for 55% of the patients with patient counselling and 41.6% for the patients without; the most common drugs stopped were: laxatives (13.5%), gastric acid suppressants (13.1%) and sedatives (7.6%); the reason for stopping these drugs was "no indication". **Limitations:** The study did not assess the impact on patient outcome after intervention. High exclusion rate, *i.e.*, patients living in nursing homes were not included in this study.			
Pippins *et al.*, 2008 [17].	Classifying and Predicting Errors of Inpatient Medication Reconciliation [17]	Prospective observational study To compare medication histories with admission and discharge orders	Country: USA 180 patients were included <50 years: 21% 50–60 years: 20% 60–75 years: 22% >75 years: 37% Number of discharge drugs: 11
Key findings: 2066 medication discrepancies were detected; 45% of these were classified as unintentional and 27% of these had potential harm for the patient. 54% of the patients had at least one potential adverse drug event (PADE). Most PADEs were due to errors in taking the preadmission medication history (72%). PADEs divided in to therapeutic categories: cardiovascular (20%), respiratory (9%), gastrointestinal (8%), lipid-lowering (6%) and antidepressant (5%) **Limitations:** Patients with a short stay at the ward were not included; this could lead to a study population with more complex medication and diseases. Study measured PADEs and not actual ADEs.			

Table 2. *Cont.*

Year	Study	Study Design	Study Population
Salanitro *et al.*, 2012 [18].	Effect of Patient- and Medication-Related Factors on Inpatient Medication Reconciliation Errors [18]	Cross-sectional analysis To identify medication-related factors that contribute to pre-admission medication list error and to test whether this error exists in the discharge medication list	Country: USA 423 patients were included Mean age: 61 years (SD 14) Mean number of preadmission drugs: 8 Mean number of discharge drugs: 10
Key findings: 158 patients (40%) had a medication error (ME) at discharge. The number of preadmission list errors and the number of medication changed during the hospitalization were significantly associated with the number of MEs identified at discharge. The number of MEs at discharge was less common for people living alone and people with cognitive impairment. **Limitations:** The pharmacist classified the severity of clinical relevant MEs, which could lead to subjective bias. This study was conducted at a hospital with electronic medical records and may differ from hospitals with a paper-based medical record.			
Paiboonvong *et al.*, 2009 [19].	Incidence of Medication Errors in Medication Reconciliation at General Medical Wards, Ramathibodi Hospital [19]	Prospective descriptive study To determine MEs through medication reconciliation during transition phases	Country: Thailand 107 patients were enrolled in this study Mean age: 57.3 years (SD 19.6) Mean number of pre-admission drugs: 6.2
Key findings: Intentional discrepancies were found in 69.5%, and unintentional discrepancies were found in 89.5% of the patients. In 16% of the patients, an ME was identified at discharge with a mean number of MEs per patient of 1.1; the class of drug most often causing MEs was anti-hyperglycaemic drugs (33.3%). Types of MEs identified at discharge: omission (55.6%) and different route, dose or frequency (44.4%) 94.4% of the MEs were prevented by the pharmacist. **Limitations:** A small study population; bias in the inclusion of patients. No interviews with patients to confirm the medication list at admission.			

Table 2. *Cont.*

Year	Study	Study Design	Study Population
Stitt *et al.*, 2011 [20].	Medication Discrepancies Identified at Time of Hospital Discharge in Geriatric Population [20]	Retrospective review of a random cohort Identify discharge medication list discrepancies	Country: USA A randomized population of 200 patients was included Mean age: 77.2 years (range 66–97) Receiving on average 13.4 medications
Key findings: In all, 1923 medication discrepancies were reported in the discharge summary, discharge orders and medication list, during the study; the most common was in relation to the route of administration. 1380 of the discrepancies were found in the physician discharge summary, whereas only 191 were found in the physician discharge orders. A linear relationship was found between the number of medications at time of discharge and the number of medication discrepancies (p-value = 0.001) 55 patients were in wards with a pharmacist, and a significantly lower number of discrepancies per patient was found for these patients. Medication discrepancies divided into therapeutic categories: central nervous system (21.1%), cardiovascular (20.8%), nutrients (13.5%), endocrine/metabolic (11.5%), gastrointestinal (8.5%), respiratory (8.4%), haematological (5.2%), renal (4.9%), anti-microbial (3.6%) and others (2.5%) **Limitations:** Retrospective design, which made it impossible to detect if a pharmacist was present for all patients during discharge at the "pharmacist-ward". During the discharge preparation time, final medication changes may occur after the medicine list has been printed, and this could lead to a change in the number of discrepancies.			
Knez *et al.*, 2011 [7].	The Need for Medication Reconciliation: A Cross-Sectional Observational Study in Adult Patients [7]	Prospective descriptive cross-sectional observational study Pre-admission therapy was compared with in-patient and discharge therapy	Country: Slovenia 101 patients were included Median age: 73 years (IQR: 65–79) Median number of pre admission drugs: 6
Key findings: Overall, the study population was prescribed 747 drugs at discharge, and it was found that 75.8% (n = 566) was in discordance with pre-admission therapy. At discharge, the percentage of MEs was 65.2%, and of this, 58.0% was rated to be clinically important. 84.2% of the patients were found to have one ME, and a median of 3 MEs per patient was recorded. Reasons for discrepancies at discharge were found to be: drug omission (28.8%), discrepancy in dose (13.8%), drug substitution (14.7%) and others (15.4%). Reasons for MEs: drug omission (40.4%), discrepancy in drug dose (15.7%) drug omission (17.9%), drug substitution (13.3%) and others (12.7%). **Limitations:** Only 101 patients were included, and it was only performed at a single site.			

Table 2. *Cont.*

Year	Study	Study Design	Study Population
Herrero-Herrero *et al.*, 2010 [21].	Medication Discrepancies at Discharge from an Internal Medicine Service [21]	Descriptive retrospective study Review on non-selected discharge reports to find discrepancies	Country: Spain Data from 790 patients corresponding to 954 discharge reports were included. Median age: 83 (SD 11) Median number of pre admission drugs: 6 Median number of discharge drugs: 7
Key findings: In 832 cases (87.2%), discrepancies were found in the reconciliation process (including justified and unjustified discrepancies). Intentional discrepancies were recorded in 828 (median 3; range 0–13 discrepancies per discharge report). Unintentional discrepancies were recorded in 52 (5.4%) discharge reports. The most frequent medication reconciliation error was drug omission (84.6%). The 5.4% with unintentional discrepancies was found to have a significantly higher number of permanent medication at admission, 7.5 medications against 6.2 (p-value = 0.005) **Limitations:** Chronic medication was not looked at when doing the medication reconciliation. This could be an explanation for the low number of errors recorded. This hospital may not be representative of all hospitals, because medication reconciliation is already an incorporated part of the work day.			
Allende Bandrés *et al.*, 2013 [1].	Pharmacist-Led Medication Reconciliation to Reduce Discrepancies in Transitions of Care in Spain [1]	Retrospective descriptive study The object was to quantify and analyse reconciliation unjustified discrepancies	Country: Spain Reviewed 1150 patients treatment Average age: 76.4 years (range 15–101)
Key findings: 1 in 5 patients had a discrepancy, and the reconciliation errors per patient w 1.93. Most frequently unjustified discrepancies (reconciliation errors): incomplete prescriptions (63.86%), omission (16.63%), different dosage/frequency/route (10.51%), wrong drug (1.85%) and other (0.35%). Therapeutic groups most often associated with medication reconciliation interventions: cardiovascular system (CVS) (34.02%) and CNS (21.85%). **Limitations:** Only unjustified discrepancies were recorded, and this could lead to an underestimate compared to other studies. Medication reconciliation at discharge was only conducted for patients taking more than 5 drugs (n = 1150); at admission, medication reconciliation was conducted for all included patients (n = 2573).			

Table 2. *Cont.*

Year	Study	Study Design	Study Population
Bjeldbak-Olesen *et al.*, 2013 [22].	Medication Reconciliation Is a Prerequisite for Obtaining a Valid Medication Review [22]	Retrospective study Comparing medication review with medication reconciliation	Country: Denmark 75 patients included in the study Mean age: 71.7 years Mean number of pre admission drugs: 5.9
Key findings: 198 discrepancies were identified during the study; 2.6 discrepancies per patient. 109 undocumented changes were found (changes where the physician did not state any reason). 86.7% of the patients had a discrepancy, and 69.3% had between 1 and 6. Types of discrepancies: omission of drug in discharge summery, extra/analogous drug in discharge summary, non-recognizable drug, uncertainty of dosage, unnecessary drug and other. **Limitations:** Categories of errors are empirically based. Small study population; a bigger study population would give the study more power and validity.			
Geurts *et al.*, 2013 [23].	Medication Reconciliation to Solve Discrepancies in Discharge Documents after Discharge from the Hospital [23]	Retrospective single-site study To evaluate the number, type and origin of discrepancies in discharge documents	Country: Netherlands 100 discharge documents (83 patients) Mean age: 63.1 years (SD 17) Mean number of pre admission drugs: 7 Mean number of discharge drugs: 8.3
Key findings: 223 discrepancies were detected, correlating to 2.2 discrepancies per discharge. 155 out of 223 (69.5%) led to a change in the discharge medicine after the pharmacy had contacted the patients' medical specialist. For each additional drug added after discharge, there was an increase of 9.8% in the number of interventions preformed. **Limitations:** Small study population. Single site study.			

Table 2. *Cont.*

Year	Study	Study Design	Study Population
Grimes *et al.*, 2011 [24]	Medication Details Documented on Hospital Discharge: Cross-Sectional Observational Study of Factors Associated with Medication Non-Reconciliation [24]	Cross-sectional observational healthcare record review survey Medication non-reconciliation, prescribing errors at discharge or lack of document for changes	Country: Ireland 1246 episodes of care were investigated Median age: 62 years (Range 16–96) Median number of pre admission drugs: 5

Key findings:

In 624 (50.1%) of the cases examined, a minimum of one medication was found; the most common reason was omission of a drug at discharge.

Patients with a chronic condition were twice as likely to experience problems with reconciliation as patients with an acute condition.

For each additional medication, a patient had a 26% increased likelihood of experiencing non-reconciliation.

Limitations:

The Hawthorne effect could lead to an underestimation of non-reconciliation.

Of the included studies, six were retrospective [1,14,20–23], and six were prospective studies [7,10,13,15,17,19]. The advantages of these types of studies include the ability to examine multiple outcomes of a single risk factor. The disadvantages of retrospective studies include: (i) if records that were not designed for the study are used, the available data may be of poor quality; (ii) there can be frequently an absence of data on potential confounding factors; and (iii) it may be difficult to identify an appropriate exposed cohort and an appropriate comparison group. Disadvantages of prospective cohort studies include: (i) having to follow large numbers of subjects for a long time; (ii) expensive and time consuming; (iii) not good for rare diseases or diseases with a long latency; and (iv) differential loss to follow up can introduce bias.

Furthermore, one study was a randomised clinical trial (RCT) [16], and two were cross-sectional observational studies [18,24]. An RCT is classified as the gold standard in the clinical setting, as it can greatly reduce the confounding factors by random assignment and, hence, make the study and control groups equivalent at study outset. This (plus any additional blinding) enables a cause and effect relationship to be established. However, the challenge with RCTs in medication reconciliation (MR) studies is that, in effect, you have to conduct MR (or a form thereof) on the controlled group to elicit medication-related problems, and so, most studies are not described as RCTs. Observational studies however reach a conclusion by comparing subjects against a control group, in cases where the researcher has no control over the experiment. One of the primary drivers for undertaking observational research is ethical concerns. One of the main challenges associated with observational studies is that the investigator has no control over the configuration of the control groups and cannot randomise the allocation of subjects. This can lead to bias and may also mask cause and effect relationships or, alternatively, suggest associations where there are none.

The number of included patients/discharges in each article varied from 60–1246. The reason for the big differences in numbers of included subjects can be explained by the fact that some of the studies were conducted at a single site and for a short period of data collection, as evidenced in the work of Vira *et al.* [15]. In contrast, the work presented by Grimes *et al.* [24] was conducted at two sites over a 29-month period. Another key difference is that in some articles, they have looked at patients, whereas other articles have looked at discharges during the study period. This means that one patient could appear in the study on more than one occasion. It is well established that increasing the sample size/study population increases the power of the study and the ability to detect with any degree of accuracy the differences between sample cohorts [25]. The mean age of the study populations for the fifteen articles varies from 56 years (standard deviation (SD) 24 years) [15] to 84 years (SD 5.8 years) in the Cornu *et al.* (2012) [14] study. The mean age in the studies included in this review is 69 (SD 9.1) years, which indicates that overall, the study population would be categorized as elderly. Due to the fact that patients taking five or more drugs are increasingly likely to be found in the older population, it is not surprising that the number of preadmission drugs are high and varies from five [24] to eight drugs per patient [18].

One of the factors identified as having a significant impact on the risk of discrepancies and ME at discharge is the number of drugs a patient is prescribed. For every additional drug, a patient is taking the risk of being exposed to discrepancies, which could lead to increased ME. Cornu *et al.* has identified this increased risk to be 47% for each additional drug prescribed [14]. Similarly, Stitt *et al.* refer to a linear relationship between the number of drugs prescribed at discharge and the volume of discrepancies at discharge [20]. A Canadian study has shown an increase in the likelihood of potential drug–drug interactions for patients aged more than 50 years due to the significant increase in the number of medication used per patient [26]. Whilst this finding is not a surprise and follows a simple proportionality association, e.g., the more drugs prescribed, the more drugs errors identified, it is worth noting that this is the case.

Ideally, the same variables would have been collected within each of the 15 studies, and the studies would have been conducted in the same way. This would ensure that a direct comparison would be possible. However, this is not the case, as there are methodological variances between the studies, which, in turn, leads to the variances in the data extracted from the each study. Specifically, the use of non-standard MR processes in Climente-Martí *et al.* (2010) [13], Cornu *et al.* (2012) [14], Paiboonvong *et al.* (2009) [19] and Herrero-Herrero *et al.* (2010) [21] is a further limitation.

One of the crucial differences between the studies is the way in which discrepancies were designated to be “intentional” or “unintentional”. In most studies, a panel including physicians and pharmacists decided if a discrepancy qualified as intentional or unintentional. This allowed for a range of healthcare professionals to be involved and, hence, is more likely to imitate usual care and take into account the views and knowledge of a range of stakeholders. In Herrero-Herrero *et al.* [21], the treating physician was solely in charge of performing the medication reconciliation, which could lead to a potential bias in the error-reporting mechanism. These differences in the classification systems and the level of consensus involved in the reporting may account for the variation of the results in between studies. To conduct a research study on medication, reconciliation guidelines regarding inclusion and exclusion of patients have to be structured. Ideally, these criteria are made to ensure that the study population reflects the population that is of interest. In the study conducted by Pippins *et al.*, patients with “short stays” at the ward were not included; the definition of a short stay was not specified in the article, but this could lead to an overestimate of discrepancies, because only those patients who were relatively more complex (and hence, had a longer stay) were included [17]. On the other hand, the exclusion of patients from nursing homes and patients taking more than five drugs could potentially lead to a significantly lower number of both MEs and discrepancies than would otherwise be the case [1,10,27].

For the six prospective studies included in this review, it is important to consider the Hawthorne effect, as suggested by Grimes *et al.* [24]. This effect can result in modified behaviour of those under observation and, hence, may distort the findings; potentially leading to an underestimate of the errors found.

By comparison of the preadmission medication list against the discharge medication list, discrepancies are identified. After a discrepancy is identified, it might lead to an ME, but this is not always the case. For example, new medications appearing on the discharge list (compared to the admissions list) would be categorised as an intentional discrepancy, but not an ME. Focusing on unintentional discrepancies only, the results of Allende Bandrés *et al.* [1] (20%) could have been unrealistically low due to the exclusion of patients taking more than five drugs at discharge and the recording of unjustified/undocumented discrepancies only. In the same way, Bjeldbak-Olsen *et al.* [22] may have overestimated the number of discrepancies by including both intentional and unintentional discrepancies, thereby reporting 86.7% discrepancies at discharge, which is higher than most studies. As the range of discrepancies varies widely and is not uniformly reported, the median value (60%) is possibly the most useful.

The variation in the inclusion and exclusion criteria of the studies examined further contributes to the wide range of reported discrepancies at discharge. If only simple (*versus* multi-morbid) patients treated with fewer than five medications are included, the number of discrepancies was lower [14]. The average number of discrepancies detected per patient varies from 1.2–5.3, although five of the seven studies that measured average discrepancy per patient found it to be around 2–3. This implies that the majority of patients who leave hospital may have more than one medication discrepancy and, therefore, could be at risk of an ME. This is supported by other studies that state that the likelihood of an ME or potential adverse drug events (PADE) increases for patients with medication discrepancies [17,28]. In addition, the variation in the geographical location of the studies under consideration may also contribute to the differences observed.

The most common discrepancy described in the literature is omission of medication. Omission was found to be the reason for discrepancies in up to 56% of the cases in one study [19]. The other major reasons for discrepancies were inaccuracies related to route/frequency/dose of medicines; one study found that these three factors were the reason for up to 44% of the discrepancies [19]. These findings are supported by other studies, where the main reasons identified for discrepancies in medical history were identified as omitted medication, as well as inconsistencies in route/frequency/dose [29,30].

The therapeutic group most frequently associated with errors regarding medication reconciliation are cardiovascular system (CVS) drugs [1]. The frequency of errors due to CVS drugs was between 20% and 34% [1,13]. The prevalence of cardiovascular diseases (CVD) worldwide is increasing, and some even describe CVD as an epidemic [31]. Many CVD patients are treated with multiple drugs, which increases the risk of ME [32]. Other therapeutic classes involved in errors during medication reconciliation are central nervous system (CNS) drugs (21%) [20] and gastrointestinal (GI) drugs (8%–20%) [10,14]. An Irish study was conducted based on the Health Service Executive (HSE)-Primary care reimbursement services (PCRS) pharmacy database. HSE-PCRS provides free or reduced health services to an estimated 1.2 million people in the Republic of Ireland (accounting for approximately 26% of the total population). This study found that the four most common therapeutic areas that patients were treated for were CVS, CNS, musculoskeletal and GI. Furthermore, this study estimated that three-quarters of the elderly population (defined in this dataset as those aged greater than 70 years) suffer from two or more chronic diseases [33]. The Institute for Safer Medication Practices (ISMP), a non-profit organization in the United States of America working for increased patient safety, has made a list of high-risk drugs according to the Anatomical Therapeutic Chemical Classification system (ATC). When looking at this list, more than 50% of the drugs on the list belong to the groups N (nervous system) and C (cardiovascular system) in the ATC drug classification system. This is due to the greater risk of causing harm if errors are made with this drugs [34]. Not all of the articles have made it clear what types of therapeutics are involved in errors. The types of drug and the frequency of discrepancy most likely change from ward to ward. Studies suggest that specialised wards, e.g., GI *versus* a general medical ward, tend to be associated with fewer errors, as they usually have a more limited range of illness-specific medicines, and staff at these wards is more experienced in their prescribing [21].

4. Conclusions

In the studies reviewed, between 20% and 87% of patients encounter discrepancies at discharge. This shows that there is a problem and one that the healthcare system needs to address. Unquestionably, the number of discrepancies per patient and the types of drugs will differ not only between hospitals, but also between wards at the hospital. A key finding is that as the number of drugs increases, so too does the risk of discrepancies, putting patients with multi-morbid conditions and receiving more than one drug at greater risk. The reasons for medical discrepancies differ, but the most common was related to omission of medication together with discrepancies in route/frequency/dose.

Author Contributions

Laura J Sahm and Paul McCague developed the initial concept in consultation with Maja Michaelsen and Colin Bradley. Maja H Michaelsen performed the article search, having defined keywords, inclusion and exclusion criteria with Laura J Sahm and Paul McCague. Results were discussed amongst all authors; Maja Michaelsen, Paul McCague, Colin Bradley and Laura J Sahm and consensus was achieved on which key results should be displayed.

Conflicts of Interest

The authors declare no conflicts of interest.

References

1. Allende Bandres, M.A.; Arenere Mendoza, M.; Gutierrez Nicolas, F.; Calleja Hernandez, M.A.; Ruiz La Iglesia, F. Pharmacist-led medication reconciliation to reduce discrepancies in transitions of care in Spain. *Int. J. Clin. Pharm.* **2013**, *35*, 1083–1090.
2. Cawthon, C.; Walia, S.; Osborn, C.Y.; Niesner, K.J.; Schnipper, J.L.; Kripalani, S. Improving care transitions: The patient perspective. *J. Health Commun.* **2012**, *17*, 312–324.
3. Andel, C.; Davidow, S.L.; Hollander, M.; Moreno, D.A. The economics of health care quality and medical errors. *J. Health Care Financ.* **2012**, *39*, 39–50.
4. Mallow, P.J.; Padya, B.; Horblyuk, R.; Kaplan, H.S. Prevalence and cost of hospital medical errors in the general and elderly United States populations. *J. Med. Econ.* **2013**, *16*, 1367–1378.
5. Ferner, R.E.; Aronson, J.K. Clarification of terminology in medication errors: definitions and classification. *Drug Saf.* **2006**, *29*, 1011–1022.
6. Bates, D.W.; Boyle, D.L.; Vander Vliet, M.B.; Schneider, J.; Leape, L. Relationship between medication errors and adverse drug events. *Gen. Intern. Med.* **1995**, *10*, 199–205.
7. Knez, L.; Suskovic, S.; Rezonja, R.; Laaksonen, R.; Mrhar, A. The need for medication reconciliation: A cross-sectional observational study in adult patients. *Respir. Med.* **2011**, *105*, S60–S66.
8. Frydenberg, K.; Brekke, M. Poor communication on patients' medication across health care levels leads to potentially harmful medication errors. *Scand. J. Primary Health Care* **2012**, *30*, 234–240.
9. Ziaeian, B.; Araujo, K.L.; van Ness, P.H.; Horwitz, L.I. Medication reconciliation accuracy and patient understanding of intended medication changes on hospital discharge. *J. Gen. Intern. Med.* **2012**, *27*, 1513–1520.

10. Karapinar-Carkit, F.; Borgsteede, S.D.; Zoer, J.; Smit, H.J.; Egberts, A.C.; van den Bemt, P.M. Effect of medication reconciliation with and without patient counseling on the number of pharmaceutical interventions among patients discharged from the hospital. *Ann. Pharmacother.* **2009**, *43*, 1001–1010.
11. Institution for Healthcare Improvment. How-to- Guide: prevent Adverse Drug Events by Implementing Medication Reconciliation. Available online: http://www.texashospitalquality.org/collaboratives/partnership_for_patients/pfp_resources/pfp_2012_conference_documents/adverse_drug_events/4_HowtoGuidePreventADEs.pdf (accessed on 16 June 2015)
12. Joint Commission on Accreditation of Healthcare Organizations, USA. Using medication reconciliation to prevent errors. *Sentin. Event Alert* **2006**, *23*, 1–4.
13. Climente-Marti, M.; Garcia-Manon, E.R.; Artero-Mora, A.; Jimenez-Torres, N.V. Potential risk of medication discrepancies and reconciliation errors at admission and discharge from an inpatient medical service. *Ann. Pharmacother.* **2010**, *44*, 1747–1754.
14. Cornu, P.; Steurbaut, S.; Leysen, T.; de Baere, E.; Ligneel, C.; Mets, T.; Dupont, A.G. Effect of medication reconciliation at hospital admission on medication discrepancies during hospitalization and at discharge for geriatric patients. *Ann. Pharmacother.* **2012**, *46*, 484–494.
15. Vira, T.; Colquhoun, M.; Etchells, E. Reconcilable differences: correcting medication errors at hospital admission and discharge. *Qual. Saf. Health Care* **2006**, *15*, 122–126.
16. Kripalani, S.; Roumie, C.L.; Dalal, A.K.; Cawthon, C.; Businger, A.; Eden, S.K.; Shintani, A.; Sponsler, K.C.; Harris, L.J.; Theobald, C.; *et al.* Effect of a pharmacist intervention on clinically important medication errors after hospital discharge: a randomized trial. *Ann. Intern. Med.* **2012**, *157*, 1–10.
17. Pippins, J.R.; Gandhi, T.K.; Hamann, C.; Ndumele, C.D.; Labonville, S.A.; Diedrichsen, E.K.; Carty, M.G.; Karson, A.S.; Bhan, I.; Coley, C.M.; *et al.* Classifying and predicting errors of inpatient medication reconciliation. *J. Gen. Intern. Med.* **2008**, *23*, 1414–1422.
18. Salanitro, A.H.; Osborn, C.Y.; Schnipper, J.L.; Roumie, C.L.; Labonville, S.; Johnson, D.C.; Neal, E.; Cawthon, C.; Businger, A.; *et al.* Effect of patient- and medication-related factors on inpatient medication reconciliation errors. *J. Gen. Intern. Med.* **2012**, *27*, 924–932.
19. Paiboonvong, T.M.; Montakantikul, P.; Chansirkarnjana, S.; Trangulpiankit, P. Incidence of Medication Errors in Medication Reconciliation at General Medical Wards, Ramathibodi Hospital. *J. Pharm. Sci.* **2009**, *36*, 44–49.
20. Stitt, D.M.; Elliott, D.P.; Thompson, S.N. Medication discrepancies identified at time of hospital discharge in a geriatric population. *Am. J. Geriatr. Pharmacother.* **2011**, *9*, 234–240.
21. Herrero-Herrero, J.I.; Garcia-Aparicio, J. Medication discrepancies at discharge from an internal medicine service. *Eur. J. Intern. Med.* **2011**, *22*, 43–48.
22. Bjeldbak-Olesen, M.; Danielsen, A.G.; Tomsen, D.V.; Jakobsen, T.J. Medication reconciliation is a prerequisite for obtaining a valid medication review. *Dan. Med. J.* **2013**, *60*, A4605.
23. Geurts, M.M.; van der Flier, M.; de Vries-Bots, A.M.; Brink-van der Wal, T.I.; de Gier, J.J. Medication reconciliation to solve discrepancies in discharge documents after discharge from the hospital. *Int. J. Clin. Pharm.* **2013**, *35*, 600–607.

24. Grimes, T.C.; Duggan, C.A.; Delaney, T.P.; Graham, I.M.; Conlon, K.C.; Deasy, E.; Jago-Byrne, M.C.; O'Brien, P. Medication details documented on hospital discharge: Cross-sectional observational study of factors associated with medication non-reconciliation. *Br. J. Clinical Pharmacol.* **2011**, *71*, 449–457.
25. Suresh, K.; Chandrashekara, S. Sample size estimation and power analysis for clinical research studies. *J. Hum. Reprod. Sci.* **2012**, *5*, 7–13.
26. Tseng, A.; Szadkowski, L.; Walmsley, S.; Salit, I.; Raboud, J. Association of age with polypharmacy and risk of drug interactions with antiretroviral medications in HIV-positive patients. *Ann. Pharmacother.* **2013**, *47*, 1429–1439.
27. Hovstadius, B.; Hovstadius, K.; Astrand, B.; Petersson, G. Increasing polypharmacy—An individual-based study of the Swedish population 2005–2008. *BMC Clin. Pharmacol.* **2010**, *10*, 16.
28. Turple, J.; MacKinnon, N.J.; Davis, B. Frequency and type of medication discrepancies in one tertiary care hospital. *Healthc. Q.* **2006**, *9*, 119–123.
29. Lisby, M.N.; Nielsen, L.P.; Mainz, J. Errors in the medication process: Frequency, type and potential clinical consequences. *Int. J. Qual. Health Care* **2005**, *17*, 15–22.
30. Nickerson, A.; MacKinnon, N.J.; Roberts, N.; Saulnier, L. Drug-therapy problems, inconsistencies and omissions identified during a medication reconciliation and seamless care service. *Healthc. Q.* **2005**, *8*, 65–72.
31. Gersh, B.S.; Sliwa, K.; Mayosi, B.M.; Yusuf, S. The epidemic of cardiovascular disease in the developing world: global implications. *Eur. Heart J.* **2010**, *31*, 642–648
32. Volpe, M.; Chin, D.; Paneni, F. The challenge of polypharmacy in cardiovascular medicine. *Fundam. Clin. Pharmacol.* **2010**, *24*, 9–17.
33. Naughton, C.; Bennett, K.; Feely, J. Prevalence of chronic disease in the elderly based on a national pharmacy claims database. *Age Ageing* **2006**, *35*, 633–636.
34. ISMPs List of High-Alert Medications. Available online: http://www.ismp.org/tools/highalertmedications.pdf (accessed on 3 March 2014).

12

The PHAR-QA Project: Competency Framework for Pharmacy Practice—First Steps, the Results of the European Network Delphi Round 1

Jeffrey Atkinson [1,*], Kristien De Paepe [2], Antonio Sánchez Pozo [3], Dimitrios Rekkas [4], Daisy Volmer [5], Jouni Hirvonen [6], Borut Bozic [7], Agnieska Skowron [8], Constantin Mircioiu [9], Annie Marcincal [10], Andries Koster [11], Keith Wilson [12] and Chris van Schravendijk [13]

[1] Pharmacology Department Lorraine University, Pharmacolor Consultants Nancy, 12 rue de Versigny, Villers 54600, France

[2] Department of Pharmaceutical and Pharmacological Sciences, Research group of In Vitro Toxicology and Dermato-Cosmetology, Vrije Universiteit Brussel, Laarbeeklaan 103, Brussels 1090, Belgium; E-Mail: kdepaepe@vub.ac.be

[3] Faculty of Pharmacy, University of Granada (UGR), Campus Universitario de la Cartuja s/n, Granada 18701, Spain; E-Mail: sanchezpster@gmail.com

[4] School of Pharmacy, National and Kapodistrian University Athens, Panepistimiou 30, Athens 10679, Greece; E-Mail: rekkas@pharm.uoa.gr

[5] Pharmacy Faculty, University of Tartu, Nooruse 1, Tartu 50411, Estonia; E-Mail: daisy.volmer@ut.ee

[6] Pharmacy Faculty, University of Helsinki, Yliopistonkatu 4, P.O. Box 33-4, Helsinki 00014, Finland; E-Mail: jouni.hirvonen@helsinki.fi

[7] Faculty of Pharmacy, University of Ljubljana, Askerceva cesta 7, Ljubljana 1000, Slovenia; E-Mail: Borut.Bozic@ffa.uni-lj.si

[8] Pharmacy Faculty, Jagiellonian University, UL, Golebia 24, Krakow 31-007, Poland; E-Mail: askowron@cm-uj.krakow.pl

[9] Pharmacy Faculty, University of Medicine and Pharmacy "Carol Davila" Bucharest, Dionisie Lupu 37, Bucharest 020021, Romania; E-Mail: constantin.mircioiu@yahoo.com

[10] European Association of Faculties of Pharmacy, Faculty of Pharmacy, Université de Lille 2, Lille 59000, France; E-Mail: annie.marcincal@univ-lille2.fr

[11] European Association of Faculties of Pharmacy, Department Pharmaceutical Sciences, Utrecht University, P.O. Box 80082, 3508 TB Utrecht, The Netherlands; E-Mail: A.S.Koster@uu.nl

[12] School of Life and Health Sciences, Aston University, Birmingham B4 7ET, UK; E-Mail: k.a.wilson@aston.ac.uk

[13] MEDINE2, Vrije Universiteit Brussel, Laarbeeklaan 103, 1090 Brussels, Belgium; E-Mail: chrisvs@vub.ac.be

* Author to whom correspondence should be addressed; E-Mail: jeffrey.atkinson@univ-lorraine.fr

Academic Editor: Yvonne Perrie

Abstract: PHAR-QA, funded by the European Commission, is producing a framework of competences for pharmacy practice. The framework is in line with the EU directive on sectoral professions and takes into account the diversity of the pharmacy profession and the on-going changes in healthcare systems (with an increasingly important role for pharmacists), and in the pharmaceutical industry. PHAR-QA is asking academia, students and practicing pharmacists to rank competences required for practice. The results show that competences in the areas of "drug interactions", "need for drug treatment" and "provision of information and service" were ranked highest whereas those in the areas of "ability to design and conduct research" and "development and production of medicines" were ranked lower. For the latter two categories, industrial pharmacists ranked them higher than did the other five groups.

Keywords: pharmacy; competence; education; practice

---

1. Introduction

Competences, and resulting learning outcomes, are more meaningful indicators than course content or duration. Furthermore, a profession such as pharmacy is defined by competences that are regularly refined in order to fulfill society's demands.

The PHAR-QA project [1] will produce a consensual, harmonized competence framework for pharmacy practice to be used as a base for a QA system for evaluation of university pharmacy education and training at the institutional, national and/or European levels. The framework is in line with the European Union (EU) directive 2013/55/EU on sectoral professions [2] and takes into account the diversity of the pharmacy profession as well as the on-going changes in healthcare systems (with an increasingly important role for pharmacists), and in the pharmaceutical industry. The varying impact of these different factors on pharmacy education in the European setting has been described in detail elsewhere [3–5].

The PHAR-QA consortium is working essentially within the context of 2 of the 5 pillars of the "pillars and foundations of quality" model of the International Pharmaceutical Federation (FIP) [6] namely "context" and "process". Regarding context, the internal environment *i.e.*, the department and university levels, is similar in Europe to that of departments in other regions like the USA, Canada or Australia. The external environment *i.e.*, the political and legal context is somewhat different. Whilst the EU directive 2013/55/EU aims at ensuring competence for pharmacy practice and gives some indications of how education can be organized to provide such competences, it also, importantly, fixes the minimum requirements for pharmacists wishing to work in a different member state country from that in which they received their education and training. This ensures the fundamental principle of the EU that is free movement across borders. EU directives are governed by comitology the process by which a directive acceptable to all members is produced. Within this context, competence frameworks are needed as a tool for international recognition when dealing with the different educational systems and programs in different EU member states. In healthcare more generally, frameworks are designed as educational and developmental tools used both in academia and in practice, both foundation formation and continuous professional development [7–10]. This is the case for competence frameworks that are being developed in individual European countries like Serbia [11], Lithuania [12], Ireland [13], and the UK [14].

The second aspect concerns the pillar "process" which in the FIP document cited above includes nine different activities from strategic planning to appraisal and development of academic staff. This article deals specifically with the seventh of these "process" activities: curricular development and improvement. The framework is intended for a European 5-year pharmacy degree.

Under the auspices of EAFP [15], PHAR-QA brought together several of the major players in pharmacy education from "old" and "new Europe", and from eastern, western, southern and northern Europe (the authors).

The methodology was based similar on that of MEDINE (Medical Education in Europe) [16] in which a framework for medical competences was proposed. Furthermore, PHAR-QA has a representative from MEDINE to help solve the many difficulties of this complex type of project.

In UK English "competence" is defined by the Oxford English Dictionary in four main ways, way 4a being "sufficiency of qualification; capacity to deal adequately with a subject" [17]. In American English, Merriam-Webster's dictionary defines "competence" as "the ability to do something well" [18]. We have used the word in this way with the additional subdivision of propositions for competences into (1) "knowledge" = "being aware of" and thus capable of applying; and (2) "ability" = "capable of doing". Thus, our definition of competence is in line with that of the American Council on Credentialing in Pharmacy [19]: "competence is the ability of a pharmacist based on his knowledge and experience to make the right decision in favor of his patient".

Stakeholders are the major EU pharmacy agencies and associations: PGEU [20], EPSA [21], EAHP [22], and EIPG [23]. PHAR-QA has made contact with pharmacy education QA agencies in the USA (ACPE [24]) and in Australia and New Zealand (PhLOS [25]). This has led to interesting and useful verbal exchange the essence of which has been transcribed into this paper.

2. Methodology

The two main phases of the PHAR-QA project were (1) 3 Delphi rounds within the consortium (authors of this paper), finishing with the development of the PHAR-QA competence framework; and (2) a European-wide survey to refine the framework in a further 2 Delphi rounds and obtain harmonized EU backing for the framework. Thus, the project uses a modified Delphi approach [26]:

(1) Initial questionnaire—round 1 questionnaire was produced by A. Sanchez-Pozo and D. Rekkas using various references [2,27–33] together with comments from the other authors.

(2) Evaluation by the consortial expert panel (the authors)—the round 1 questionnaire was modified in three Delphi rounds, the panel providing rankings and comments on what was unclear, missing, or in duplicate, *etc.*, so producing the fourth version. Nine out of thirteen of the panel

(authors) are practicing pharmacists in addition to being academics. Several have more than 20 years of experience as practicing pharmacists. Twelve out of thirteen have a long experience of university teaching of pharmacy, in most cases of 25 years or more. One is an expert in medical education. Once terminology issues were resolved there was widespread consensus on the different visions of pharmacy practice.

(3) The fourth version of the questionnaire consisting of 68 propositions for competences for pharmacy practice in 13 clusters was submitted to a large expert panel (academics, students, and pharmacists from all areas of the profession ($n = 1245$).

(4) The analysis of ranking data and comments on the fourth version, gathered using a *surveymonkey* questionnaire [34], will lead to the production of the fifth version. The ranking data and comments on the fourth version are presented in this article. The *surveymonkey* questionnaire (Figure 1) was available online from 14 February 2014 through 1 November 2015 *i.e.*, 8.5 months. Such a long period was required in order to achieve (a modicum of) balance in the distribution of respondents (by occupation, country, age…).

(5) A future second evaluation by the large European wide expert panel will lead to the production of the final QA framework.

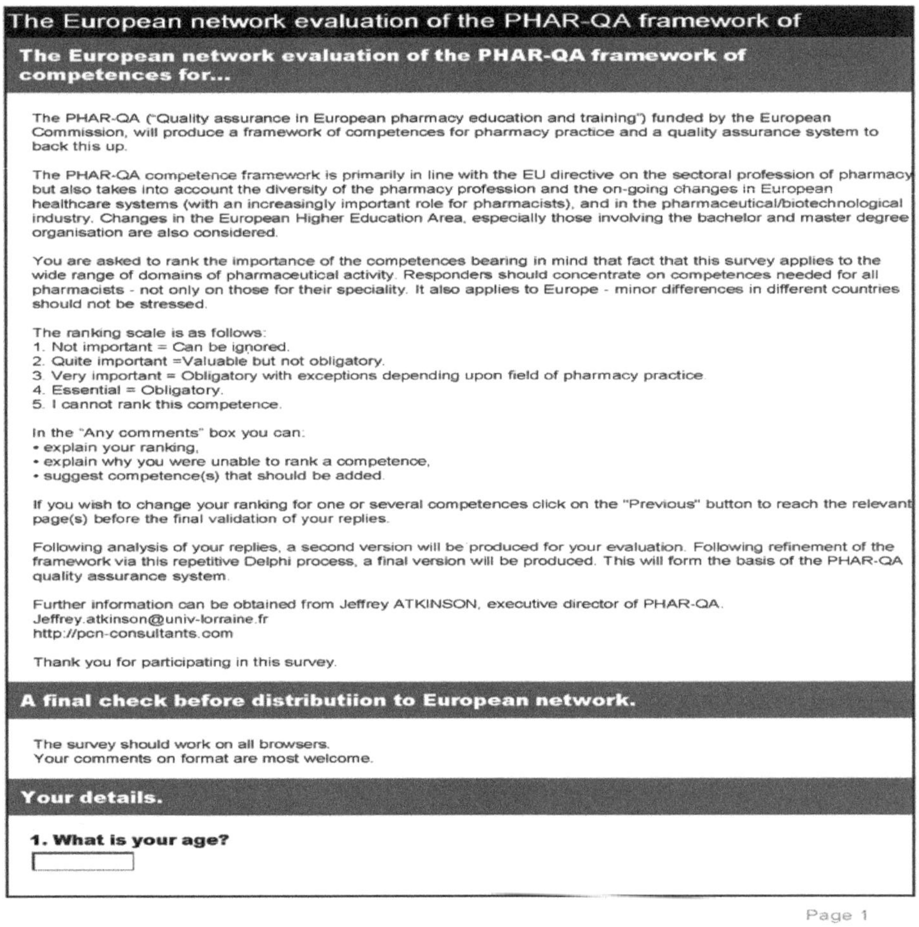
The European network evaluation of the PHAR-QA framework of

The European network evaluation of the PHAR-QA framework of competences for...

The PHAR-QA ("Quality assurance in European pharmacy education and training") funded by the European Commission, will produce a framework of competences for pharmacy practice and a quality assurance system to back this up.

The PHAR-QA competence framework is primarily in line with the EU directive on the sectoral profession of pharmacy but also takes into account the diversity of the pharmacy profession and the on-going changes in European healthcare systems (with an increasingly important role for pharmacists), and in the pharmaceutical/biotechnological industry. Changes in the European Higher Education Area, especially those involving the bachelor and master degree organisation are also considered.

You are asked to rank the importance of the competences bearing in mind that fact that this survey applies to the wide range of domains of pharmaceutical activity. Responders should concentrate on competences needed for all pharmacists - not only on those for their speciality. It also applies to Europe - minor differences in different countries should not be stressed.

The ranking scale is as follows:
1. Not important = Can be ignored.
2. Quite important =Valuable but not obligatory.
3. Very important = Obligatory with exceptions depending upon field of pharmacy practice.
4. Essential = Obligatory.
5. I cannot rank this competence.

In the "Any comments" box you can:
- explain your ranking,
- explain why you were unable to rank a competence,
- suggest competence(s) that should be added.

If you wish to change your ranking for one or several competences click on the "Previous" button to reach the relevant page(s) before the final validation of your replies.

Following analysis of your replies, a second version will be produced for your evaluation. Following refinement of the framework via this repetitive Delphi process, a final version will be produced. This will form the basis of the PHAR-QA quality assurance system.

Further information can be obtained from Jeffrey ATKINSON, executive director of PHAR-QA.
Jeffrey.atkinson@univ-lorraine.fr
http://pcn-consultants.com

Thank you for participating in this survey.

A final check before distributiion to European network.

The survey should work on all browsers.
Your comments on format are most welcome.

Your details.

1. What is your age?

Page 1

Figure 1. The introductory page of the *surveymonkey* questionnaire.

It should be noted that the first phase of this Delphi process consists in the production of a concerted, harmonious, position paper by a group of experts; this is the essence of the Delphi process [35]. The second phase—the European wide survey—is aimed at producing a harmonized European position on general competence framework.

There were six questions on the profile of the respondent:

(1) Age
(2) Country of residence
(3) Current occupation: community, hospital or industrial pharmacist, pharmacist working on other area, student, academic
(4) If you are a student, what is your year of enrolment?
(5) If you are a professional (licensed practitioner, academic staff...), how long have you been practicing?
(6) Job title

These were followed by 13 clusters in two major domains with a total in all of 68 competences (see Appendix). Questions in clusters 7 through 11 were concerned with personal competences and in clusters 12 through 19 with patient care competences:

Personal competences

(1) Learning and knowledge.
(2) Values.
(3) Communication and organizational skills.
(4) Knowledge of different areas of the science of medicines.
(5) Understanding of industrial pharmacy.

Patient care competences

(6) Patient consultation and assessment.
(7) Need for drug treatment.
(8) Drug interactions.
(9) Provision of drug product.
(10) Patient education.
(11) Provision of information and service.
(12) Monitoring of drug therapy.
(13) Evaluation of outcomes.

Most of those competencies are the same as described in Global Competency Framework, which was published by the FIP [6].

Respondents were asked to rank the proposals for competences with a Likert scale:

(1) Not important = Can be ignored.
(2) Quite important =Valuable but not obligatory.
(3) Very important = Obligatory with exceptions depending upon field of pharmacy practice.
(4) Essential = Obligatory.

The assessment methodology was based on that used by the MEDINE [36]; the even-numbered Likert scale was the same as that used by MEDINE. A pilot MEDINE experiment using a 5-point Likert scale, with a rank 3 = "neutral", showed that respondents tended to "opt out" by replying with rank 3 throughout (M.T. Ross and A. Cummins, MEDINE, personal communication, 2012).

Respondents had the possibility to opt for "I cannot rank this competence" or to leave the answer blank. Finally, they could add their comments.

The distribution of surveymonkey to potential respondents was organized by the PHAR-QA regional directors, *viz* for northern Europe J. Hirvonen, for eastern B. Bozic, for western D. Rekkas, and for southern: A. Sanchez-Pozo. The stakeholders (EPSA, PGEU, EAHP, and EIPG) also distributed the questionnaire to their members. More than one-off emailing was required to obtain some balance in distribution of the profiles of the respondents; numerous telephone contacts and personal contacts were also made. The numbers of respondents snowballed through individual, local contacts.

Results are presented here in the form of scores based on the methodology used in MEDINE: score = (frequency rank 3 + frequency rank 4) as % total.

For example: data for community pharmacists ranking competence number 1:

Rank		Frequency
1		3
2		121
3		480
4		622
Total = 1226	$f3 + f4 = 1102$	Score = (1102/1226) × 100 = 90%

Scores give more granularity and a better pictorial representation; they represent "obligatory" rankings. A comparison with medians and means is given in the annex.

3. Statistical Analysis

Data presented in this paper are for:

- Overall rankings by six groups of respondents. These are given as means and scores. Although the parametric use of means was probably robust enough under the circumstances, means are given as an indication only and differences were determined using non-parametric methods (see below).
- Comparisons of ranking by community pharmacists with that of the 5 other professional groups of respondents

The differences between rankings of competences or between rankings by different categories of respondents were determined by the chi-square test (confidence level 95%).

Estimated sample size was calculated with a 95% confidence interval and a 10% error [37]. The confidence interval (also called margin of error) is the "plus-or-minus". The confidence level is a measure of confidence. It is expressed as a percentage and represents how often the true percentage of the population who would pick an answer lies within the confidence interval. Most researchers use the 95% confidence level. For example: for community pharmacists (estimated population size: 400,000, 95% confidence interval and 10% confidence interval (margin of error)), the minimal sample size is 97. With a sample of 258 out of 400,000, a confidence level of 95% and a 10% error, for a score of 90% the confidence interval is 4, thus giving a score range of 86%–94%.

4. Results

There were 1613 entries in the *surveymonkey* questionnaire. Of these 1613, 1245 (77%) went beyond the profile description questions (first 6 questions on occupation, *etc.*) and ranked the competence ranking questions (competence clusters 7 through 19).

The numbers of the respondents in the 6 groups are given in Table 1. The relative size of the professional groups was: students > community pharmacists = academics > hospital pharmacists = industrial pharmacists > pharmacists working in other professions. The "other" group included pharmacists working in government agencies (regulatory affairs…), in wholesale, in marketing and sales, *etc.* In all groups sample sizes were well above calculated minimal sampling size (Table 1).

Table 1. Respondents by professional group, and sampling rates.

Professional Groups	Number of Respondents	%	Estimated EUROPEAN POPULATION (× 1000)	Calculated Minimal Sample Size (95% Confidence Level, 10% Error)
Community pharmacists	258	20.7	400 (PGEU)	97
Hospital pharmacists	152	12.2	12 (EAHP)	96
Industrial pharmacists	135	10.8	10 (EIPG)	96
Others	77	6.2	?	?
Breakdown of "others"				
Regulatory affairs, government	27	-	?	?
Consultancy	10	-	?	?
Wholesale, marketing, distribution	10	-	?	?
Lobbyist, NGO	6	-	?	?
Pharmacy chamber, society, association	5	-	?	?
Healthcare insurance agency	1	-	?	?
Not specified	18	-	-	-
Students	382	30.7	200 (PHARMINE)	96
Academics	241	19.4	10 (PHARMINE)	96
Total	1245	100	400 + 12 + 10 + 200 + 10 = 632	97

The ranking of the majority of the 1245 respondents (rank 3 + rank 4: 69.7%, Table 2) showed that the respondents considered the proposed competences were obligatory for pharmacy practice. 12% considered that competences were not important (rank 1), could not rank or left blanks. 9% either could not rank or left blanks.

Figure 2 shows the ranking of the 68 competences by the 6 groups of respondents. There was overall agreement between groups. Scores greater than 90% were observed for competences in groups 7, 8, 9, 10, 14, 15 and 17, and scores less than 50% for competences in groups 7, 9, 10, 11 and 12. These results indicate that some competences are not considered important although the group in general it is.

Table 2. Global ranking for entire population of respondents, $n = 1245$.

Rank	Number	%
1	2470	2.9
2	14,933	17.6
3	30,132	35.6
4	29,194	34.1
Cannot rank	1764	2.1
Blank	6167	7.3
Theoretical total	=68 × 1245 = 84,660	100%

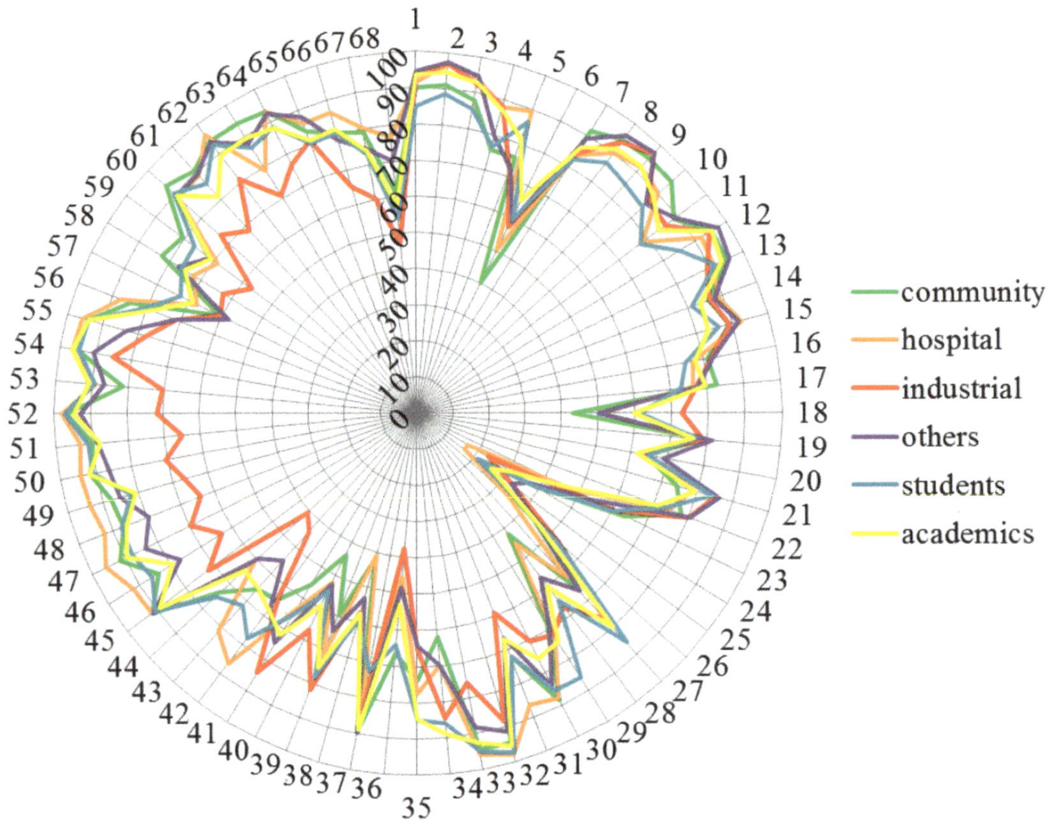

Figure 2. Ranking of the 68 competences by the 6 groups of respondents (community pharmacists: green, industrial pharmacists: red, hospital pharmacists: orange, others: purple, students; blue, academics: yellow). Numbers on the circumference refer to competences (1 through 68). Numbers on the vertical axis refer to % score (0 through 100).

Comparisons between community pharmacists and other groups are given below.

Figure 3 shows that there was little difference in the rankings of hospital and community pharmacists. Ranking for competences 23, 24, 36 and 63 was community > hospital, and for competences 42, 43 and 68 community < hospital.

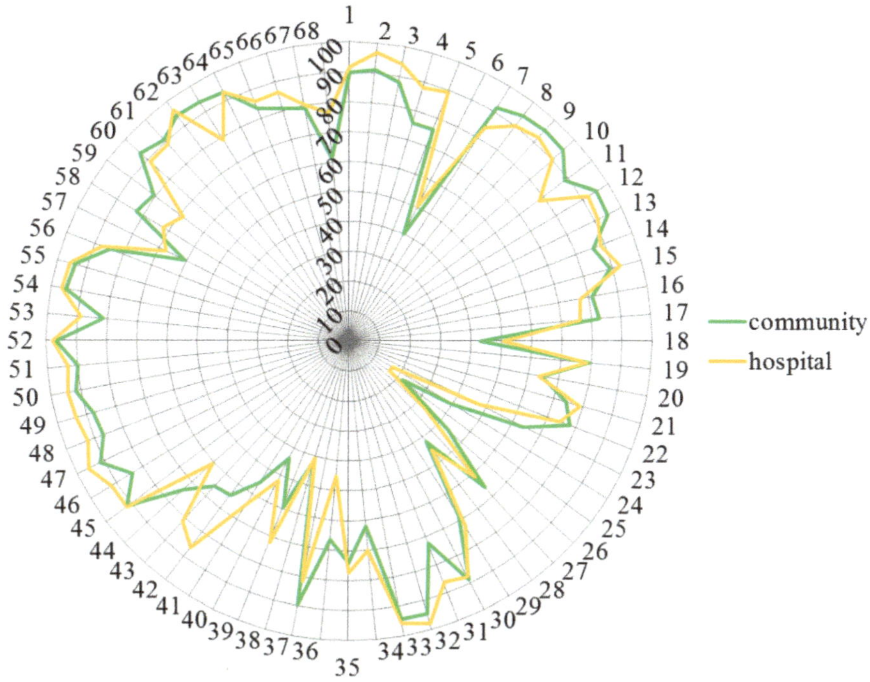

Figure 3. Comparisons of rankings by hospital (orange) and community pharmacists (green). Numbers on the circumference refer to competences (1 through 68). Numbers on the vertical axis refer to % scores (0 through 100).

Figure 4 shows that industrial pharmacists scored differently from community pharmacists. Ranking for competences 24, 30, 33, 36, 43–52, 55, 58, 60, 61, 63, 64, 66 and 67 was community > industrial, and for competences 6, 18, 28, 34 and 38–41 community < industrial.

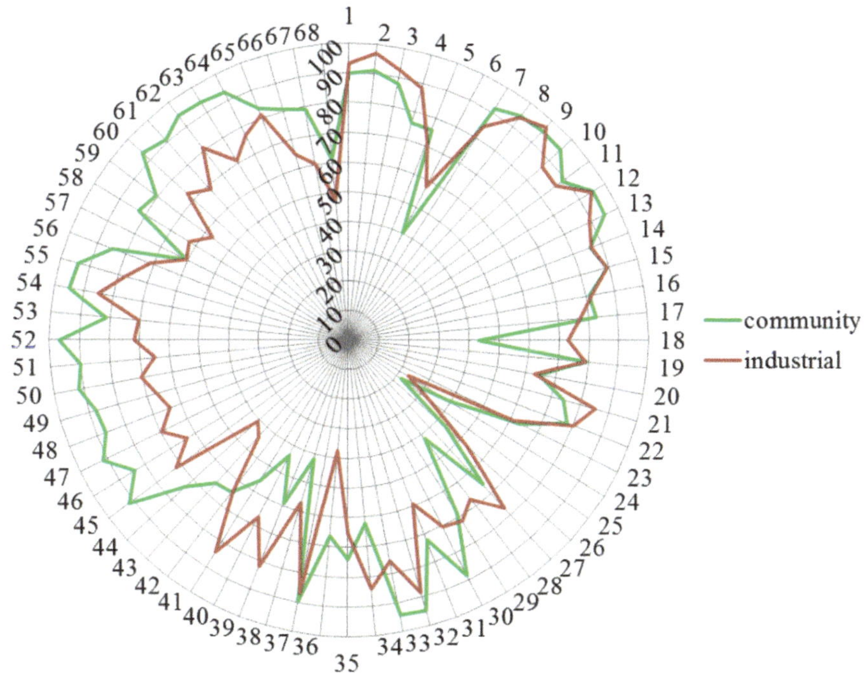

Figure 4. Comparisons of rankings by industrial (red) and community pharmacists (green).Numbers on the circumference refer to competences (1 through 68). Numbers on the vertical axis refer to % score (0 through 100).

Figure 5 shows that pharmacists working in professions other than community, industrial or hospital pharmacy gave scores similar to those of community pharmacists. Ranking for competence 36 was community > industrial, and for competences 6, 28 and 41 community < industrial.

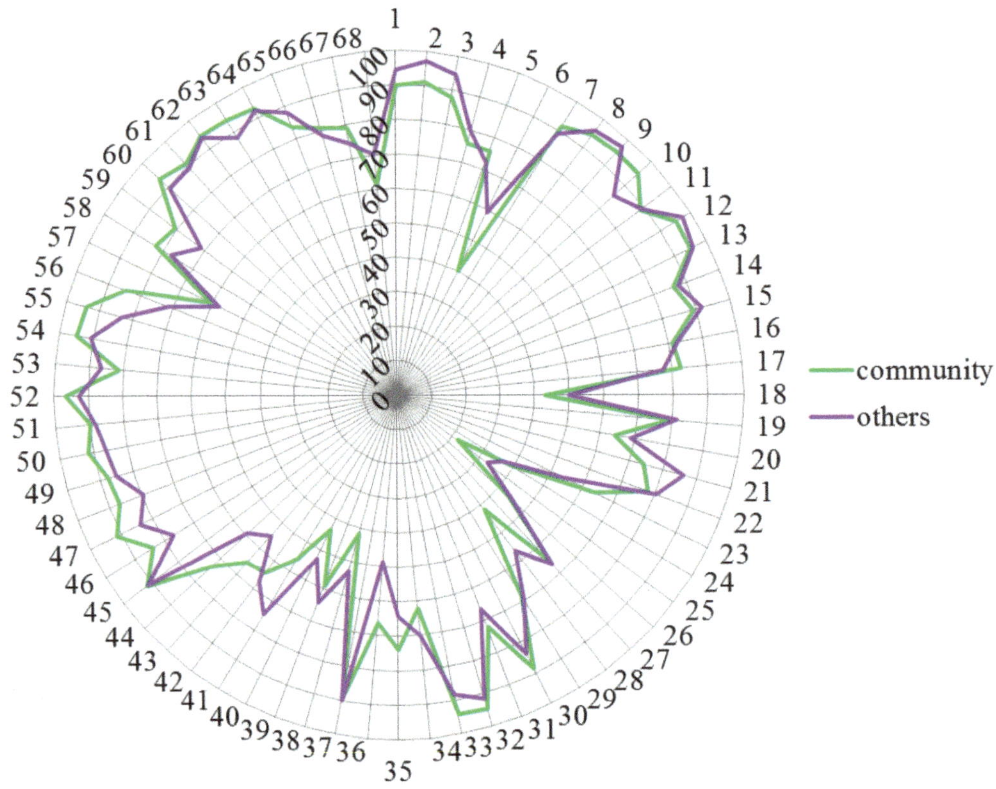

Figure 5. Comparisons of rankings by pharmacists working in other professions (purple) and community pharmacists (green). Numbers on the circumference refer to competences (1 through 68). Numbers on the vertical axis refer to % score (0 through 100).

Figure 6 shows that students often gave higher scores than community pharmacists. Ranking for competence 37 was community > students, and for competences 6, 18, 27–29, 34, 38 and 39 community < students.

Academics often scored higher than community pharmacists. Figure 7 shows that ranking for competence 23 was community > academics, and for competences 6, 18, 28, 34 and 38–41 community < academics.

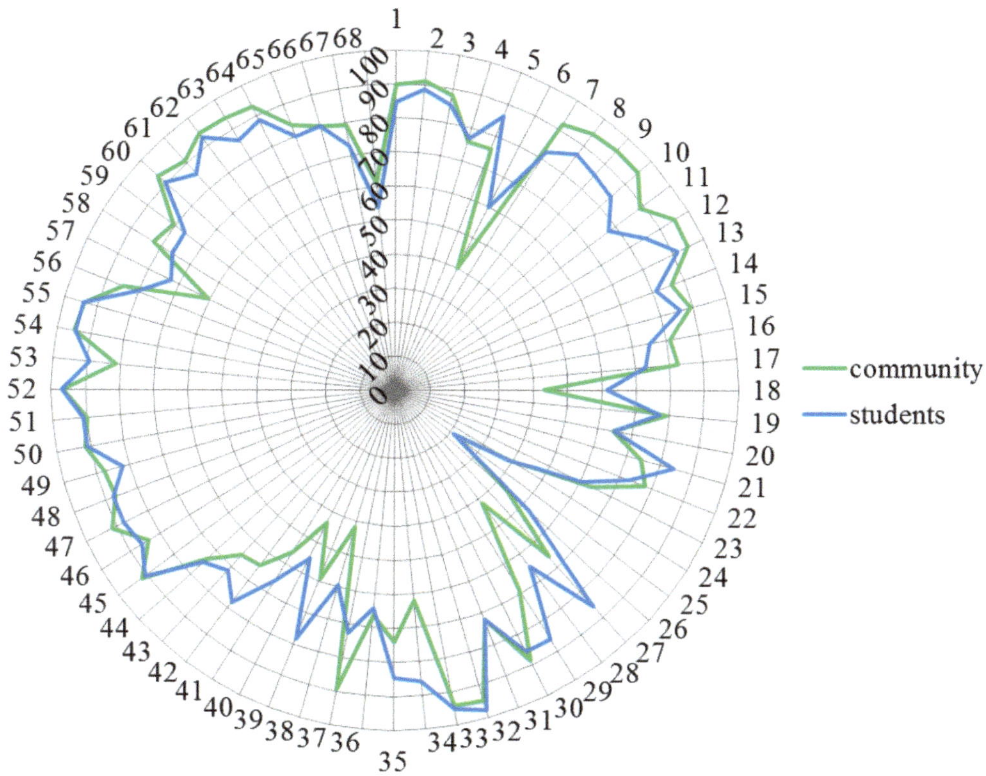

Figure 6. Comparisons of rankings by students (blue) and community pharmacists (green).

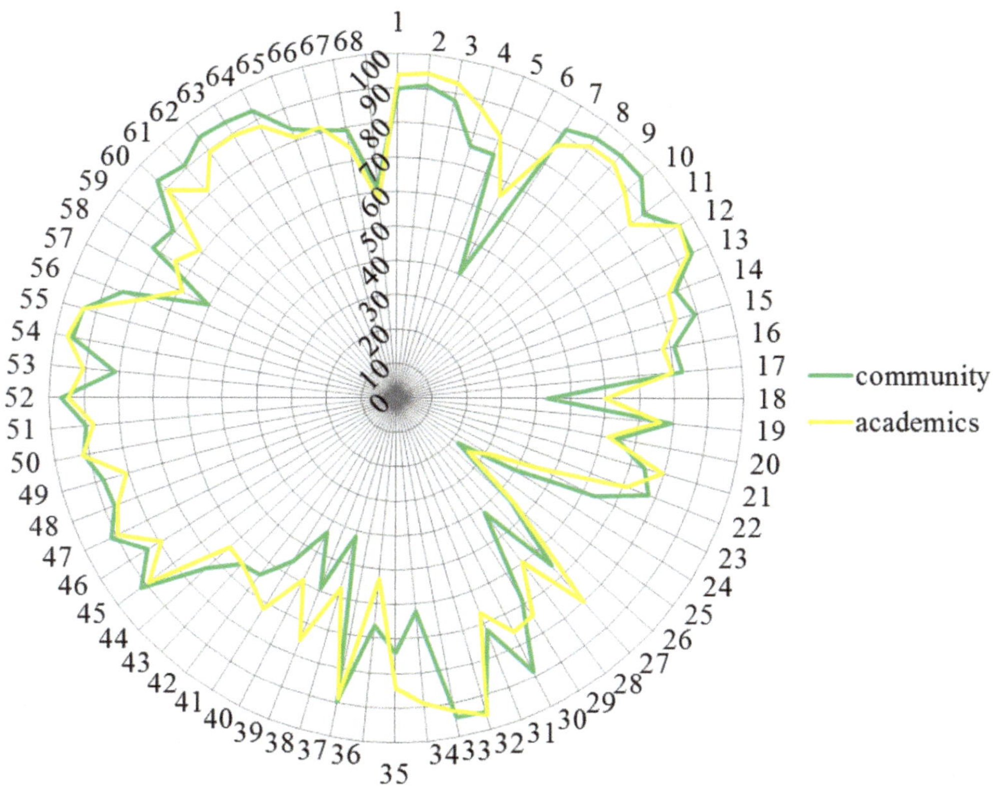

Figure 7. Comparisons of rankings by academics (yellow) and community pharmacists (green). Numbers on the circumference refer to competences (1 through 68). Numbers on the vertical axis refer to % score (0 through 100).

The *surveymonkey* text analysis tool allows the frequency of key words and key terms to be determined thus illustrating the relative importance of the terms. In Figure 8, the font size is proportional to number of citations.

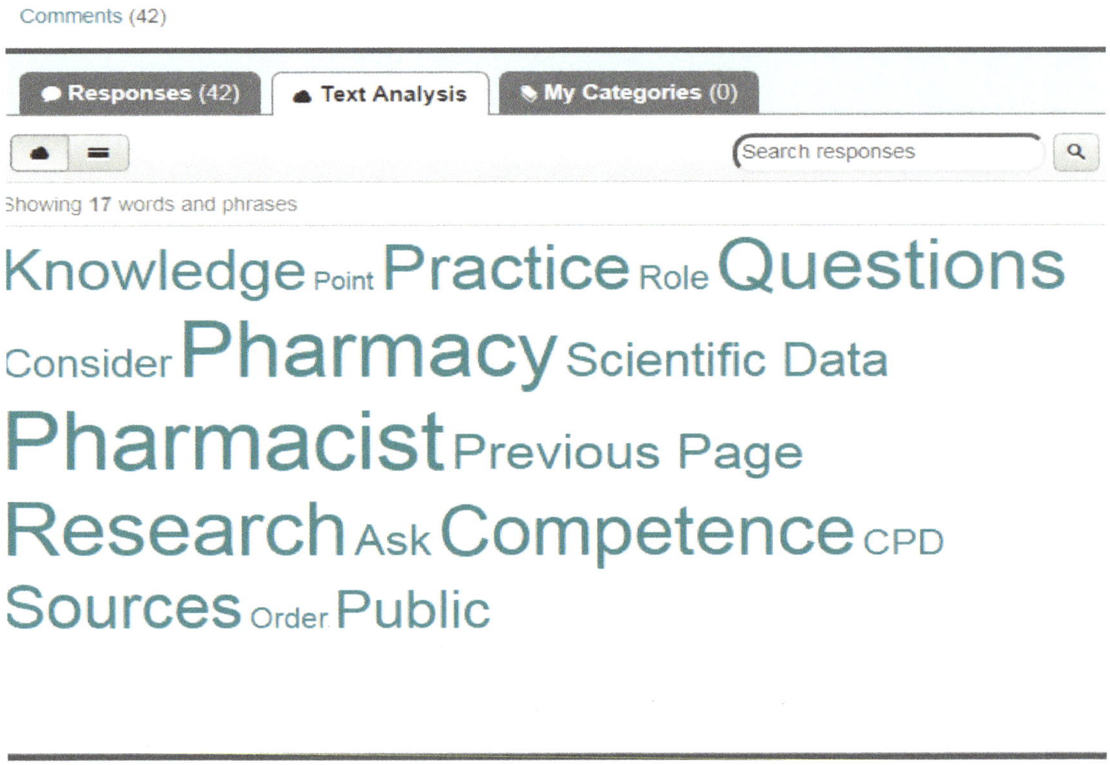

Figure 8. The *surveymonkey* text analysis tool (example for profile question group 10: Personal competences: learning and knowledge).

Comments that occurred frequently included:

- Target audience
    - "…refer to daily work in a community pharmacy"
    - "focus on practicing pharmacists"
    - "for specialists"
    - "Not really the role of primary care, but important for some knowledge and awareness."
    - "Things that every pharmacist should be familiar with and even more in patient care fields, as in hospital or community pharmacy."
    - "For community pharmacists the above are essential, but for other pharmacists less."
    - "Can imagine it to be important in hospitals..."
    - "For clinical and hospital pharmacists."
- University level
    - "Competences recorded as 'very important' cannot be fully obtained on pre-graduate level and also postgraduate training is needed."
    - "Competence 66 cannot be fully achieved during the pre-graduate training and requires also postgraduate education."

- Difficulties in application
    - "Are subject areas professional competences?"
    - "If not commercially available I would contend that we should change what we are prescribing. I do not believe in 'specials' which in the UK are abused and contribute hugely and inappropriately to our drugs bill."
    - "There are always people who need some special drug which is not commercially available."
    - "Not sure how most pharmacists would be able to manufacture?"
    - "General information on diet or exercise is important but the specific recommendations for the patient should be made by the experts in those areas (e.g. dietician or physiotherapist)."
    - "Information should be basically provided by doctors, before pharmacists."
    - "I am not sure that pharmacists know current clinical guidelines. If medicine is prescribed we give it to patient."
- Suggestions for further inclusions, *etc.*
    - "Acquire other competencies for new services like vaccinations in the pharmacy, screening tests (colon cancer, heart disease, COPD, *etc.*) Public Health services in general, NCD (non-communicable diseases)"
    - "Services like vaccinations, screenings (colon cancer, kidney, COPD, Heart disease, *etc.*) and others should become essential in the curriculum in order to be able to perform the services in the future."
    - "Pharmacist should also provide information about medical devices and other items available in the pharmacy."
    - "The knowledge on drug therapies and reactions on failing therapies are core fields for pharmacists."
    - "Radio-pharmacy"
- Technical difficulties with the survey
    - "In my browser section 6 appears blank"
    - "Never ask 2 things in the same question…"
    - "No possibility of open-ended questions…"
- Language difficulties
    - "Too complicated for my simple English…"
    - "I cannot rank this competence for I do not fully understand the meaning of the competence."

5. Discussion

The results show that competences in the areas of "drug interactions", "need for drug treatment" and "provision of information and service" were ranked highest whereas those in the areas of "ability to design and conduct research" and "development and production of medicines" were ranked lower. For the latter two competences one out of six categories—industrial pharmacists—ranked higher than the other 5 groups. The impact of the professional group status on the ranking will be dealt with in a future paper.

The six groups were formed following the end of data collection from respondents. There was no prior separation into sampling groups and no selection. Comments received during European-wide data collection (unpublished) suggested that snowballing was occurring with respondents being recruited by colleagues and friends. Furthermore, the identity of the respondents was unknown; only the computer IP numbers were collected; several respondents could use the same computer. Thus, the requirement for anonymity in Delphi studies was maintained in the second phase *i.e.*, the European-wide survey. This was not the case in the first phase *i.e.*, the elaboration of the survey by three Delphi rounds within the consortium.

Another question that scored low was that concerned with the subject area "physics". This, however, is not a competence as such. They were included as they are part of the EU directive on the sectoral profession of pharmacy [2]. The question to be asked here was more accurately "adequate knowledge of the following areas (physics…) in the science of medicines is necessary to support pharmaceutical practice" but once again one is not dealing with competences for practice. Perhaps the best way to consider this is to take the teaching of certain subject areas as an essential, integral part of the acquirement of given competences for practice. This is the position taken by FIP (2012 reference) when they propose that the foundations of quality in pharmacy education are science (or knowledge), practice and ethics. The two aspects "knowledge" and "practice" are well separated and several papers have dealt with the question of how practice relates to knowledge (e.g., Waterfield) and whether pharmacy is a knowledge/science-based profession. The European answer to this question would be "yes" with the proviso that the way in which individual member state countries link practice to knowledge/science is their responsibility and not that of the European Commission.

This freedom of action is also reflected in the issue that organization and management competencies are not included in the framework, nor are time management, financial issues, responsibility for processes and decisions, new tools in the pharmacy profession, such as marketing, category management, procurement, and reimbursement for services. It is judged that such issues are more national than European. Albeit, a question is asked on the "ability to identify the need for new services" with the possibility to develop the answer in the comments box. Several comments were received on future developments in pharmacy practice.

The main difference of the PHAR-QA with the PHARMINE survey is that the former is shorter and more concise. It is intended that the PHAR-QA framework—compared to other national frameworks for example in the UK (CoDEG cited above)—be short and concise and represent a harmonized European version that can be adapted to the national situation in a given member state. The use of the second phase Delphi process ensured that the PHAR-QA framework is consensual and harmonized throughout European countries. This was done by using extensive, random, snowballing recruitment. As stated above, the recruitment was not entirely random as it was distributed by PHAR-QA regional directors and stakeholders—all pharmaceutical in nature—and was thus aimed at a specific population. The survey aimed at balance throughout European countries, professional and age groups. This was largely attained although some groups (e.g., students) and some countries (e.g., Germany) were over-represented in terms of the number of actual respondents compared to the number of potential respondents.

There was a relatively large number of respondents who did not go beyond the profile questions (23%). These were mainly students and this may be related to issues with the English language. The question can be asked as to whether the respondents were suitably armed to reply to the questionnaire. It is unfortunate that 23% of respondents did not go beyond the first six profile questions. However of the 1245 respondents × 68 questions = 84,660 potential replies there were "only" 2.1% "cannot rank" and 7.3% blanks.

The number of respondents (1245) far exceeded the sample size number of 100 respondents estimated for a total population of 632,000 potential respondents. As the numbers in all six categories are large this will allow inter- and intra-group comparisons. In this article, we presented comparisons between ranking by community pharmacists and the ranking by the other 5 professional groups. Many other comparisons are possible such as 1st year students *versus* 5th/6th year students, academics with students, different age groups, *etc*. These will be the subject of further publications. One particular comparison is of great interest: that concerning the ranking in different countries. Ever since the pioneering work of Bourlioux and the founder members of the EAFP [38] there has been a move to harmonization of pharmacy education throughout the EU driven partly by the publication of EU directives on the sectoral profession of pharmacy [39]. It will be interesting to know whether professionals in different member states have (or have not) similar views on the importance of the different competences for practice.

Regarding statistics, as the ordinal data of the Likert scale has only 4 units (1, 2, 3 or 4), the score was an attempt to introduce more granularity into the results than can be obtained with the use of medians. Scores measure the degree to which competences are considered "obligatory" (ranks 3 and 4). Although this adds granularity it does not convert the ordinal data into ratio data.

The comments from the respondents raised several issues on English phraseology and idiom and these have been corrected in the second version. Words that have a loose definition such as "familiarity" were also removed. Questions that asked 2 separate sub-questions such as "ability to perform and interpret medical laboratory tests" were simplified.

6. Conclusions

The results show that competences in the areas of "drug interactions", "need for drug treatment" and "provision of information and service" were ranked highest whereas those in the areas of "ability to design and conduct research" and "development and production of medicines" were ranked lower.

This PHAR-QA framework does not, however, replace member state law or the EU directive on qualifications for the sectoral profession of pharmacy. The PHAR-QA framework simply represents the consensual opinion of several hundred European pharmacy professionals, academics and students.

7. Perspectives

The project started in October 2012 and will finish in March 2016, thus it is now entering its critical, final stage.

On the basis of the results above PHAR-QA has now produced a fifth version of the competence framework taking into account:

- The ranking of the fourth version of the framework presented in this paper
- The comments of the respondents, namely
    - Need for simplified construction of questions
    - Attention given to use of easy to understand English

- The question "did we miss anything?" with suggestions for competences to be included (open-ended question)

The revised version of the question is available and readers are invited to respond [40].

The final PHAR-QA framework will be exploited by EAFP that will propose its use in European pharmacy departments and suggest the modalities through which it could be introduced. In a later stage efforts will be made to introduce this competence framework approach to other aspects of education such as continuing professional development and to monitoring of practice.

Acknowledgments

With the support of the Lifelong Learning programme of the European Union: 527194-LLP-1-2012-1-BE-ERASMUS-EMCR.

This project has been funded with support from the European Commission. This publication reflects the views only of the author; the Commission cannot be held responsible for any use which may be made of the information contained therein.

Author Contributions

Jeffrey Atkinson designed, constructed, ran and analysed the survey, and wrote the paper. Kristien De Paepe ran the PHAR-QA consortium. Constantin Mircioiu played a major role in the statistical analyses of the data. Antonio Sánchez Pozo and Dimitrios Rekkas developed the questionnaire. Antonio Sánchez Pozo, Dimitrios Rekkas, Jouni Hirvonen, Borut Bozic, Annie Marcincal and Agnieska Skowron helped with distribution of the survey. Antonio Sánchez Pozo and Borut Bozic provided useful criticism and suggestions during revision of the manuscript. Chris van Schravendijk assured the contacts with MEDINE2.

Conflicts of Interest

The authors declare no conflict of interest.

Appendix

Table A1. Ranking data for 68 competences (n = 1245 respondents).

	Number of Competence	Mean Ranking	Median Ranking	Score 3% + 4%
7. Personal competences: learning and knowledge.				
1. Ability to identify learning needs and to learn independently (including continuous professional development (CPD)).	1	3.4	4	89.89
2. Analysis: ability to apply logic to problem solving, evaluating pros and cons and following up on the solution found.	2	3.5	4	92.70
3. Synthesis: capacity to gather and critically appraise relevant knowledge and to summarize the key points.	3	3.4	4	89.70
4. Capacity to evaluate scientific data in line with current scientific and technological knowledge.	4	3.2	3	81.38

Table A1. *Cont.*

	Number of Competence	Mean Ranking	Median Ranking	Score 3% + 4%
5. Ability to interpret preclinical and clinical evidence-based medical science and apply the knowledge to pharmaceutical practice.	5	3.2	3	81.02
6. Ability to design and conduct research using appropriate methodology.	6	2.7	3	55.47
7. Ability to maintain current knowledge of relevant legislation and codes of pharmacy practice.	7	3.3	3	85.96
8. Personal competences: values.				
1. Demonstrate a professional approach to tasks and human relations.	8	3.4	4	91.09
2. Demonstrate the ability to maintain confidentiality.	9	3.5	4	91.74
3. Take full personal responsibility for patient care and other aspects of one's practice.	10	3.4	4	88.43
4. Inspire the confidence of others in one's actions and advice.	11	3.2	3	82.84
5. Demonstrate high ethical standards.	12	3.6	4	91.88
9. Personal competences: communication and organizational skills.				
1. Effective communication skills (both orally and written).	13	3.4	4	92.60
2. Effective use of information technology.	14	3.1	3	84.63
3. Ability to work effectively as part of a team.	15	3.3	3	87.76
4. Ability to identify and implement legal and professional requirements relating to employment (e.g., for pharmacy technicians) and to safety in the workplace.	16	3.1	3	78.43
5. Ability to contribute to the learning and training of staff.	17	3.0	3	77.46
6. Ability to design and manage the development processes in the production of medicines.	18	2.7	3	56.59
7. Ability to identify and manage risk and quality of service issues.	19	3.1	3	77.99
8. Ability to identify the need for new services.	20	2.8	3	64.00
9. Ability to communicate in English and/or locally relevant languages.	21	3.2	3	80.67
10. Ability to evaluate issues related to quality of service.	22	2.9	3	75.07
11. Ability to negotiate, understand a business environment and develop entrepreneurship.	23	2.7	3	56.62
10. Personal competences: knowledge of different areas of the science of medicines.				
1. Plant and animal biology.	24	2.2	2	32.87
2. Physics.	25	2.0	2	23.65

Table A1. *Cont.*

	Number of Competence	Mean Ranking	Median Ranking	Score 3% + 4%
3. General and inorganic chemistry.	26	2.5	2	46.50
4. Organic and medicinal/pharmaceutical chemistry.	27	3.1	3	75.26
5. Analytical chemistry.	28	2.7	3	56.29
6. General and applied biochemistry (medicinal and clinical).	29	3.0	3	75.74
7. Anatomy and physiology; medical terminology.	30	3.2	3	82.86
8. Microbiology.	31	2.9	3	71.21
9. Pharmacology including pharmacokinetics.	32	3.7	4	95.21
10. Pharmacotherapy and pharmaco-epidemiology.	33	3.6	4	91.98
11. Pharmaceutical technology including analyses of medicinal products.	34	3.2	3	78.24
12. Toxicology.	35	3.1	3	77.92
13. Pharmacognosy.	36	2.7	3	56.07
14. Legislation and professional ethics.	37	3.3	3	83.13
11. Personal competences: understanding of industrial pharmacy.				
1. Current knowledge of design, synthesis, isolation, characterization and biological evaluation of active substances.	38	2.6	3	52.39
2. Current knowledge of good manufacturing practice (GMP) and of good laboratory practice (GLP).	39	3.0	3	72.60
3. Current knowledge of European directives on qualified persons (QPs).	40	2.6	3	54.44
4. Current knowledge of drug registration, licensing and marketing.	41	2.9	3	67.36
5. Current knowledge of good clinical practice (GCP).	42	3.0	3	71.96
12. Patient care competences: patient consultation and assessment.				
1. Ability to perform and interpret medical laboratory tests.	43	2.9	3	66.46
2. Ability to perform appropriate diagnostic or physiological tests to inform clinical decision making e.g., measurement of blood pressure.	44	2.8	3	66.27
3. Ability to recognize when referral to another member of the healthcare team is needed because a potential clinical problem is identified (pharmaceutical, medical, psychological or social).	45	3.4	4	88.86
13. Patient care competences: need for drug treatment.				
1. Retrieval and interpretation of relevant information on the patient's clinical background.	46	3.2	3	82.23

Table A1. *Cont.*

	Number of Competence	Mean Ranking	Median Ranking	Score 3% + 4%
2. Retrieval and interpretation of an accurate and comprehensive drug history if and when required.	47	3.4	4	87.83
3. Identification of non-adherence and implementation of appropriate patient intervention.	48	3.3	3	84.80
4. Ability to advise to physicians and—in some cases—prescribe medication.	49	3.2	3	83.10
14. Patient care competences: drug interactions.				
1. Identification, understanding and prioritization of drug-drug interactions at a molecular level (e.g., use of codeine with paracetamol).	50	3.5	4	89.35
2. Identification, understanding, and prioritization of drug-patient interactions, including those that preclude or require the use of a specific drug (e.g., trastuzumab for treatment of breast cancer in women with HER2 overexpression).	51	3.4	4	87.51
3. Identification, understanding, and prioritization of drug-disease interactions (e.g., NSAIDs in heart failure).	52	3.6	4	93.61
15. Patient care competences: provision of drug product.				
1. Familiarity with the bio-pharmaceutical, pharmacodynamic and pharmacokinetic activity of a substance in the body.	53	3.3	3	85.62
2. Supply of appropriate medicines taking into account dose, correct formulation, concentration, administration route and timing.	54	3.6	4	94.03
3. Critical evaluation of the prescription to ensure that it is clinically appropriate and legal.	55	3.5	4	91.87
4. Familiarity with the supply chain of medicines and the ability to ensure timely flow of drug products to the patient.	56	3.1	3	80.26
5. Ability to manufacture medicinal products that are not commercially available.	57	2.9	3	66.57
16. Patient care competences: patient education.				
1. Promotion of public health in collaboration with other actors in the healthcare system.	58	3.1	3	75.53
2. Provision of appropriate lifestyle advice on smoking, obesity, *etc.*	59	3.0	3	73.07
3. Provision of appropriate advice on resistance to antibiotics and similar public health issues.	60	3.3	3	88.66

Table A1. *Cont.*

	Number of Competence	Mean Ranking	Median Ranking	Score 3% + 4%
17. Patient care competences: provision of information and service.				
1. Ability to use effective consultations to identify the patient's need for information.	61	3.2	3	84.84
2. Provision of accurate and appropriate information on prescription medicines.	62	3.5	4	91.81
3. Provision of informed support for patients in selection and use of non-prescription medicines for minor ailments (e.g., cough remedies...).	63	3.4	4	86.09
18. Patient care competences: monitoring of drug therapy.				
1. Identification and prioritization of problems in the management of medicines in a timely manner and with sufficient efficacy to ensure patient safety.	64	3.3	3	89.01
2. Ability to monitor and report to all concerned in a timely manner, and in accordance with current regulatory guidelines on Good Pharmacovigilance Practices (GVPs), Adverse Drug Events and Reactions (ADEs and ADRs).	65	3.2	3	82.35
3. Undertaking of a critical evaluation of prescribed medicines to confirm that current clinical guidelines are appropriately applied.	66	3.1	3	79.88
19. Patient care competences: evaluation of outcomes.				
1. Assessment of outcomes on the monitoring of patient care and follow-up interventions.	67	3.0	3	74.14
2. Evaluation of cost effectiveness of treatment.	68	2.7	3	59.60

References

1. The PHAR-QA Project: Quality Assurance in European Pharmacy Education and Training. Available online: http://www.phar-qa.eu (accessed on 12 November 2015).
2. The European Commission. The EU Directive 2013/55/EU on the Recognition of Professional Qualifications. Available online: http://eur-lex.europa.eu/LexUriServ/LexUriServ.do?uri=OJ:L:2005:255:0022:0142:EN:PDF (accessed on 18 March 2014).
3. Atkinson, J.; Rombaut, B. The PHARMINE paradigm—matching the supply of pharmacy education and training to demands. *Eur. Ind. Pharm.* **2010**, *6*, 4–7.
4. Atkinson, J.; Rombaut, B. The PHARMINE study on the impact of the European Union directive on sectoral professions and of the Bologna declaration on pharmacy education in Europe. *Pharm. Pract.* **2011**, *9*, 169–187.
5. Atkinson, J.; Rombaut, B.; Sánchez Pozo, A.; Rekkas, D.; Veski, P.; Hirvonen, J.; Bozic, B.; Skowron, A.; Mircioiu, C.; Marcincal, A.; *et al.* Systems for Quality Assurance in Pharmacy Education and Training in the European Union. *Pharmacy* **2014**, *2*, 17–26.

6. International Pharmaceutical Federation. FIP Education Initiative. In *Quality Assurance of Pharmacy Education: The FIP Global Framework*, 2nd ed.; 2014. Available online: https://www.fip.org/files/fip/PharmacyEducation/Quality_Assurance/QA_Framework_2nd_Edition_online_version.pdf (accessed on 12 November 2015).
7. Bruno, A.; Bates, I.; Brock, T.; Anderson, C. Towards a global competency framework. *Am. J. Pharm. Educ.* **2010**, *74*, 56.
8. Govaerts, M.J. Educational competencies or education for professional competence? *Med. Educ.* **2008**, *42*, 234–236.
9. Mestrovic, A.; Stanicic, Z.; Ortner-Hadziabdic, M.; Mucalo, I.; Bates, I.; Duggan, C.; Carter, S.; Bruno, A.; Košiček, M. Individualized education and competency development of Croatian community pharmacists using the General Level Framework. *Am. J. Pharm. Educ.* **2012**, *76*, 23.
10. Dorman, T.; Miller, B.M. Continuing medical education: The link between physician learning and health care outcomes. *Acad. Med.* **2011**, *86*, 1339.
11. Svetlana1, S.; Ivana, T.; Tatjana, C.; Duskana, K.; Bates, I. Evaluation of Competences at the Community Pharmacy Settings. *Ind. J. Pharm. Edu. Res.* **2014**, *48*, 22–30.
12. The Association of Lithuanian Serials. Center of Competence of Healthcare and Pharmacy Specialists. Available online: http://serials.lt/news/ (accessed on 12 November 2015.
13. The Pharmaceutical Society of Ireland. Core Competency Framework. Available online: http://www.thepsi.ie/gns/pharmacy-practice/core-competency-framework.aspx (accessed on 12 November 2015).
14. The Competency Development and Evaluation Group (CoDEG). The CoDEG General Level Framework (GLF). Available online: http://www.codeg.org/frameworks/general-level-practice/ (accessed on12 November 2015).
15. European Association of Faculties of Pharmacy (EAFP). Available online: http://www.eafponline.eu/ (accessed on12 November 2015).
16. The TUNING Network. Competences: Medical Doctors. Available online: http://www.unideusto.org/tuningeu/subject-areas/medicine.html (accessed on12 November 2015);
17. Oxford English Dictionary. Definition of "Competence". Available online: http://www.oed.com/view/Entry/37567?redirectedFrom=competence#eid (accessed on12 November 2015).
18. Merriam-Webster's Dictionary. Definition of "Competence". Available online: http://www.merriam-webster.com/dictionary/competence (accessed on12 November 2015).
19. The Council on Credentialing in Pharmacy. Credentialing in Pharmacy. *Am. J. Health Syst. Pharm.* **2001**, *58*, 69–76.
20. PGEU—Pharmaceutical Group of the European Union. Available online: http://www.pgeu.eu/ (accessed on 12 November 2015).
21. EPSA—European Pharmaceutical Students Association online. Available online: http://www.epsa-online.org/ (accessed on12 November 2015).
22. EAHP—European Association of Hospital Pharmacists. Available online: http://www.eahp.eu/ (accessed on 12 November 2015.
23. EIPG—European Industrial Pharmacists Group. Available online: http://www.eipg.eu/ (accessed on 12 November 2015).

24. ACPE—Accreditation Council for Pharmacy Education. Available online: https://www.acpe-accredit.org/ (accessed on 12 November 2015).
25. Stupans, I.; McAllister, S.; Clifford, R.; Hughes, J.; Krass, I.; March, G.; Owen, S.; Woulfe, J. Nationwide collaborative development of learning outcomes and exemplar standards for Australian pharmacy programmes. *Int. J. Pharm. Pract.* **2014**. Available online: http://onlinelibrary.wiley.com/doi/10.1111/ijpp.12163/pdf (accessed on 12 November 2015).
26. Hsu, C.C.; Sandford, B.A. The Delphi Technique: Making Sense of Consensus. *Pract. Assess. Res. Eval.* **2007**, *12*, 1–8.
27. A Competency Framework for Pharmacy Practitioners General Level (CoDEG): General Level Framework, September, 2010. Available online: http://www.codeg.org/frameworks/general-level-practice/ (accessed on 12 November 2015).
28. World Federation for Medical Education (WFME) Global Standards for Quality Improvement in Basic Medical Education BME in English. Available online: http://wfme.org/standards/bme (accessed on 12 November 2015).
29. PHARMINE WP3 Final Report Identifying and Defining Competences for Pharmacists. Available online: http://www.pharmine.org/wp-content/uploads/2014/05/PHARMINE-WP3-Final-ReportDEF_LO.pdf (accessed on 12 November 2015).
30. Medical Education in Europe (MEDINE). Available online: http://medine2.com/archive/medine1/ (accessed on 12 November 2015).
31. International Medical School IMS2020 Report 2011. Available online: http://www.ims-2020.eu/ (accessed on 12 November 2015).
32. Association for Dental Education in Europe ADEE 2009. Available online: http://www.adee.org/ (accessed on 12 November 2015).
33. Eurohealth 2012 Volume 18/2. Available online: http://www.euro.who.int/en/about-us/partners/observatory/publications/eurohealth/gender-and-health (accessed on 12 November 2015).
34. SurveyMonkey (Online Survey Development Cloud). Available online: https://www.surveymonkey.com/ (accessed on 12 November 2015).
35. Goodman, C. The Delphi technique: A critique. *J. Adv. Nurs.* **1987**, *12*, 729–734.
36. Marz, R.; Dekker, F.W.; van Schravendijk, C.; O'Flynn, S.; Ross, M.T. Tuning research competences for Bologna three cycles in medicine: Report of a MEDINE2 European consensus survey. *Perp. Med. Educ.* **2013**, *2*, 181–195.
37. Survey Software—The Survey System. Available online: http://www.surveysystem.com/sscalc.htm (accessed on 12 November 2015).
38. Bourlioux, P. Erasmus subject evaluations. Studies in pharmacy in Europe. Available online: http://www.phar-qa.eu/wp-content/uploads/2015/04/P_Bourlioux_Erasmus-subject-evaluations-1995.pdf (accessed on 12 November 2015).
39. EUA Briefing Note on Directive 2013/55/EU, Containing the Amendments to Directive 2005/36/EC on the Recognition of Professional Qualifications. Available online: http://www.eua.be/Libraries/Higher_Education/EUA_briefing_note_on_amended_Directive_January_2014.sflb.ashx (accessed on 12 November 2015).

40. The consortium evaluation of the PHAR-QA framework of competences for pharmacists—revised version. Available online: https://www.surveymonkey.com/r/pharqa2 (accessed on 12 November 2015).

13

Expectations do not Influence the Response to Phosphosdiesterase Type 5 Inhibitor Therapy for Erectile Dysfunction

Connie C. J. Louizos and Peter K. Knight *

School of Medical Sciences, University of Sydney, Sydney NSW 2006, Australia;
E-Mail: conniecj@tpg.com.au

* Author to whom correspondence should be addressed; E-Mail: Peter.knight@sydney.edu.au

Academic Editor: Maree Donna Simpson

Abstract: It has been reported that patients frequently discontinue treatment for erectile dysfunction (ED) with phosphodiesterase type 5 inhibitors (PDE5Is) despite apparently good therapeutic results. Because expectations have been shown to affect patients' appraisals of many drugs, the purpose of this study was to determine whether expectations affected the therapeutic response to PDE5Is in men with apparent psychogenic ED. An unvalidated questionnaire was used to collect data on expectations in 80 men commencing PDE5I therapy, and after three and six months of treatment. At the same time, subjects completed the International Index of Erectile Function (IIEF), the Sexual Excitation/Inhibition Scale (SIS/SES) and Beck's Depression Inventory (BDI). No evidence of an effect on expectations on changes in IIEF or BDI scores could be identified. Although changes in IIEF, and BDI scores from recruitment to three months were indicative of improved sexual function and less depression, scores for most items on the expectations scale decreased, suggesting that expectations were not being met. The items for which scores decreased were the expectation to be prescribed a drug, that the drug would restore the sexual function to normal, would work within 30 minutes of administration, improve patients confidence to engage in sexual activity, and that the medication was the best treatment for ED across the three data collection points. The findings of this study indicate that improvements in erectile function did not translate into changes in medication expectations that suggested user satisfaction.

Keywords: patient expectations; erectile dysfunction; phosphodiesterase Type 5 inhibitors; questionnaire

1. Introduction

Phosphodiesterase Type 5 Inhibitors (PDE5Is) are an established first line treatment for erectile dysfunction (ED). However, discontinuation rates ranging from 15% to 57% have been reported amongst PDE5I users, often despite good therapeutic outcomes [1–5]. The reasons for the high discontinuation rates have not been fully explained.

Expectations and beliefs contribute to the therapeutic effect in patients being treated with a variety of drugs for many different conditions [6], and may therefore play a role in determining the response to PDE5Is. Expectations and beliefs, which reflect the patient's perceptions of the aetiology, likely duration, and personal consequences of the condition being treated, can have positive or negative impacts on drug effects at several stages in the therapeutic process [7,8]. Evidence supporting the importance of expectations in shaping the response to medication comes from studies that have examined the placebo effect. A number of randomised controlled trials of PDE5Is have identified placebo responses in ED patients [9–13]. The positive placebo responses may have resulted from anticipation of future positive outcomes, reductions in anxiety or the activation of reward mechanisms [14]. However, high expectations may adversely impact a patient's ongoing appraisal of a drug, affecting compliance and discontinuation rates. The decision to discontinue use can be explained by the disconfirmation theory, which states that consumers compare their pre-use expectations of products, including medications, with subsequent perceived performance [15,16]. A mismatch results in disconfirmation, which is an important trigger of dissatisfaction [17]. It has been shown that patients may respond to disconfirmation by changing medications or discontinuing their use [17–20]. Excessively high expectations may result in a perceived lack of efficacy which underpins the decision of the patient to discontinue use of the medication [21]. This may be particularly relevant to PDE5Is, as most patients have high, often unrealistic, expectations of the benefits of the medications [22].

Given that patient expectations of treatment have been shown to influence the therapeutic response to some drugs, the purpose of this study was to the explicitly explore whether the therapeutic response to PDE5Is could be predicted by an assessment of a patient's expectations at the beginning of treatment. A second aim was to examine how expectations change over a period of treatment, as changing expectations may impact on a patient's decision to continue to use the drug in the long term.

2. Experimental Section

2.1. Materials and Methods

Approval for this study was obtained from the University of Sydney Human Research Ethics Committee (approval 2012/458). The participants in this study, who gave informed written consent to participate, were patients of 13 medical general practitioners (GPs) practicing in Australia. The GPs had identified themselves as having a special interest in the treatment of erectile problems by enrolling on the online register of practitioners maintained by Impotence Australia [23]. There are no requirements for registration, and the register is available to the public.

All men who consulted a participating GP and met the inclusion criteria were invited to enrol in the study. In order to be included, men had to be diagnosed with psychogenic ED and to have never previously been treated with PDE5Is. The clinical diagnosis was based on the absence of evidence of any vasculogenic or other physical cause of ED, and was reached using the protocols normally followed by the examining GPs. The diagnosis was not based on the results of tests conducted as part of a specialist investigation, nor did it specifically comply with the requirements for a diagnosis of psychogenic ED specified in the Diagnostic and Statistical Manual of Mental Disorders. Men who at the time of recruitment were identified as having any comorbidity that could contribute to ED, including use of specific medications, known drug or alcohol dependence, cardiovascular diseases or previously identified endocrinological abnormalities were excluded from the study. Participants were required to be between the ages of 18 and 70 years, in a stable heterosexual relationship of at least six months duration, and be fluent in English. There was no requirement for participants to be making a minimum number of attempts to achieve intercourse over the course of the study.

Recruitment continued until the target of 100 enrolled subjects was reached. Each GP was asked to recruit as many men as possible. At recruitment, each participant completed the expectations questionnaire described below. They also completed the International Index of Erectile Function (IIEF) [24], the Sexual Inhibition/Sexual Excitation Scale (SIS/SES) [25], Becks Depression Inventory (BDI) [26], and a general questionnaire eliciting basic demographic information.

The IIEF is a 15 item self-report questionnaire that has been used extensively in the assessment of erectile dysfunction. IIEF items are categorised into five domains: erectile function (IIEF-EF), orgasmic function (IIEF-OF), sexual desire (IIEF-SD), intercourse satisfaction (IIEF-IS), and overall satisfaction (IIEF-OS). The SIS/SES is a 45 item self-administered questionnaire that examines responses to stimuli that could elicit sexual inhibition and sexual excitation. The questions describe hypothetical situations, some of which incorporate elements of threat. The SIS/SES yields three total scores: Sexual Excitation (SES), Sexual Inhibition 1 (SIS1—threat of performance failure), and Sexual Inhibition 2 (SIS2—threat of consequences). The BDI is a self-report 21-item scale that assesses the severity of symptoms associated with depression to enable a numerical depression score to be calculated.

At the completion of the first visit, participants were issued a prescription for a PDE5I and appointments were made for repeat consultations to occur three and six months after the date of recruitment. At these consultations the questionnaires were again completed.

2.2. Expectations Questionnaire

A search of the Medline database using combinations of the keywords erectile dysfunction, satisfaction, expectations, phosphodiesterase type 5 inhibitors and questionnaires failed to identify any questionnaires suitable for investigating expectations for PDE5I therapy. Consequently, it was necessary to develop a new instrument.

The process began with the generation of an initial list of questions by the authors that was based on the themes identified in the literature search. Questions examining general attitudes towards medications, and the subjects' perceived understanding of how PDE5Is should be used were included as such knowledge has been shown to influence satisfaction with other drugs [27]. The initial list contained 19 questions, seven of which were removed following an initial review which assessed relevance and overlap in content between questions which was conducted by the authors. The 12 remaining questions (expectation items) were formatted as 5-point Likert scales, with responses assigned a numerical value for analysis. The response options (with the value assigned to them) were: strongly disagree (1), disagree (2), neutral/unsure (3), agree (4), and strongly agree (5).

The questionnaire was tested by administering it to 10 ED patients visiting a GP, who were asked to provide written feedback on its ease of use and suggestions for how the clarity of questions or instructions could be improved. The only suggestion received was to simplify the instructions for completing the questionnaire. The final items in the questionnaire are shown in Table 1.

Table 1. Items on the expectations questionnaire with mean (± sd) scores at recruitment and after three and six months of PDE5I treatment.

		Recruitment	3 months	6 months
1	I expected to be prescribed a drug when I decided to visit the doctor with this problem.	3.49 ± 1.07	3.14 ± 1.06 [b]	1.49 ± 0.55 [b,d]
2	Erectile dysfunction is having a significant adverse effect on my life.	1.73 ± 0.57	1.83 ± 0.85	1.48 ± 0.53 [a,c]
3	I expect that this medication will restore my sexual function to normal.	3.13 ± 0.79	2.76 ± 1.12[a]	1.34 ± 0.58 [b,d]
4	I expect that this medication will work within 30 minutes of taking it.	2.06 ± 1.11	1.93 ± 1.05	1.36 ± 0.51 [b,d]
5	I expect that this medication is the best treatment available for erectile dysfunction.	3.10 ± 0.84	2.83 ± 1.06 [a]	1.78 ± 0.91 [b,d]
6	I expect that the effects of this medication will last long enough for me to complete intercourse.	3.09 ± 0.77	2.74 ± 0.92 [a]	2.99 ± 0.95
7	I expect that this medication will increase my confidence to engage in sexual activity	2.02 ± 0.66	1.82 ± 0.48 [a]	1.44 ± 0.91 [a,c]
8	I expect that my partner will be satisfied with the effects of my treatment.	1.93 ± 1.09	1.74 ± 1.02 [b]	2.71 ± 1.30 [b,d]
9	In the past, I have had generally good experiences and results with medications.	2.05 ± 0.59	1.67 ± 0.53 [a]	1.69 ± 0.57
10	I believe that I have sufficient understanding of how the medication is used.	1.31 ± 0.67	1.20 ± 0.43	1.51 ± 0.60 [a,c]
11	I believe that I have sufficient understanding of the medication's effects.	1.85 ± 0.51	1.61 ± 0.51 [a]	1.84 ± 0.93
12	I believe it is better to do without medications.	1.40 ± 0.80	1.28 ± 0.55	1.27 ± 0.55

Notes: [a] Significantly different from recruitment score $P < 0.05$; [b] Significantly different from recruitment score $P < 0.01$; [c] Significantly different from 3-month score $P < 0.05$; [d] Significantly different from 3-month score $P < 0.01$.

The initial decision to recruit 100 participants was arbitrary. The decision was tested using a post hoc power analysis (G Power 3.1) assessing the ability to detect a 6-point change in IIEF-EF score, which is considered the smallest change to be clinically relevant [24].

Due to difficulty in recruiting participants for the study, it was not possible to validate the questionnaire before administration, as validation requires a unique group of subjects whose results cannot be used in the experimental study.

2.3. Statistical Analysis

All statistical analyses were conducted using IBM SPSS version 20. Descriptive statistics (mean and standard deviation) were calculated for responses obtained from the expectations, IIEF, SIS/SES, BDI and demographic questionnaires. Skewness and kurtosis were also calculated as indicators of the normality of the data distribution. Data that were not normally distributed were log transformed before analysis. All means and standard deviations reported below are for untransformed results.

Recruitment IIEF, SIS/SES and BDI scores for subjects prescribed sildenafil and tadalfil were compared using unpaired t tests. As no difference was found between groups, the results were pooled for analysis. In order to minimise heterogeneity of the subjects, only those receiving the highest possible dose were included in the analyses reported below.

Pearson product-moment correlation coefficients were calculated for items on the expectations scale. Correlations between the following data sets were calculated: expectation, IIEF and BDI scores at recruitment; expectations scores at recruitment and IIEF and BDI changes 0–3 months; expectations scores at recruitment and IIEF and BDI changes 0–6 months; changes in expectations scores and changes in IIEF and BDI scores 0–3 months; and changes in expectations scores and changes in IIEF and BDI scores 3–6 months. Changes in SIS/SES scores were not analysed in this way, as the scale may measure underlying traits rather than time specific patient states [25].

Repeated measures ANOVA was used to identify significant changes in scores for the expectations, IIEF, SIS/SES and BDI scales between the three data collection points.

For all analyses described above, statistical significance was defined by $\alpha < 0.05$.

3. Results

3.1. Descriptive Statistics

Details of the specific PDE5I prescribed and the dose rate at which it was to be used were not obtained for 17 men. All but three of the remaining 83 subjects were initially prescribed, and continued to use, the highest dose of PDE5I, with 59 men receiving 100 mg sildenafil and 21 men 20 mg tadalafil. Results for the 17 recruited subjects for whom drug information was not available, and the three that did not receive the highest dose were not included in the analyses.

The mean age at recruitment of the 80 subjects included in the study was 52.2 ± 6.2 years (range 40–67 years). Mean scores on the IIEF, SIS/SES and BDI at recruitment, and the IIEF and BDI at the 3- and 6-month data collections are shown in Table 2. There was a significant increase in scores in each of the IIEF domains from recruitment to the 3-month data collection, and a further increase from 3–6 months. Significant decreases in BDI scores were observed from recruitment to three months, and from 3–6 months.

Table 2. Mean (±sd) scores on the IIEF, SIS/SES and BDI scales at recruitment and after three and six months of PDE5I treatment.

	Recruitment	3 months	6 months
IIEF-EF	8.77 ± 2.16	16.33 ± 4.65 [a]	21.41 ± 2.73 [a,c]
IIEF-OF	3.73 ± 1.21	4.98 ± 1.73 [a]	6.29 ± 0.88 [a,c]
IIEF-SD	3.41 ± 1.43	5.55 ± 1.77 [a]	7.59 ± 1.01 [a,c]
IIEF-IS	2.81 ± 0.91	5.23 ± 1.74 [a]	9.38 ± 1.61 [a,c]
IIEF-OS	2.56 ± 0.57	5.23 ± 1.59 [a]	6.22 ± 0.94 [a,c]
BDI	23.26 ± 7.35	11.68 ± 4.72 [a]	10.19 ± 3.18 [a,b]
SES	53.87 ± 4.11		
SIS1	38.77 ± 4.06		
SIS2	35.35 ± 4.00		

[a] Significantly different from recruitment score $p < 0.01$; [b] Significantly different from 3-month score $p < 0.05$; [c] Significantly different from 3-month score $p < 0.01$

At recruitment, 75% of participants had BDI scores in the range 19–29, indicating moderately severe depression, with a further 12% scoring 30 or greater—indicative of severe depression [28]. At three months, 6% of participants had scores in the moderate range, with none in the severe range. At six months, 40% of participants scored in the moderate range, and 5% in the severe range. The percentage of participants whose scores indicated that they were not depressed increased from 9% at recruitment to 33% at three months and 44% at six months.

Mean scores for the expectations items at the three data collection points are shown in Table One. Significant decreases in scores from recruitment to three months were observed for all questions except 2, 10 and 12. At six months, scores for questions 1, 2, 3, 4 and 5 were significantly lower than the 3-month scores, whereas the scores for questions 8 and 10 were significantly higher. The score for question 10 was also higher than at recruitment.

3.2. Correlations

Because of the large number of correlation analyses conducted, only significant results are presented here.

The following correlations were observed between expectations item scores and questionnaire scores at recruitment: Item 2 and SIS2 (0.30, $p < 0.01$); Item 8 and IIEF-EF (0.27, $p < 0.05$); Item 8 and BDI (−0.28, $p < 0.05$); Item 10 and SES (0.28, $p < 0.05$); and Item 12 and BDI (−0.40, $p < 0.01$).

The change in IIEF-SD score from 0–3 months was correlated with recruitment scores for Item 1 ($r = -0.24$, $p < 0.01$); Item 3 ($r = 0.23$, $p < 0.01$); Item 8 ($r = 0.35$, $p < 0.01$); Item 10 ($r = 0.23$, $p < 0.01$) and Item 12 ($r = 0.25$, $p < 0.01$). The change in IIEF-IS score from recruitment three months correlated with the recruitment score for Item 4 ($r = 0.24$, $p < 0.05$) as was the change in IIEF-OS score ($r = 0.25$, $p < 0.05$). The change in BDI score from recruitment to three months was correlated with the recruitment scores for items Item 5 ($r = 0.40$, $p < 0.01$); Item 6 ($r = 0.33$, $p < 0.01$) and Item 12 ($r = 0.30$, $p < 0.01$).

The change in IIEF-SD score over the six months of the study correlated with the recruitment scores for Items 1 ($r = -0.34$, $p < 0.01$) and 8 ($r = 0.27$, $p < 0.05$). The change in IIEF-OS was correlated with recruitment scores for Items 4 ($r = 0.40$, $p < 0.01$) and 11 ($r = -0.26$, $p < 0.05$); and the change in BDI with Items 5 ($r = 0.28$, $p < 0.05$) and 12 ($r = 0.34$, $p < 0.01$).

The only significant correlation between changes in expectation item and questionnaire scores from 0–3 months was IIEF-SD and Item 2 ($r = -0.28$, $p < 0.05$). The following significant correlations were identified between changes in scores for expectations items and changes in questionnaire between three and six months: IIEF-EF and Item 10 ($r = 0.29$, $p < 0.05$); IIEF-OF and Item 6 ($r = 0.35$, $p < 0.01$); IIEF-SD and Item 4 ($r = 0.35$, $P < 0.01$); IIEF-IS and Items 4 ($r = 0.33$, $p < 0.01$) and 11 ($r = 0.25$, $p < 0.05$).

We originally intended to perform multiple linear regression is in order to identify predictors of the changes occurring in response to treatment. However the low number of significant correlations between variables rendered the data unsuitable for this analysis.

3.3. Power Analysis

The post hoc power analysis yielded a value of 73%, with a minimum detectable difference of 5.75 and a required sample size of 58.

4. Discussion

This paper reports findings relevant to the prescription of PDE5Is in general medical practice and reflects routine clinical practice at the GP level of care. It is important to emphasise that the diagnosis of ED was based on IIEF cutoffs, and that a definitive diagnosis of psychogenic ED was not made. Rather, the diagnosis was presumptive and based on the absence of causes of ED that were identifiable on routine clinical examination. The diagnosis therefore depended on the examination conducted by each of the doctors, which could not be controlled. Although there are established guidelines for the investigation of ED, there is little evidence confirming that these are adhered to in general practice. One study found that GPs treating men presenting with ED took a sexological history in only 85% of cases, and requested laboratory tests in 13.6% [29]. The authors suggested that this lack of thorough investigation may reflect the fact that "men may in many cases request a drug prescription from their GP and may not be interested in a physical examination". A separate study found that 83.9% of GPs believed that only selected patients required extensive diagnostic evaluations for ED [30]. Even amongst urologists there is evidence that investigations of conditions potentially contributing to ED are often abbreviated or deferred [31].

The first aim of this study was to determine whether expectations influence the response to PDE5Is. The paucity of correlations between expectations and measures of sexual function meant we were unable to fully explore this question, nor to address the question of what influences expectations. On the basis of the results of this study there is no evidence to support the view that expectations influence the therapeutic response to PDE5Is.

Across the period of the study, the increases in IIEF scores indicated improved erectile function and sexual satisfaction. The mean increase in IIEF scores from recruitment to three months exceeded the six point increase that is considered necessary for clinical significance [24]. While it is important to recognize that patient satisfaction with the medication was not directly measured, overall agreement with items 5, 6, 7 and 8 on the expectations questionnaire decreased from recruitment to three months (during which time overall sexual satisfaction measured on the IIEF-OS scale increased significantly). Given the nature of the questions, and interpreting these findings in terms of disconfirmation theory suggests that the changes in erectile function were insufficient to satisfy the patients. One possible explanation of the observed findings is that patient expectations for the effects of medication were excessively high. This is reflected in the response to the statement "I expect that this medication will restore my sexual function to normal" which had the second highest level of agreement of all statements at recruitment. It is likely that this is an unrealistic expectation, especially amongst men with apparent psychogenic ED, a condition for which combined psychological and pharmaceutical therapy gives better outcomes than medication use alone [32].

Hypothesising that expectations were excessively high raises the question of "how high is too high?". Only four items at recruitment had expectation scores greater than 3 (indicating overall agreement). It therefore appears that low expectation scores do not preclude the possibility that expectations will be too high to be met. An alternative approach is to ask "how much improvement in erectile function is required before patients are satisfied"—a question that cannot be answered from this study but which may be important in improving satisfaction with PDE5I use.

Expectations had not stabilised after three months of treatment. Between three and six months, the expectation to be prescribed a medication, the expectation that sexual function would be restored to normal and the expectation that the medication was the best treatment for ED all decreased. This suggests an ongoing loss of confidence in the drug despite improving erectile function, and may provide some explanation for the reported high discontinuation rates for PDE5Is [33].

In the 3–6 month period there were significant increases in scores for items 8 and 10 which relate to the patient's perception of partner satisfaction and understanding of drug use. Agreement with both statements was higher at six months than at either of the earlier data collection times. At three months, agreement with the statement that "ED is having a significant adverse effect on my life" was higher than at recruitment, but by six months agreement was significantly lower than the recruitment score. This change mirrors the change in agreement with the statement on perceived partner satisfaction. Taken together, the findings show that although the initial response to ED medication may be disappointing, there is scope for improvement in some domains if treatment is continued for long enough. However, with the exception of IIEF-EF, the size of the changes in domain scores required for a clinically significant outcome are unknown, and it is therefore impossible to determine whether the observed changes are of significance to the patient. The low scores for item 10 indicate that patient education was less than optimal, and that to some extent, men appear to learn how to use the medications by experience.

A review of the correlations between items sheds some light on the relationships between expectations and sexual confidence in this group of men. There was strong negative correlation between the expectation that the drug would restore sexual function to normal and that it would increase the users' confidence to engage in sexual activity. This suggests that improved physical capacity for intercourse was less important than other factors in generating their sexual confidence, and supports the view that in cases of psychogenic ED, the use of medications to restore erectile function should not be the only therapeutic strategy employed [34]. The importance of a rapid onset of action is reflected in its moderate positive correlation with the expectation that the drug will increase sexual confidence—in other words, a faster acting drug will have a greater beneficial effect on confidence. However, a rapid onset of action is more strongly correlated with expectations that partner satisfaction will increase.

A large number of participants met the BDI criteria for depression. Despite receiving no specific pharmacological or psychological treatment for depression, mean BDI scores decreased from recruitment to three months, with a further decrease from three to six months. The finding that men in this study were depressed is in accordance with other studies that have reported a relationship between depression and ED [35,36]. However, the nature of the relationship between the two conditions is unclear as ED may contribute to, or be a consequence of, depression [37]. The fact that the changes in IIEF-EF and BDI scores were not correlated suggests that depression was not a significant contributor to the aetiology of ED in these men. This contrasts with the previously reported negative correlation between changes in IIEF-EF and depression scores in men with ED who received treatment with PDE5Is [36]. However, men with ED of any aetiology were included in that study, and it is possible that the relationship between ED and depression varies according to the underlying cause of the ED. A positive effect of PDE5I therapy on depression has also been previously reported. Significantly greater reductions in symptoms of depression were reported in ED patients being treated with vardenafil compared with subjects in placebo groups [36,38] and changes in IIEF scores were negatively correlated with changes in scores on a depression scale in men with ED who received treatment with PDE5Is [36]. However, there is evidence of a placebo effect on changes in BDI. At the end of a six week double-blind study 73.2% of subjects treated with sildenafil, who were clinically depressed at recruitment, had a BDI score indicative of no or minimal depression. However, 47.1% of the placebo were not depressed at the end of the study [39]. Orr *et al.* [40] observed a positive effect of sildenafil on depressive symptoms independent of changes in EF. They suggested that these could be due to the effects of the drug on the autonomic nervous system or hippocampal neurogenesis. Whilst the findings of the present study have again shown a relationship between treatment with PDE5Is and a decrease in depressive symptom, they do not shed further light on the mechanism by which this effect is mediated. Changes in IIEF variables were not correlated with the observed improvement in BDI score, supporting the view that changes in EF are not principally responsible for improvements in depressive symptoms.

The study has several limitations that must be considered. The first is the fact psychogenic ED was a diagnosis of exclusion, with none of the subjects undergoing the full battery of tests necessary to achieve a definitive diagnosis. The results of the study do however reflect routine non-specialist medical management of ED patients. The study was observational with no control group, and patient history and clinical intervention could not be controlled. The possibility of a participation bias cannot be excluded. Because recruitment was limited to subjects diagnosed with apparent psychogenic ED, we do not suggest that the findings would be translatable to men with other types of ED.

A second important limitation is the fact that the expectations questionnaire was not validated. The decision not to validate the questionnaire was a practical one, based on the difficulty of recruiting sufficient subjects to complete both validation and experimental phases.

5. Conclusions

In conclusion, although expectations did not predict the response to therapy, the significant changes in expectations that were identified suggest the need for better patient management and counselling. Specifically, although erectile function improved with PDE5I use, agreement with statement that men understood how to use the drug remained low throughout the study. The study has shown the importance of advising men that initial dissatisfaction with the effects of PDE5Is on anticipated partner satisfaction and life impacts can be reversed if they persevere with treatment. There is a need to re-establish sexual norms after a period of ED, and initial attempts at intercourse are frequently associated with excessive anxiety [23]. As IIEF, BDI and several expectations scores changed from three to six months, it appears that men should persevere with PDE5I use for at least six months. A second important finding is that even after six months of use, agreement with the idea that the patient has sufficient knowledge of how PDE5Is are used remains low. Further examination of educational needs and how these can be met appears warranted.

Author Contributions

Connie C. J. Louizos and Peter K. Knight conceived and designed the experiments, Connie C. J. Louizos conducted the experiments and analyzed the data, Connie C. J. Louizos and Peter K. Knight wrote the paper.

Conflicts of interest

The authors declare no conflict of interest.

References

1. Carvalheira, A.A.; Pereira, N.M.; Maroco, J.; Forjaz, V. Dropout in the treatment of erectile dysfunction with PDE5: A study on predictors and a qualitative analysis of reasons for discontinuation. *J. Sex. Med.* **2012**, *9*, 2361–2369.
2. Ljunggren, C.; Hedelin, H.; Salomonsson, K.; Ströberg, P. Giving patients with erectile dysfunction the opportunity to try all three available phosphodiesterase type 5 inhibitors contributes to better long-term treatment compliance. *J. Sex. Med.* **2008**, *5*, 469–475.
3. Klotz, T.; Mathers, M.; Klotz, R.; Sommer, F. Why do patients with erectile dysfunction abandon effective therapy with sildenafil (Viagra)? *Int. J. Impot. Res.* **2005**, *17*, 2–4.
4. Son, H.; Park, K.; Kim, S.C.; Paick, J. Reasons for discontinuation of sildenafil citrate after successful restoration of erectile function. *Asian J. Androl.* **2004**, *6*, 117–120.
5. Jiann, B.; Yu, C.; Su, C.; Tsai. J. Compliance of sildenafil treatment for erectile dysfunction and factors affecting it. *Int. J. Impot. Res.* **2006**, *18*, 146–149.
6. Mondloch, M.V.; Cole, D.C.; Frank, J.W. Does how you do depend on how you think you'll do? A systematic review of the evidence for a relation between patients' recovery expectations and health outcomes. *CMAJ.* **2001**, *165*, 174–179.
7. Horne, R. Patients' beliefs about treatment: The hidden determinant of treatment outcome? *J. Psychosom. Res.* **1999**, *47*, 491–495.
8. Phatak, H.M.; Thomas, J. Relationships between beliefs about medications and nonadherence to prescribed chronic medications. *Ann. Pharmacother.* **2006**, *40*, 1737–1742.
9. Goldstein, I.; Lue, T.F.; Padma-Nathan, H.; Rosen, R.C.; Steers, W.D.; Wicker, P.A. Oral sildenafil in the treatment of erectile dysfunction. *N. Engl. J. Med.* **1998**, *338*, 1397–1404.
10. Dinsmore, W.W.; Hodges, M.; Hargreaves, C.; Osterloh, I.H.; Smith, M.D.; Rosen, R.C. Sildenafil citrate (Viagra) in erectile dysfunction: near normalization in men with broad-spectrum erectile dysfunction compared with age-matched healthy control subjects. *Urology* **1999**, *53*, 800–805.

11. Montorsi, F.; McDermott, T.E.D.; Morgan, R.; Olsson, A.; Schultz, A.; Kirkeby H.J.; Osterloh, I.H. Efficacy and safety of fixed-dose oral sildenafil in the treatment of erectile dysfunction of various etiologies. *Urology* **1999**, *53*, 1011–1018.
12. Young, J.M.; Feldman, R.A.; Auerbach, S.M.; Kaufman, J.M.; Garcia, C.S.; Shen, W.; Murphy, A.I.; Beasley, C.M.; Hague, J.A.; Ahuja, S. Tadalafil Improved Erectile Function at Twenty-Four and Thirty-Six Hours After Dosing in Men With Erectile Dysfunction: US Trial. *J. Androl.* **2005**, *26*, 310–318.
13. Rubio-Aurioles, E.; Casabé, A.; Torres, L.O.; Quinzaños, L.; Glina, S.; Filimon, I.; Kopernicky, V.; Leñero, E. Efficacy and safety of tadalafil in the treatment of Latin American men with erectile dysfunction: Results of integrated analyses. *J. Sex. Med.* **2008**, *5*, 1965–1976.
14. Benedetti, F. Placebo and the new physiology of the doctor-patient relationship. *Physiol. Rev.* **2013**, *93*, 1207–1246.
15. Oliver, R.L. A cognitive model of the antecedents and consequences of satisfaction decisions. *J. Mark. Res.* **1980**, *17*, 460–469.
16. Ho, F.N.; Mursch, J.D.; Ong, B.S.; Peittula, B. Consumer satisfaction with OTC drugs: An analysis using the confirmation/disconfirmation model. *Health Mark. Q.* **1998**, *15*, 103–117.
17. Dolovich, L.; Nair, K.; Sellors, C.; Lohfeld, L.; Lee, A.; Levine, M. Do patients' expectations influence their use of medications? Qualitative study. *Can. Fam. Physician* **2008**, *54*, 384–393.
18. Kumar, R.N.; Kirking, D.M.; Hass, S.L.; Vinokur, A.D.; Taylor, S.D.; Atkinson, M.J.; McKircher, P.L. The association of consumer expectations, experiences and satisfaction with newly prescribed medications. *Qual. Life Res.* **2007**, *16*, 1127–1136.
19. Weaver, M.; Patrick, D.L.; Markson, L.E.; Martin, D.; Frederic, I.; Berger, M. Issues in the measurement of satisfaction with treatment. *Am. J. Manag. Care* **1997**, *3*, 579–594.
20. Atkinson, M.J.; Sinha, A.; Hass, S.L.; Colman, S.S.; Kumar, R.N.; Brod, M.; Rowland, C.R. Validation of a general measure of treatment satisfaction, the Treatment Satisfaction Questionnaire for Medication (TSQM), using a national panel study of chronic disease. *Health Qual. Life Outcomes* **2004**, *2*, 12, doi:10.1186/1477-7525-2-12.
21. Conaglen, H.M.; Conaglen, J.V. Couples' Reasons for Adherence to, or Discontinuation of, PDE Type 5 Inhibitors for Men with Erectile Dysfunction at 12 to 24-Month Follow-Up after a 6-Month Free Trial. *J. Sex Med.* **2012**, *9*, 857–865.
22. Kendirci, M.; Tanriverdi, O.; Trost, L.; Hellstrom, W.J. Management of sildenafil treatment failures. *Curr. Opin. Urol.* **2006**, *16*, 449–459.
23. Impotence Australia. Available online: http://www.impotenceaustralia.com.au (accessed on 4 November 2015).
24. Rosen, R.C.; Riley, A.; Wagner, G.; Osterloh, I.H.; Kirkpatrick, J.; Mishra, A. The international index of erectile function (IIEF): A multidimensional scale for assessment of erectile dysfunction. *Urology* **1997**, *49*, 822–830.
25. Janssen, E.; Vorst, H.; Finn, P.; Bancroft J. The Sexual Inhibition (SIS) and Sexual Excitation (SES) Scales: I. Measuring sexual inhibition and excitation proneness in men. *J. Sex. Res.* **2002**, *39*, 114–126.
26. Beck, A.T.; Ward, C.H.; Mendelson, M.; Mock, J.; Erbaugh, J. An inventory for measuring depression. *Arch. Gen. Psychiatry* **1961**, *4*, 561–571.

27. Rajpurkar, A.; Dhabuwala, C.B. Comparison of satisfaction rates and erectile function in patients treated with sildenafil, intracavernous prostaglandin E1 and penile implant surgery for erectile dysfunction in urology practice. *J. Urol.* **2003**, *170*, 159–163.
28. Beck, A.T.; Steer, R.A.; Garbin, M.G. Psychometric properties of the Beck Depression inventory. Twenty-five years of evaluation. *Clin. Psych. Review* **1988**, *8*, 77–100.
29. Kedde, H.; Donker, G.; Leusink, P.; Kruijer, H. The incidence of sexual dysfunction in patients attending Dutch general practitioners. *Int. J. Sex. Health* **2011**, *23*, 269–277.
30. De Berardis, G.; Pellegrini, F.; Franciosi, M.; Pamparana, F.; Morelli, P.; Tognoni, G.; Nicolucci, A. Management of erectile dysfunction in general practice. *J. Sex. Med.* **2009**, *6*, 1127–1134.
31. Schnetzler, G.; Marfatia, A.; Zou, K.H.; Muniain, J.; Symonds, T. Current erectile dysfunction management: A survey among delegates of the 2008 annual EAU congress in Milan. *Eur. Urol. Suppl.* **2009**, *8*, 212, doi:10.1016/S1569-9056(09)60370-5.
32. Banner, L.L.; Anderson, R.U. Integrated sildenafil and cognitive-behavior sex therapy for psychogenic erectile dysfunction: A pilot study. *J. Sex. Med.* **2007**, *4*, 1117–1125.
33. Otero, J.R.; Gómez, B.G.; Polo, J.M.; Alcaide, E.J.; Cruz, E.G.; Font, A.S.; Antolín, A.R. Evaluation of current errors within the administration of phosphodiesterase-5 inhibitors after more than 10 years of use. *Urology* **2014**, *83*, 1334–1338.
34. Schmidt, H.M.; Munder, T.; Gerger, H.; Frühauf, S.; Barth, J. Combination of psychological intervention and phosphodiesterase-5 inhibitors for erectile dysfunction: A narrative review and meta-analysis. *J. Sex. Med.* **2014**, *11*, 1376–1391.
35. Araujo, A.B.; Durante, R.; Feldman, H.A.; Goldstein, I.; McKinlay, J.B. The relationship between depressive symptoms and male erectile dysfunction: cross-sectional results from the Massachusetts male aging study. *Psychosom. Med.* **1998**, *60*, 458–465.
36. Rosen, R.; Shabsigh, R.; Berber, M.; Assalian, P.; Menza, M.; Rodriguez-Vela, L. Efficacy and tolerability of vardenafil in men with mild depression and erectile dysfunction: the depression-related improvement with vardenafil for erectile response study. *Am. J. Psychiatry* **2006**, *163*, 79–87.
37. Shim, Y.S.; Pae, C.U.; Cho, K.J.; Kim, S.W.; Kim, J.C.; Koh, J.S. Effects of daily low-dose treatment with phosphodiesterase type 5 inhibitor on cognition, depression, somatization and erectile function in patients with erectile dysfunction: A double-blind, placebo-controlled study. *Int. J. Impot. Res.* **2014**, *26*, 76–80.
38. Hatzichristou, D.; Cuzin, B.; Martin-Morales, A.; Buvat, J.; Porst, H.; Laferriere, N. Vardenafil improves satisfaction rates, depressive symptomatology, and self-confidence in a broad population of men with erectile dysfunction. *J. Sex. Med.* **2005**, *2*, 109–116.
39. Kennedy, S.H.; Dugré, H.; Defoy, I. A multicenter, double-blind, placebo-controlled study of sildenafil citrate in Canadian men with erectile dysfunction and untreated symptoms of depression, in the absence of major depressive disorder. *Int. Clin. Psychopharmacol.* **2011**, *26*, 151–158.
40. Orr, G.; Seidman, S.N.; Weiser, M.; Gershon, A.A.; Dubrov, Y.; Klein, D.F. An open-label pilot study to evaluate the efficacy of sildenafil citrate in middle-aged men with late-onset dysthymia. *J. Nerv. Ment. Dis.* **2008**, *196*, 496–500.

14

Does the Subject Content of the Pharmacy Degree Course Influence the Community Pharmacist's Views on Competencies for Practice?

Jeffrey Atkinson [1,2,*], Kristien De Paepe [3], Antonio Sánchez Pozo [4], Dimitrios Rekkas [5], Daisy Volmer [6], Jouni Hirvonen [7], Borut Bozic [8], Agnieska Skowron [9], Constantin Mircioiu [10], Annie Marcincal [11], Andries Koster [12], Keith Wilson [13], Chris van Schravendijk [14] and Jamie Wilkinson [15]

[1] Pharmacology Department, Lorraine University, 5 rue Albert Lebrun, 54000 Nancy, France

[2] Pharmacolor Consultants Nancy, 12 rue de Versigny, Villers 54600, France

[3] Department of Pharmacy, Vrije Universiteit Brussel, Laarbeeklaan 103, Brussels 1090, Belgium; E-Mail: kdepaepe@vub.ac.be

[4] Faculty of Pharmacy, University of Granada (UGR), Campus Universitario de la Cartuja s/n, Granada 18701, Spain; E-Mail: sanchezp@ugr.es

[5] School of Pharmacy, National and Kapodistrian University Athens, Panepistimiou 30, Athens 10679, Greece; E-Mail: rekkas@pharm.uoa.gr

[6] Pharmacy Faculty, University of Tartu, Nooruse 1, Tartu 50411, Estonia; E-Mail: daisy.volmer@ut.ee

[7] Pharmacy Faculty, University of Helsinki, Yliopistonkatu 4, P.O. Box 33-4, Helsinki 00014, Finland; E-Mail: jouni.hirvonen@helsinki.fi

[8] Faculty of Pharmacy, University of Ljubljana, Askerceva cesta 7, Ljubljana 1000, Slovenia; E-Mail: Borut.Bozic@ffa.uni-lj.si

[9] Pharmacy Faculty, Jagiellonian University, UL, Golebia 24, Krakow 31-007, Poland; E-Mail: askowron@cm-uj.krakow.pl

[10] Pharmacy Faculty, University of Medicine and Pharmacy "Carol Davila" Bucharest, Dionisie Lupu 37, Bucharest 020021, Romania; E-Mail: constantin.mircioiu@yahoo.com

[11] European Association of Faculties of Pharmacy, Faculty of Pharmacy, Université de Lille 2, Lille 59000, France; E-Mail: annie.marcincal@pharma.univ-lille2.fr

[12] European Association of Faculties of Pharmacy, Department Pharmaceutical Sciences, Utrecht University, PO Box 80082, 3508 TB Utrecht, The Netherlands; E-Mail: A.S.Koster@uu.nl

[13] School of Life and Health Sciences, Aston University, Birmingham, B4 7ET, UK; E-Mail: k.a.wilson@aston.ac.uk

[14] Vrije Universiteit Brussel, Laarbeeklaan 103, 1090 Brussels, Belgium; E-Mail: chrisvs@vub.ac.be

[15] Pharmaceutical Group of the European Union (PGEU), Rue du Luxembourg 19, 1000 Brussels, Belgium; E-Mail: j.wilkinson@pgeu.eu

* Author to whom correspondence should be addressed; E-Mail: jeffrey.atkinson@univ-lorraine.fr

Academic Editor: Reem Kayyali

Abstract: Do community pharmacists coming from different educational backgrounds rank the importance of competences for practice differently—or is the way in which they see their profession more influenced by practice than university education? A survey was carried out on 68 competences for pharmacy practice in seven countries with different pharmacy education systems in terms of the relative importance of the subject areas chemical and medicinal sciences. Community pharmacists were asked to rank the competences in terms of relative importance for practice; competences were divided into personal and patient-care competences. The ranking was very similar in the seven countries suggesting that evaluation of competences for practice is based more on professional experience than on prior university education. There were some differences for instance in research-related competences and these may be influenced, by education.

Keywords: pharmacy; education; community; practice; competence

1. Introduction

In 1985, the then European Economic Community (EEC) published a directive [1] on pharmacy practice that assumed that pharmacy education in the EEC was broadly comparable and, thus, that the European education system was producing pharmacists with similar competences. In the early 1990s, the European Association of Faculties of Pharmacy (EAFP) [2] questioned these assumptions [3]. EAFP surveyed pharmacy courses in the 11 EEC members and found that although the emphasis in most faculties was on chemical sciences, there was great variability in pharmacy degree courses in the EEC regarding the percentages of time spent on different subjects [4].

At that time it was hoped that European integration would produce greater harmonization in pharmacy education and therefore in competences for practice. In 2011, the PHARMINE ("*PHARMacy Education IN Europe*") project [5] revisited this problem. In the 20-year interval between the two studies there was a shift in several countries from chemical to medicinal sciences, albeit, overall variability in degree courses from country to country had not decreased [6]. PHARMINE reflected upon whether differences in pharmacy degrees could be minored by expressing content as competences rather than subjects.

As a follow-up to PHARMINE, a second study, the PHAR-QA ("*Quality Assurance in European PHARmacy-Education and Training*") project [7], again funded by the European Commission, asked community pharmacists to rank competences for pharmacy practice.

This paper combines the results of the PHARMINE and PHAR-QA studies. It looks at whether the nature of the degree course (in terms of the relative importance of the subject areas chemical and medicinal sciences taken as an indication of a more "scientific" or a more "clinical" course) has any influence on the way in which community pharmacists ranked the competences they consider are required for practice. The paper evaluates to what extent university education or professional experience can influence the way in which practicing community pharmacists judge their *métier* and how the balance between these two factors could be altered by the introduction of competence-based education.

2. Experimental Section

In the PHARMINE project, country profiles for pharmacy education and training were drawn up with the help of academics, students, professional pharmacists, and their organizations, as well as representatives of different governmental bodies concerned with pharmacy in the 47 countries of the European Higher Education Area [8]. Amongst others, one of the areas explored in the country profiles was the structure of the pharmacy degree course that was divided into six subject areas: chemical sciences, medicinal sciences, biological sciences, pharmaceutical technology, and law and societal issues. A subject area course index was calculated as: ((percentage of contact hours spent on medicinal subjects/percentage of contact hours spent on chemical subjects) x 100) using data from the PHARMINE study, as given in the 2014 paper on heterogeneity of pharmacy education cited above [6].

In the PHARMINE study, "medicinal subjects" included contact hours in the subjects of anatomy, physiology, medical terminology, pathology, histology, nutrition, pharmacology/pharmacotherapy, toxicology, hematology, immunology, parasitology, hygiene, emergency therapy, non-pharmacological treatment, clinical chemistry/bio-analysis, radiochemistry, dispensing process, drug prescription, prescription analysis (detection of adverse effects and drug interactions), generic drugs, planning, running and interpretation of the data, of clinical trials, medical devices, orthopedics, over the counter medicines, complementary therapy, at-home support and care, skin illness and treatment, homeopathy, phyto-therapy, drugs in veterinary medicine, pharmaceutical care, pharmaceutical therapy of illness, and disease. "Chemical subjects" included contact hours in the subjects of general and inorganic chemistry, medical physico-chemistry, organic chemistry, pharmacopeia analysis, analytical chemistry, and pharmaceutical chemistry including analysis of medicinal products.

Ranking data on competences for practice were taken from the PHAR-QA *surveymonkey* [9] questionnaire that was available online from 14 January 2014 to 1 November 2014 *i.e.*, 8.5 months. Contacts were made by electronic and other means with the same groups as in the PHARMINE study (see previously). *Post hoc* analysis of the data allowed the creation of six subgroups: academics, students, community pharmacists, hospital pharmacists, industrial pharmacists, and pharmacists working in other areas. Here we will present the data for community pharmacists; data for other professional categories will be presented elsewhere [10].

The first six questions of the PHAR-QA survey were on the profile of the respondent asking, amongst others, country of residence, current occupation, and duration of activity.

Questions seven through 19 asked about 13 groups of competences with a total of 68 competences (see annex). Questions in groups seven through 11 were concerned with personal competences and in groups 12 through 19 with patient care competences.

Respondents were asked to rank the proposals for competences with a Likert scale:

1. Not important = Can be ignored.
2. Quite important = Valuable but not obligatory.
3. Very important = Obligatory with exceptions depending upon field of pharmacy practice.
4. Essential = Obligatory.

Results are presented in the form of "scores" based on the methodology used in MEDINE2 [11]: score = (frequency rank 3 + frequency rank 4) as % of total frequency. Scores give more granularity and a better pictorial representation than the basic Likert data. Data were obtained from 39 European countries. Data presented here are from the seven European Union member states in which the number of respondents was > 10 (Table 1). Analysis was limited to the European Union as its 28 member states come under the directive on sectoral professions such as pharmacy [12]. One of the annexes of this directive lists the subject areas that are to be taught in the pharmacy degree course in the European Union. Of the 28 member states only seven provided 10 or more community pharmacists respondents.

Statistical Analysis

Results are also expressed as medians with 25 and 75% percentiles; differences among countries were analyzed using the Kruskal-Wallis test followed by Dunn's multiple comparisons test. All statistics were performed using GraphPad software [13].

3. Results and Discussion

In Table 1 are the medians for duration of practice. Kruskal-Wallace analysis showed a significant effect of country ($P = 0.0014$) and the Dunn's multiple comparisons test showed that the duration of practice of the respondents from the Czech Republic was lower than that of respondents from Germany, Ireland or Spain. None of the other comparisons were significant.

Table 1 also shows the medicinal sciences/chemical sciences scores. In Germany the degree course is more "chemical"; in Belgium, the Czech Republic, and Spain the importance of the two subject areas is equal; in The Netherlands and the United Kingdom there is a more "medicinal" course, and this is even more pronounced in Ireland. The medicinal/chemical ratio varies almost four-fold from Germany (0.7) to Ireland (2.6).

Finally, Table 1 shows overall the median rankings for competences ($n = 68$). The Kruskal-Wallis test showed a significant difference amongst countries ($P = 0.0006$) with a significantly higher median for Spain compared to Belgium, Germany, and Ireland. None of the other multiple comparisons amongst countries reached statistical significance.

Table 1. Characteristics of the seven countries, the medicinal sciences/chemical sciences indices (latter data from the PHARMINE study), and the rankings for competences.

Country	Number of respondents	Duration of activity (years; median, 25% and 75% percentiles)	Medicinal sciences %	Chemical sciences %	Medicinal/chemical score	Ranking of competences (median, 25% and 75% percentiles, $n = 68$)
Belgium	25	10/5/20	24	27	1.1	81/63/91
Czech Republic	15	5/5/15	19	17	1.1	84/67/92
Germany	13	30/15/30	28	40	0.7	82/67/92
Ireland	13	20/10/33	36	14	2.6	77/55/92
Spain	27	15/10/30	28	24	1.2	91/82/96
The Netherlands	18	20/5/23	31	20	1.6	82/57/94
United Kingdom	48	10/5/20	24	14	1.7	87/59/96

Figure 1 shows the ranking by the seven countries of the 68 competences. This is presented as a radar chart. Radar charts are a useful way to display multivariate observations with an arbitrary number of variables. It allows one to find clusters and also to identify outliers [14]. This radar chart presentation allows an easy overview of the global rankings of competences. It underlines the fact that overall the global rankings by the different countries are similar, with similar highs and lows. This is especially true for the left-hand side of the Figure that represents the rankings for the patient care competences (number 43 through 68). Opinions of the relative importance of such competences appear to be formed by work experience rather than university education. In answer to the question "do community pharmacists coming from different educational backgrounds rank the importance of competences for practice differently" the answer would be no in the case of patient care competences. Examination of Figure 1 shows that the ranking of competences for practice is very similar in seven countries that have different systems of pharmacy education. It should be noted that the ranking score is based on a combination of ranks 3 and 4 that specify that competences are "obligatory".

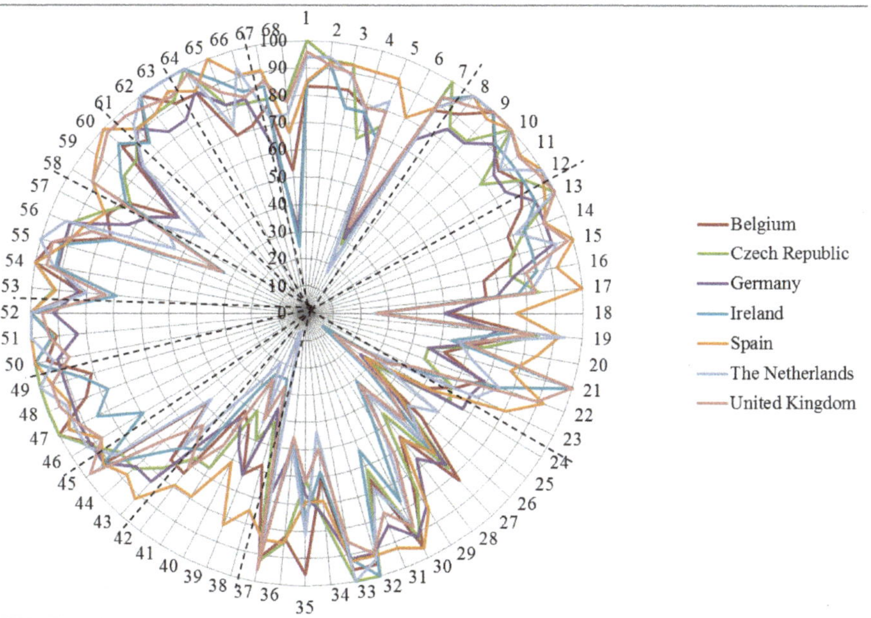

Figure 1. Radar chart of the ranking scores (on the central vertical axe, 0%–100%) for the 68 competences (on the circumference) by the seven countries (in different colours). Dotted lines separate the 13 competence groups (see annex) in Figure 1 are given the ranking scores for the 68 competences by the seven countries.

There are more differences in the right-hand side of the Figure that represents personal competences. Competence 6 is an interesting case. The difference between minimum and maximum for country rankings in group 7 ("personal competences: learning and knowledge") competence 6 ("ability to design and conduct research using appropriate methodology") was large (63, see Table A1); Spain, which has a "balanced" course with a medicinal sciences/chemical sciences index of 1.2, ranked highest with 80%. Ireland and the Netherlands which have more "medical" indices of 2.6 and 1.6, respectively, showed the lowest rankings for competence 6: 18 and 17%, respectively. Spain also ranked highest for all competences. In the research-related group 11 ("personal competences: understanding of industrial pharmacy") Spain scored highest for all 5 competences. Thus differences for Spain may be influenced by education rather than professional experience, albeit, Germany, which has a more "chemical" index (0.7), did not rank competence 6 or the competences in group 11 particularly high.

Several provisos should be added. It is possible that differences in ranking scores are related to duration of practice (*i.e.,* numbers of years since leaving university) rather than to course content. With the median years of practice being significantly different it could very well be that older pharmacists in a given country took a very different course of study 30–40 years ago than younger pharmacists from the same country. Furthermore, it is likely the mix of medicinal/chemical subjects would have differed within countries for participants dependent on when they studied especially as there has been a move towards more medicinal sciences in the past 20 years (see introduction). This cannot be tested, however, as numbers in the different groups do not allow the creation of subgroups based on duration of practice. Some comments can be made on the basis of the existing data. The community pharmacist respondents from the Czech Republic were younger than in several other countries, but the Czech Republic community pharmacists did not show any marked differences with other countries as far as ranking of competences was concerned. Spanish community pharmacists did show a specific pattern of ranking in several groups of competences but their median duration of practice was mid-range.

The conclusion of this paper relies on the fact that the curricula investigated are as different as possible in the relative importance of "medicinal" versus "chemical" sciences component. The seven countries selected were selected on the basis of providing more than 10 respondents. Nonetheless they do represent a significantly wide range of scores. Ireland has the highest value of the 26 European Union member states that have pharmacy departments (1st/26), and Germany the 3rd from the lowest (23rd/26)[vi].

The PHARMINE study cited above showed that a competence approach is rarely used in pre-graduate pharmacy education in Europe. There have been several studies on the use of a competence framework to monitor and improve pharmacy practice in a working environment. A study using the general level framework with Singaporean hospital pharmacists showed that all but eight of the 63 behavioral descriptors improved in nine months [15]. A similar study with hospital pharmacists in Queensland showed an improvement in 35 out of 61 competences [16]. Studies have also been conducted in Canada [17]. and elsewhere. The results of all these studies are that competence frameworks are useful tools to monitor and improve performance.

4. Conclusions

This study shows that community pharmacists largely form their opinions on the importance of competences of the basis of work experience rather than university education. The move to harmonize European pharmacy practice expressed in the 1980s seems to have been successful, as judged from the similar way in which community pharmacists from different countries rank competences for practice. However this is less the result of harmonization of pharmacy education that still shows wide diversity.

The short-term perspective of this work is the modification of the existing questionnaire according to the results obtained and the endorsement of the modified version.

The long-term perspective is the introduction of competence-based learning into the university curriculum for pharmacy. This is being discussed in Australia and New Zealand [18] and elsewhere. It now needs to be considered in Europe. Our results suggest that differences in university pharmacy programs are not crucial in the development of specific competencies (at least in the field of community pharmacy, where the majority of pharmacists work). Thus, we do not need a very stringent and tight framework for curricula of pharmacy education. Academia provides graduates with competencies as "novices" (according to five-stage model of competencies proposed by Dreyfus and Dreyfus, 1980 [19]). Thus, competence-based learning in universities would provide a sound foundation allowing graduates to gather experience through practical training in the real job environment. Furthermore, academic freedom as to course content should be incorporated into quality assurance of pharmacy education especially when EU directive is "translated" into national frameworks.

Acknowledgements

With the support of the Lifelong Learning programme of the European Union: 527194-LLP-1-2012-1-BE-ERASMUS-EMCR. This project has been funded with support from the European Commission. This publication reflects the views only of the author; the Commission cannot be held responsible for any use which may be made of the information contained therein.

Author Contributions

Jeffrey Atkinson designed, constructed, ran and analysed the survey and wrote the paper. Kristien De Paepe ran the PHAR-QA consortium. Constantin Mircioiu played a major role in the statistical analyses of the data. Antonio Sánchez Pozo and Dimitrios Rekkas developed the questionnaire. Antonio Sánchez Pozo, Dimitrios Rekkas, Jouni Hirvonen, Borut Bozic, Annie Marcincal and Agnieska Skowron helped with distribution of the survey. Antonio Sánchez Pozo, Daisy Volmer and Kristien De Paepe provided useful criticism and suggestions during revision of the manuscript. Chris van Schravendijk assured the contacts with MEDINE. Jamie Wilkinson played a major role in distributing the survey to community pharmacists.

Conflicts of Interest

The authors declare no conflict of interest.

Appendix

Table A1. Ranking of competences by countries.

Seq.	Competence	Belgium	Czech Republic	Germany	Ireland	Spain	The Netherlands	United Kingdom	Min.	Max.	Range: max–min.
	Group 7. Personal competences: learning and knowledge										
1	1. Ability to identify learning needs and to learn independently (including continuous professional development (CPD)).	83	100	85	85	85	94	96	83	100	17
2	2. Analysis: ability to apply logic to problem solving, evaluating pros and cons and following up on the solution found.	83	93	92	92	93	94	92	83	94	11
3	3. Synthesis: capacity to gather and critically appraise relevant knowledge and to summarise the key points.	83	93	77	77	93	89	90	77	93	16
4	4. Capacity to evaluate scientific data in line with current scientific and technological knowledge.	78	67	77	77	92	78	79	67	92	25
5	5. Ability to interpret preclinical and clinical evidence-based medical science and apply the knowledge to pharmaceutical practice.	63	73	62	69	92	83	79	62	92	31
6	6. Ability to design and conduct research using appropriate methodology.	33	29	31	18	80	17	36	17	80	63
7	7. Ability to maintain current knowledge of relevant legislation and codes of pharmacy practice.	88	100	75	92	89	89	93	75	100	25
	Group 8. Personal competences: values										
8	1. Demonstrate a professional approach to tasks and human relations.	92	86	85	100	100	100	96	85	100	15
9	2. Demonstrate the ability to maintain confidentiality.	100	86	85	100	96	100	100	85	100	15
10	3. Take full personal responsibility for patient care and other aspects of one's practice.	92	100	92	92	100	100	100	92	100	8

Table A1. *Cont.*

Seq.	Competence	Belgium	Czech Republic	Germany	Ireland	Spain	The Netherlands	United Kingdom	Min.	Max.	Range: max–min.
11	4. Inspire the confidence of others in one's actions and advice.	87	79	85	92	96	88	96	79	96	18
12	5. Demonstrate high ethical standards.	92	93	85	92	100	100	98	85	100	15
	Group 9. Personal competences: communication and organisational skills.										
13	1. Effective communication skills (both orally and written).	87	100	92	92	96	100	100	87	100	13
14	2. Effective use of information technology.	78	85	92	85	92	81	92	78	92	14
15	3. Ability to work effectively as part of a team.	78	77	92	85	100	94	98	77	100	23
16	4. Ability to identify and implement legal and professional requirements relating to employment (e.g., for pharmacy technicians) and to safety in the workplace.	65	75	77	85	92	88	81	65	92	27
17	5. Ability to contribute to the learning and training of staff.	65	85	69	77	100	81	83	65	100	35
18	6. Ability to design and manage the development processes in the production of medicines.	52	25	50	25	76	25	26	25	76	51
19	7. Ability to identify and manage risk and quality of service issues.	82	85	69	75	92	94	83	69	94	25
20	8. Ability to identify the need for new services.	62	67	62	54	85	56	59	54	85	31
21	9. Ability to communicate in English and/or locally relevant languages.	52	46	46	100	77	63	100	46	100	54
22	10. Ability to evaluate issues related to quality of service.	68	46	69	75	92	75	90	46	92	46
23	11. Ability to negotiate, understand a business environment and develop entrepreneurship.	61	58	67	50	81	69	43	43	81	37
	Group 10. Personal competences: knowledge of different areas of the science of medicines.										
24	1. Plant and animal biology.	52	62	67	31	54	27	35	27	67	40

Table A1. *Cont.*

Seq.	Competence	Belgium	Czech Republic	Germany	Ireland	Spain	The Netherlands	United Kingdom	Min.	Max.	Range: max–min.
25	2. Physics.	26	31	25	8	27	60	13	8	60	52
26	3. General and inorganic chemistry.	57	46	42	31	46	50	39	31	57	26
27	4. Organic and medicinal/pharmaceutical chemistry.	83	77	75	69	69	63	53	53	83	29
28	5. Analytical chemistry.	57	46	67	31	58	38	33	31	67	36
29	6. General and applied biochemistry (medicinal and clinical).	74	77	83	46	85	56	62	46	85	38
30	7. Anatomy and physiology; medical terminology.	96	92	92	77	96	88	88	77	96	19
31	8. Microbiology.	65	62	83	54	92	69	78	54	92	38
32	9. Pharmacology including pharmacokinetics.	96	100	92	100	92	94	91	91	100	9
33	10. Pharmacotherapy and pharmaco-epidemiology.	96	100	92	92	92	100	85	85	100	15
34	11. Pharmaceutical technology including analyses of medicinal products.	61	77	75	58	69	44	50	44	77	33
35	12. Toxicology.	96	62	67	75	69	81	62	62	96	34
36	13. Pharmacognosy.	83	85	50	46	85	50	46	46	85	39
37	14. Legislation and professional ethics.	91	92	67	92	85	88	96	67	96	29
	Group 11. Personal competences: understanding of industrial pharmacy.										
38	1. Current knowledge of design, synthesis, isolation, characterisation and biological evaluation of active substances.	58	42	36	25	75	7	28	7	75	68
39	2. Current knowledge of good manufacturing practice (GMP) and of good laboratory practice (GLP).	63	50	64	25	83	43	42	25	83	58
40	3. Current knowledge of European directives on qualified persons (QPs).	47	40	55	25	61	20	27	20	61	41

Table A1. *Cont.*

Seq.	Competence	Belgium	Czech Republic	Germany	Ireland	Spain	The Netherlands	United Kingdom	Min.	Max.	Range: max–min.
41	4. Current knowledge of drug registration, licensing and marketing.	42	67	45	33	79	27	57	27	79	53
42	5. Current knowledge of good clinical practice (GCP).	74	67	55	63	79	40	71	40	79	39
	Group 12. Patient care competences: patient consultation and assessment.										
43	1. Ability to perform and interpret medical laboratory tests.	73	77	83	67	92	67	56	56	92	36
44	2. Ability to perform appropriate diagnostic or physiological tests to inform clinical decision making e.g., measurement of blood pressure.	48	85	83	77	88	47	69	47	88	41
45	3. Ability to recognise when referral to another member of the healthcare team is needed because a potential clinical problem is identified (pharmaceutical, medical, psychological or social).	91	85	92	92	92	87	98	85	98	13
	Group 13. Patient care competences: need for drug treatment.										
46	1. Retrieval and interpretation of relevant information on the patient's clinical background.	91	92	92	69	88	93	87	69	93	24
47	2. Retrieval and interpretation of an accurate and comprehensive drug history if and when required.	100	100	92	85	96	93	91	85	100	15
48	3. Identification of non-adherence and implementation of appropriate patient intervention.	86	100	91	77	92	93	96	77	100	23
49	4. Ability to advise to physicians and—in some cases—prescribe medication.	81	100	91	85	96	100	96	81	100	19
	Group 14. Patient care competences: drug interactions.										

Table A1. *Cont.*

Seq.	Competence	Belgium	Czech Republic	Germany	Ireland	Spain	The Netherlands	United Kingdom	Min.	Max.	Range: max–min.
50	1. Identification, understanding and prioritisation of drug-drug interactions at a molecular level (e.g., use of codeine with paracetamol).	95	100	92	100	100	93	87	87	100	13
51	2. Identification, understanding, and prioritisation of drug-patient interactions, including those that preclude or require the use of a specific drug (e.g., trastuzumab for treatment of breast cancer in women with HER2 overexpression).	91	92	83	92	100	100	93	83	100	17
52	3. Identification, understanding, and prioritisation of drug-disease interactions (e.g., NSAIDs in heart failure).	100	100	92	100	100	100	96	92	100	8
	Group 15. Patient care competences: provision of drug product.										
53	1. Familiarity with the bio-pharmaceutical, pharmacodynamic and pharmacokinetic activity of a substance in the body.	82	92	83	69	91	80	73	69	92	22
54	2. Supply of appropriate medicines taking into account dose, correct formulation, concentration, administration route and timing.	100	100	92	92	100	93	96	92	100	8
55	3. Critical evaluation of the prescription to ensure that it is clinically appropriate and legal.	95	92	92	92	91	100	96	91	100	9
56	4. Familiarity with the supply chain of medicines and the ability to ensure timely flow of drug products to the patient.	76	92	92	75	87	93	83	75	93	18
57	5. Ability to manufacture medicinal products that are not commercially available.	81	83	73	33	82	53	34	33	83	50
	Group 16. Patient care competences: patient education.										

Table A1. *Cont.*

Seq.	Competence	Belgium	Czech Republic	Germany	Ireland	Spain	The Netherlands	United Kingdom	Min.	Max.	Range: max–min.
58	1. Promotion of public health in collaboration with other actors in the healthcare system.	77	75	67	77	91	60	91	60	91	31
59	2. Provision of appropriate lifestyle advice on smoking, obesity, *etc.*	59	83	58	85	96	47	93	47	96	49
60	3. Provision of appropriate advice on resistance to antibiotics and similar public health issues.	90	83	82	92	100	80	98	80	100	20
	Group 17. Patient care competences: provision of information and service.										
61	1. Ability to use effective consultations to identify the patient's need for information.	86	92	92	85	91	93	98	85	98	13
62	2. Provision of accurate and appropriate information on prescription medicines.	100	92	83	100	91	100	95	83	100	17
63	3. Provision of informed support for patients in selection and use of non-prescription medicines for minor ailments (e.g., cough remedies...)	90	92	83	100	96	100	93	83	100	17
	Group 18. Patient care competences: monitoring of drug therapy.										
64	1. Identification and prioritisation of problems in the management of medicines in a timely manner and with sufficient efficacy to ensure patient safety.	90	100	91	100	91	100	98	90	100	10
65	2. Ability to monitor and report to all concerned in a timely manner, and in accordance with current regulatory guidelines on Good Pharmacovigilance Practices (GVPs), Adverse Drug Events and Reactions (ADEs and ADRs).	70	82	82	92	100	73	87	70	100	30
66	3. Undertaking of a critical evaluation of prescribed medicines to confirm that current clinical guidelines are appropriately applied.	71	80	82	85	91	93	82	71	93	22

Table A1. *Cont.*

Seq.	Competence	Belgium	Czech Republic	Germany	Ireland	Spain	The Netherlands	United Kingdom	Min.	Max.	Range: max–min.
	Group 19. Patient care competences: evaluation of outcomes.										
67	1. Assessment of outcomes on the monitoring of patient care and follow-up interventions.	78	80	60	85	90	73	87	60	90	30
68	2. Evaluation of cost effectiveness of treatment.	53	80	30	25	67	73	78	25	80	55

Seq.: sequential numbering (as in Figure 1); Min.: minimum; Max.: maximum; Note that the numbering of the groups of competences starts at 7, *i.e.*, after the 6 questions on profile.

References

1. The European Union. The Council Directive of 16 September 1985 concerning the coordination of provisions laid down by law, regulation or administrative action in respect of certain activities in the field of pharmacy. Available online: http://eur-lex.europa.eu/legal-content/EN/TXT/PDF/?uri=CELEX:31985L0432&from=EN (accessed on 28 August 2015).
2. European Association of Faculties of Pharmacy (EAFP). Available online: http://www.eafponline.eu/ (accessed on 28 August 2015).
3. The European Commission. ERASMUS Subject Evaluations: Summary Reports of the Evaluation Conferences by Subject Area. Volume 1 pharmacy. Available online: http://eafponline.eu/wp-content/uploads/2013/04/EAFP-report-prepared-In-European-Commission.-Erasmus-Subject-Evaluations-1995.pdf (accessed on 28 August 2015).
4. BERLIN Humboldt University. 2nd European meetings of the faculties, schools and institutes of pharmacy. 27 September 1994. Available online: http://www.pharmine.org/wp-content/uploads/2014/05/2nd-EU-meeting-of-the-faculties-of-pharmacy-Berlin-1994.pdf (accessed on 28 August 2015).
5. Pharmine: pharmacy education in Europe. Available online: http://www.pharmine.org/ (accessed on 28 August 2015).
6. Atkinson, J. Heterogeneity of pharmacy education in Europe. *Pharmacy* **2014**, *2*, 231–243. Available online: http://www.mdpi.com/2226-4787/2/3/231 (accessed on 28 August 2015).
7. PHAR-QA. The PHAR-QA project: Quality Assurance in European Pharmacy Education and Training. Available online: www.phar-qa.eu (accessed on 28 August 2015).
8. Bologna Process-European Higher Education Area. History. Available online: http://www.ehea.info/article-details.aspx?ArticleId=3 (accessed on 28 August 2015).
9. Surveymonkey survey creation system. Available online: https://www.surveymonkey.com/ (accessed on 28 August 2015).
10. Atkinson, J.; De Paepe, K.; Sánchez Pozo, A.; Rekkas, D.; Volmer, D.; Hirvonen, J.; Bozic, B.; Skowron, A.; Mircioiu, C.; Marcincal, A.; Koster, A.; Wilson, K.; van Schravendijk, C. The PHAR-QA project: Quality Assurance in European Pharmacy Education and Training. *Results of the Eur. Netw. Delphi*. **2015**, in press.
11. Marz, R.; Dekker, F.W.; Van Schravendijk, C.; O'Flynn, S.; Ross, M.T. Tuning research competences for Bologna three cycles in medicine: Report of a MEDINE2 European consensus survey. *Perp. Med. Educ.* 2013. Available online: http://www.ncbi.nlm.nih.gov/pmc/articles/PMC3792236/ (accessed on 28 August 2015).
12. European University Association (EUA). EUA Briefing Note on Directive 2013/55/EU, containing the amendments to Directive 2005/36/EC on the Recognition of Professional Qualifications. Available online: http://www.eua.be/Libraries/Higher_Education/EUA_briefing_note_on_amended_Directive_January_2014.sflb.ashx (accessed on 28 August 2015).
13. GraphPad statistical pack. Available online: http://www.graphpad.com/ (accessed on 28 August 2015).

14. Chambers, J.; Cleveland, W.; Kleiner, B.; Tukey, P. Graphical Methods for Data Analysis. *J. Appl.* Stat. **1984** *11*, 233–234. Available online: http://www.tandfonline.com/doi/abs/10.1080/02664768400000024?journalCode=cjas20#.VciiCocbCpo (accessed on 28 August 2015).
15. Rutter, V.; Wong, C.; Coombes, I.; Cardiff, L.; Duggan, C.; Yee, M.-L.; Lim, K.W.; Bates, I. Use of a General Level Framework to Facilitate Performance Improvement in Hospital Pharmacists in Singapore. *Am. J. Pharm. Educ.* **2012**, *76*, 1–10. Available online: http://www.ajpe.org/action/doSearch?AllField=bates (accessed on 28 August 2015).
16. Coombes, I.; Avent, M.; Cardiff, L.; Bettenay, K.; Coombes, J.; Whitfield, K.; Stokes, J.; Davies, G.; Bates, I. Improvement in Pharmacist's Performance Facilitated by an Adapted Competency-Based General Level Framework. *J. Pharm. Pract. Res.* **2010,** *40*, 111–118. Available online: http://onlinelibrary.wiley.com/doi/10.1002/j.2055-2335.2010.tb00517.x/abstract (accessed on 28 August 2015).
17. Winslade, N.E.; Tamblyn, R.M.; Taylor, L.K.; Schuwirth, L.W.T.; Van der Vleuten, C.P.M. Integrating Performance Assessment, Maintenance of Competence, and Continuing Professional Development of Community Pharmacists. *Am. J. Pharm. Educ.* **2007**, *71*, 1–9.
18. Stupans, I.; McAllister, S.; Clifford, R.; Hughes, J.; Krasse, I.; March, G.; Owen, S.; Woulf, J. Nationwide collaborative development of learning outcomes and exemplar standards for Australian pharmacy programmes. *Int. J. Pharm. Pract.* **2014**, *24*, 1–9.
19. Dreyfus, S.E.; Dreyfus, H.L. *A Five-Stage Model of the Mental Activities Involved in Directed Skill Acquisition*; Storming Media: Washington, USA, 1980.

15

Views of English Pharmacists on Providing Public Health Services

Catherine Dewsbury, Ruth M Rodgers and Janet Krska *

Medway School of Pharmacy, The Universities of Greenwich and Kent, Central Avenue, Chatham Maritime, Kent ME4 4TB, UK; E-Mail: c.dewsbury@kent.ac.uk (C.D.); r.m.rodgers@kent.ac.uk (R.M.R.)

* Author to whom correspondence should be addressed; E-Mail: j.krska@kent.ac.uk

Academic Editor: Reem Kayyali

Abstract: Locally-commissioned pharmacy public health services have developed in England over the last 20 years. Few studies have sought pharmacist views on commissioning and provision of public health services in general. This study sought views of community pharmacists (n = 778) in 16 areas of England on services provided, decisions about services, support, promotion and future developments, using a postal questionnaire with two reminders. Response rate was 26.5% (206). Funded public health services provided most frequently were: emergency contraception (71%), smoking cessation (62%), and supervised drug consumption (58%). Blood pressure monitoring was provided by 61% and was considered to be one of the services pharmacists perceived as being most valued by customers, but was not National Health Services (NHS)-funded. Motivation for providing public health services was professional not financial, particularly from those working in independent pharmacies. Only 35% were personally involved in deciding which services to deliver, and fewer than 20% based decisions on local public health reports. Pharmacists had positive attitudes towards providing public health services, but mixed views on support for services and their promotion. Most thought services would increase in future, but were concerned about commissioning. Both national and local support is needed to ensure future commissioning of pharmacy public health services.

Keywords: community pharmacy; public health; commissioning; primary care; pharmacist opinions

1. Introduction

A succession of governments in England has acknowledged the potential contribution of community pharmacy in supporting public health [1–5]. Public health services are also supported by pharmacy contractor representatives and professional bodies [6–10]. A wide range of pharmacy public health services have developed over the last 20 years, with public health being embedded into the revision of the National Health Services (NHS) pharmacy contractual framework in 2005 [11]. Since then, enhanced services, such as needle exchange schemes and supervised consumption of medicines for drug misusers, minor ailment schemes, smoking cessation services and some sexual health services have become widespread nationally, but were commissioned by local health organisations—Primary Care Trusts (PCTs).

Pharmacists working within PCTs contributed to the decisions of these commissioning organisations to develop specific services, based on local needs. The need for services was identified by PCT staff using information provided in Local Health Profiles, published by Public Health Observatories, reports from Directors of Public Health (DPH) and a Joint Strategic Needs Assessment (JSNA), which incorporates information from a Pharmaceutical Needs Assessment (PNA). Each area would thus be expected to commission different services, dependent on the health needs of the local population.

The commissioners normally negotiate the terms of service provision with a Local Pharmaceutical Committee (LPC), which represents the community pharmacy contractors in the area, however, since the 2005 revision of the contractual framework, there is no longer a requirement to do so. A study showed that despite this, both Directors of Public Health and pharmacists working in PCTs thought the revised contractual framework would strengthen pharmacists' public health role, but felt this could be constrained by lack of funding [12]. The implementation of the revised contract was evaluated two years after its introduction, and showed that over half of community pharmacies had increased their public health activities: most were offering health promotion and over 85% were providing at least one public health service, most frequently smoking cessation (44%), medicine supply through patient group directions (written instructions for the supply or administration of medicines to groups of patients who may not be individually identified before presentation for treatment) (42%) and supervised administration of medicines (39%) [11]. Other work suggested that services were provided with differing frequencies depending on location and ownership [13].

Since then, the Healthy Living Pharmacy (HLP) concept was developed, which provides a framework for commissioning public health services through three levels of increasing complexity and the expertise required of pharmacy staff [14]. Early work evaluating this programme suggested that HLPs saw more clients for public health services than other pharmacies in the same geographical area [15] and a larger evaluation, published in 2013, found that HLPs delivered a wider range of services than other pharmacies [16].

However, major changes to the structure of primary care in England in April 2013 resulted in the abolition of PCTs, and responsibility for local public health was moved to local government. Commissioning of primary care services thus became the responsibility of the NHS Commissioning

Board (known as NHS England) and locally-based Clinical Commissioning Groups, the latter comprising mostly general practitioners [17]. This re-structuring was anticipated to result in changes to the commissioning and provision of pharmacy public health services, which could either suffer or be enhanced. This study determined the views of community pharmacists on public health services in general and their perceptions of the future, immediately prior to the implementation of this significant change.

Much research has shown that community pharmacists have positive attitudes towards providing specific public health services, but studies suggest that while most pharmacists see these as important and part of their role, they are considered secondary to medicine-related roles [18]. Moreover, most studies seeking pharmacist views look at individual public health services [18,19] with very little work having obtained views on public health services in general and/or policies driving these [13]. The changes in commissioning mechanisms presented an opportunity to seek the views of English pharmacists on provision of public health services in general, to form a baseline for future comparison and to enable comparison with previous work [13].

It may be anticipated that pharmacists working in areas where many different services are commissioned could have more positive views of their role in public health and that pharmacists with managerial responsibilities or pharmacy owners may welcome the opportunity to increase income through these commissioned services. The aims were thus: (i) to obtain information about public health service provision and the views of community pharmacists in England on providing these services; and (ii) to assess whether service provision and views differed depending on the pharmacy ownership, pharmacist role and the number of PCT-reported commissioned pharmacy public health services.

2. Methods

The study was approved by a University Research ethics committee and conducted in November 2012, prior to implementation of the NHS reorganisation in April 2013.

2.1. Questionnaire Development

A random sample of 20 pharmacists from one PCT, which was randomly selected from those reported to be providing two or three public health services, were invited to take part in a telephone interview. Eleven agreed and were interviewed, the findings of which informed the content of the questionnaire. The questionnaire was piloted by postal distribution to the remaining pharmacists in this area, who were also asked to evaluate the content, ease of use and time taken to complete.

The final questionnaire covered service provision, selection of services and views on public health service commissioning, provision and importance. Questions on service provision included: a list of 26 potential services mentioned in interviews from which respondents could select those they considered as public health services, those they provided and those which were NHS-funded; reasons for public health service delivery in general and service selection, using options derived from interview data; open-ended questions seeking the three public health services pharmacists viewed as most valued by customers and any other services respondents wished to provide. Selection of services was determined using: closed questions seeking reasons for providing public health services; perceptions of who made decisions about service provision; awareness and use of four local (PNA, JSNA, DPH report and Local Health Profile) and two national documents (Pharmacy in England 2008, Choosing Health through

Pharmacy) in selecting services. Views on public perceptions, promotion, support and the future of pharmacy public health services, were sought using 5-point semantic differential scales, plus four statements accompanied by 5-point Likert response options, covering the areas raised by pharmacist in interviews. Demographic data collected covered pharmacist gender, years qualified, role in pharmacy, plus pharmacy ownership, location and HLP status.

2.2. Questionnaire Distribution

PCTs were selected from annual returns of NHS General Pharmaceutical Services provision for the year April 2010–March 2011 [20], excluding those not providing an annual return. The remainder were stratified dependent on whether 1, 2, 3 or ≥ 4 of the following services were reported as being commissioned: minor ailment schemes; needle exchange services; services under Patient Group Direction (PGD); screening; stop smoking; supervised administration of medicines. NHS data were not available for any other pharmacy public health services. A 10% sample from each stratum was randomly selected using a random number generator. All pharmacies in each PCT were sent a questionnaire by post, accompanied by an information sheet, plus a freepost envelope for return of the completed questionnaire. One postal reminder was sent and a reminder telephone call made to non-responders.

2.3. Data Analysis

Data were analysed using SPSS version 20. Pharmacist roles were collapsed into owner/superintendent and manager/second pharmacist/locum to enable data analysis, which used Chi-squared tests and t-tests to assess differences between sub-groups.

3. Results and Discussion

Of the 151 PCTs in England in financial year 2010/11, an annual return of service provision was available for 147. From this list 17 were selected, one reporting two commissioned services, for questionnaire development and piloting, and 16 for the questionnaire distribution. The latter reported 1 (4 PCTs), 2 (6), 3 (4) or ≥4 (2) commissioned services and included 778 pharmacies in total (Table 1).

3.1. Response Rate

The overall response rate was 206 (26.5%), ranging from 15.1% to 35.9% between PCTs (Table 1). Response rate was unrelated to the number of reported commissioned services. Two-thirds of responses were received after the first mailing (138; 67%), with a further 56 (27%) following the second mailing and 12 (6%) after the telephone reminder.

Table 1. Number of pharmacies, reported public health services commissioned and questionnaire return rate for the 16 Primary Care Trust areas in the study. NHS—National Health Services; PCT—Primary Care Trusts.

Number of NHS-reported public health services	Number of pharmacies in PCT	Number (%) of questionnaires returned
1	34	10 (29.4%)
	51	11 (21.6%)
Sub-total	85	21 (24.7%)
2	64	12 (18.8%)
	52	17 (32.7%)
	44	11 (25.0%)
	49	10 (20.4%)
Sub-total	209	50 (23.9%)
3	27	8 (29.6%)
	73	17 (23.4%)
	53	8 (15.1%)
	49	12 (24.5%)
	77	15 (19.5%)
	46	7 (15.2%)
Sub-total	325	67 (20.6%)
4	69	16 (23.2%)
	39	14 (35.9%)
	66	18 (27.3%)
	64	20 (31.3%)
Sub-total	238	68 (28.6%)
Total	778	206 (26.5%)

3.2. Demographic Characteristics

The characteristics of both the pharmacist responders and their pharmacies are shown in Table 2. Approximately half the respondents had qualified within the previous ten years, two-thirds were managers, 10% owners and 62% were working in multiples (defined as > 6 pharmacies). Twenty-nine (14.1%) indicated their pharmacy was designated as a Healthy Living Pharmacy (HLP), but 34 (16.5%) did not know and four (0.2%) did not respond. The 29 HLPs were across areas with differing levels of commissioned services and 23 were in multiple ownership.

Table 2. Characteristics of pharmacist responders and pharmacies ($n = 206$).

Characteristic		**Number (Proportion of total)**
Gender (203) *	Female	91 (44.8)
	Male	112 (55.2)
Years qualified (196) *	5 or fewer	49 (25.0)
	5 to 10	51 (26.0)
	More than 10	96 (49.0)
Role in pharmacy (205) *	Manager	134 (65.7)
	Second pharmacist	18 (8.8)
	Locum	17 (8.3)
	Superintendent	14 (6.9)
	Owner	22 (10.3)
Type of pharmacy	Multiple (> 5 pharmacies)	128 (62.1)
	Independent pharmacy	78 (37.9)
Location of pharmacy	High street/suburban	80 (38.8)
	Shopping precinct/out of town centre	19 (9.3)
	Village	43 (20.9)
	Supermarket	14 (6.8)
	Attached to GP surgery	22 (10.7)
	Other (city centre, secondary parade, residential, other)	28 (13.6)

* Missing data excluded.

3.3. Public Health Service Provision

Respondents self-reported a median of six locally commissioned public health services (range 0 to 26; mean ± SD = 6.44 ± 3.8). The mean number of services respondents indicated they provided was not related to the number of commissioned services reported by the PCTs in which their pharmacy was located. Pharmacists from areas with only one PCT-reported public health service claimed they delivered a mean of 8.1 services; the equivalent for PCTs reporting two, three and four services was 7.2/pharmacy, 6.5/pharmacy and 5.3/pharmacy respectively. There was no statistically significant difference in the mean number of public health services provided by the 29 HLPs (6.7 ± 3.9) compared to the remaining pharmacies (6.3 ± 3.3) ($t = 0.58$; $p = 0.56$). Nor were there differences in the mean number of services provided by 78 pharmacies classed as independent (6.2 ± 3.6) compared to the 128 multiples (6.6 ± 3.9) ($t = 0.65$; $p = 0.514$).

The most common service provided through a patient group direction which was NHS-funded was emergency contraception, but some pharmacies provided other medicines which were non-NHS-funded, particularly antimalarial treatment and orlistat (Figure 1). However not all were viewed as public health, particularly medicines provision for emergency planning.

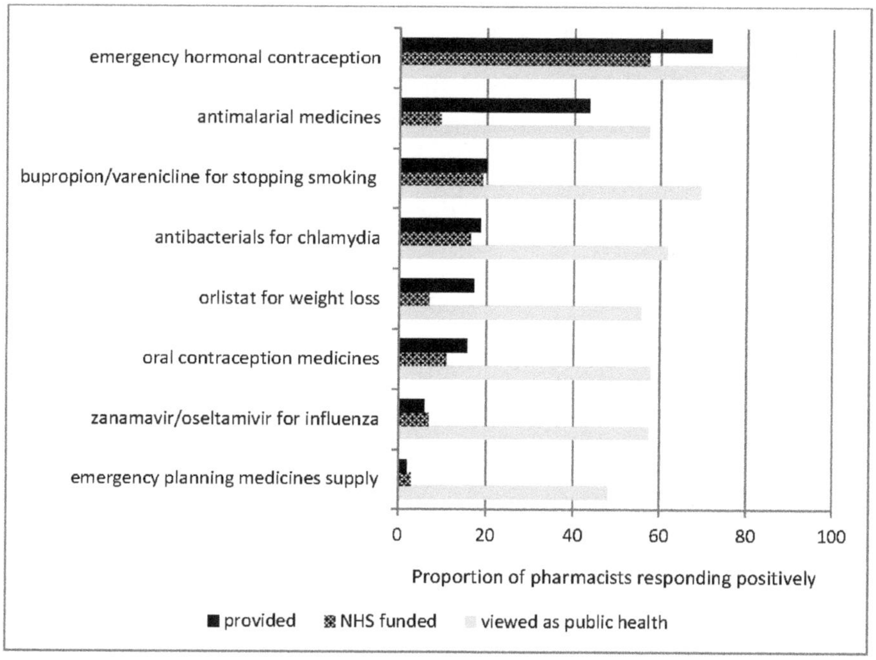

Figure 1. Self-reported provision of medicines supply under group direction.

Among other services not involving medicines supply under a patient group direction, stop smoking support was most frequently provided, followed by blood pressure monitoring, although while the former was primarily NHS-funded, the latter was not (Figure 2). Other services provided which were reported as not being NHS-funded were: influenza vaccination, weight management support, cholesterol testing and travel vaccination.

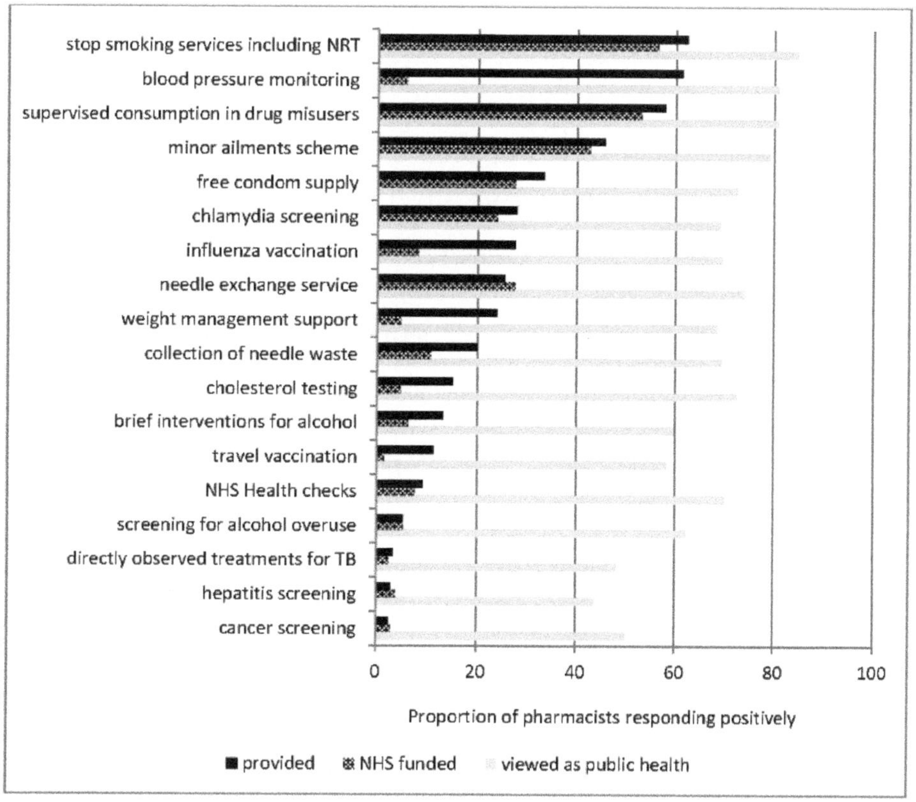

Figure 2. Self-reported provision of other public health services.

The public health services perceived by pharmacist respondents as being most valued by customers were smoking cessation support (cited by 97/188; 51.6%), emergency contraception (72; 38.3%) and minor ailments (49; 26.1%), all NHS-funded services, with blood pressure monitoring also rated as being valued by 31 (16.5%). Forty-one respondents (19.9%) indicated a desire to provide more services, 30 of whom indicated examples of these, the most frequent being anticoagulant services (4; 13%).

3.4. Reasons for Providing Public Health Services

From the range of potential reasons for providing public health services included in the questionnaire, those most frequently cited were professional responsibility (151; 76.6%), patient satisfaction (147; 74.6%) and personal satisfaction (131; 66.5%). Personal satisfaction was cited more frequently by respondents from independently-owned pharmacies compared to multiples (55/73; 75.3% *vs.* 76/124; 61.3%; Pearson's chi-square = 4.01; $p = 0.03$) and among owners/superintendents compared to managers/second pharmacists (28/33; 84.8% *vs.* 102/162; 63.0%; Pearson's chi-square = 5.91; $p = 0.01$). Financial incentives were selected by relatively few, with profit margin chosen by only 46 (23.4%) and bonus payments by even fewer (28; 14.2%), with no differences relating to pharmacy ownership or pharmacist role. Pressure from head office was cited by 62, 57 of whom described their pharmacy as a multiple (Pearson's chi-square = 32.6; $p < 0.001$ compared to independent).

Requests from patients/the public was cited by approximately a third of respondents (66; 33.5%) as a reason for providing services, with a similar proportion (69; 35.2%) also selecting this as a reason for choosing which services to provide. More frequently cited reasons for choosing services were the needs of patients/the public (157; 80.1%) and competence (95; 48.5%). Profit margin and performance targets were again less important, selected by 50 (25.5%) and 57 (29.1%) respectively.

Respondents' perceptions of who made decisions on which services to provide were most frequently that it was a combination of individuals/organisations (73; 35.4%), but many also considered these decisions were made entirely by the company/superintendent pharmacist (50; 24.3%) or by the PCT (26; 12.6%). Only 70 (34.0%) felt personally involved in decisions about service provision, most of whom (68) were either managers or owners/superintendents. Overall 82 (39.8%) considered the PCT were involved and only 11 (5.3%) the LPC.

There were 126 respondents (64.0%) who agreed/strongly agreed with the statement: "public health services are based on the needs of my local population". However, awareness of documents outlining need for services ranged from 40.9% for local health profiles to 74.7% for PNAs (Table 3). Fewer than half claimed to have read these documents, with the PNA being most widely read, but fewer than 20% had used one of them to help decide on services, again the most common being the PNA. Overall slightly more owners/superintendents claimed to have read the PNA, but HLP status or number of PCT-commissioned services did not affect use of these documents.

Table 3. Awareness and use of local information relating to population needs ($n = 206$)

Document	Number (proportion) of pharmacists who...		
	Are aware of	Have read	Used to help decide on services
Pharmaceutical needs assessment (PNA)	148 (74.7%)	96 (48.5%)	33 (16.7%)
Joint Strategic Needs Assessment (JSNA)	104 (52.5%)	36 (18.2%)	11 (5.6%)
Direct of Public Health report	100 (50.5%)	29 (14.6%)	7 (3.5%)
Local health profile	81 (40.9%)	21 (10.6%)	7 (3.5%)
Pharmacy in England	119 (60.1%)	85 (42.9%)	10 (5.1%)
Choosing Health through Pharmacy	106 (53.5%)	51 (25.8%)	8 (4.0%)

3.5. Views on Commissioning, Promotion and Support for Public Health Services

Responses to the statements covering commissioning, promotion of and support for pharmacy-based public health services are shown in Table 4. The large majority of respondents were positive about the value of these services to both the public and to their pharmacies. In addition, responses to further statements showed that 148 respondents (75.1%) agreed/strongly agreed that: "public health services are vital for my pharmacy's business" and 106 (53.5%) disagreed/strongly disagreed that: "I do not focus on public health services because dispensing volume is more important". There were no differences in these proportions relating to pharmacy ownership, number of commissioned services or pharmacist role.

Table 4. Pharmacists' views on current commissioning, promotion and support for pharmacy public health services.

Statement	Anchor	Frequency of responses (% of total responding)					Anchor
Pharmacy-based public health services are...	not valued by the public	2.6	10.7	21.4	37.8	27.6	valued by the public
The public is...	unaware of these services	8.6	24.7	40.9	20.2	5.6	aware of these services
Promotion of these services needs to ...	increase	55.6	21.2	12.6	7.1	3.5	decrease
Promoting pharmacy-based public health services is ...	a local responsibility	9.1	8.1	21.8	20.3	40.6	a national responsibility
Promotion of these services is the responsibility of...	the profession	8.6	11.7	43.7	18.8	17.3	the government
Promotion of these services is...	my responsibility	13.1	17.2	51.5	10.6	7.6	someone else's responsibility
In my local area pharmacy public health services are...	increasing	13.1	26.3	36.9	11.1	12.6	decreasing
Providing public health services is...	a waste of my time	2.0	6.6	24.9	36.0	30.5	highly valuable for me
My local GPs are...	unsupportive of pharmacy based public health services	17.4	27.4	34.3	14.4	6.5	supportive of pharmacy public health services
The local director of public health is...	supportive of pharmacy based public health services	11.1	18.2	51.5	12.6	6.6	unsupportive of pharmacy public health services

Table 4. *Cont.*

Statement	Anchor	Frequency of responses (% of total responding)					Anchor
The pharmacists at our PCT are the…	barrier to developing public health services	5.5	9.0	33.8	33.8	17.9	advocates of developing public health services
My Local Pharmaceutical Committee…	aids local service development	22.9	31.8	30.3	9.0	6.0	hinders local service development

A high proportion of respondents viewed local PCT staff as supportive, although fewer indicated that local GPs supported pharmacy public health services, with no differences dependent on the number of PCT-reported commissioned services. Most respondents (76.8%) also considered there was a need for increased promotion of services, but there was less clarity about whose role this was, with 60.9% indicating that responsibility was national, but 43.7% were unsure whether this responsibility lay with the profession or the government. Moreover, only 30.3% felt that promotion of pharmacy public health services was their responsibility, with just over half selecting the mid-point option. There was also uncertainty about the extent to which the Director of Public Health was supportive.

3.6. Future Development of Public Health Services

Most respondents (69.9%) felt they would need a lot of support during the period of change to service commissioning, with only 14.8% indicating they felt fully informed about the changes to the NHS. However, 69.8% indicated that the NHS changes could put the commissioning of pharmacy public health services at risk (Table 4). Results suggest uncertainty about whether these changes would increase or decrease opportunities to provide public health services and whether local or national support would be needed.

Public health services were viewed as being of increasing importance in the future, with 44.8% of respondents indicating they were looking forward to public health services being the main focus of their work, 83.7% being of the view that provision of public health advice would increase in future and 54.2% that profit from public health services would be more important than profit from dispensing in future (Table 5). Moreover, 150 (72.1%) also agreed/strongly agreed with the statement: "I would focus on public health services more if demand from the public increased".

3.7. Summary of Main Findings

This survey involved community pharmacists in 16 areas spread throughout England, selected on the basis of differing numbers of PCT-reported locally commissioned public health services. It is the first national survey to seek pharmacist views on reasons for providing public health services and the local and national support for these. Respondents self-reported offering a wider range of services than indicated by NHS data, indeed the number of self-reported services was unrelated to the number in NHS returns. There were no differences in the number of services provided dependent on pharmacy ownership or HLP status, although the latter were few in number. Smoking cessation, blood pressure monitoring and supervised drug consumption were provided by over 50% of respondents. Blood pressure monitoring was identified as one a service which was highly valued by customers, but was not generally offered as an NHS-funded service.

Table 5. Pharmacists' views on NHS reorganisation and the future of pharmacy public health services.

Statement	Anchor	Frequency of responses (% of total responding)					Anchor
The NHS is about to undergo major reorganisation and I feel…	uninformed about the proposed changes	15.3	34.5	35.5	12.8	2.0	fully informed about these changes
With the coming changes in local commissioning of public health services in my area I will require...	little support to help me through these changes	2.5	5.4	22.2	37.9	32.0	a lot of support to help me through these changes
During this time of change in the NHS I will look for support from…	local pharmacy bodies such as the LPC	18.3	15.8	35.1	17.3	13.4	national pharmacy bodies such as the RPS or PSNC
I believe the commissioning of pharmacy based public health services...	will be unaffected by the planned changes to the NHS	1.0	4.0	25.2	33.7	36.1	is at risk as a result of planned changes in the NHS
Changes in commissioning of pharmacy services may...	remove opportunities for me to develop my public health practice	13.4	18.3	40.6	19.8	7.9	provide further opportunities for me to develop my public health practice
If demand for these services increased…	I would not cope with the extra work	9.1	21.7	28.8	21.7	18.7	I would welcome the extra work
I am looking forward to public health services being …	removed from my day to day work to let me focus on dispensing	1.0	7.5	46.8	26.9	17.9	the main focus of my day to day work now that dispensing can be undertaken by qualified technicians
My role in dispensing medicines for patients will	increase	10.3	12.3	26.6	34.5	16.3	decrease
My role in providing health advice to the public	increase	38.9	44.8	8.9	5.4	2.0	decrease
Profit from these services will be…	less important that profit from dispensing	3.4	8.9	33.5	27.6	26.6	more important than profit from dispensing
My role in provision of these services	increase	39.1	40.1	14.9	4.0	2.0	decrease

Motivation for providing public health services was professional not financial, particularly in independent pharmacies. However only 35% indicated personal involvement in decisions regarding which services should be delivered, with less than a fifth of pharmacists having used local public health reports to inform these decisions. While most respondents were positive about providing public health services and viewed them as potentially increasing in future, there were mixed views concerning local and national support for service provision and promotion, plus a desire for support in relation to changes which could affect service commissioning. Many respondents selected neutral options in relation to statements concerning promotion of, support for and the future of pharmacy public health services. This may be a reflection of the lack of awareness of local priorities, the content of local documents and what impact the re-structuring would have on service commissioning.

3.8. Strengths and Limitations

The questionnaire used was developed using data from interviews conducted with community pharmacists providing public health services, thus covered issues relevant to service commissioning and provision. We did not seek views on the provision of privately-funded public health services. The survey included all pharmacies in a stratified random sample of PCTs, which ensured that for the areas included the number of commissioned services varied. However, only 16 of the 151 total PCTs in England at the time of the study, thus findings may not be nationally representative. All pharmacies within each PCT were included in the survey, but it achieved a low response rate, despite two reminders. Respondents were thus potentially biased towards providers of public health services, perhaps also with positive views. Service provision and use of documents were self-reported, thus subject to potential social desirability and recall bias. Our definition of multiple pharmacy ownership was six or more pharmacies, thus our findings are not directly comparable to other work using different ownership options.

3.9. Relation to Literature/Implications for Policy and Practice

The findings confirm those of many studies reporting pharmacists' views towards individual public health services, in that the profession in England has positive views about public health [18,19]. Our work differs from most previous work in that the target population was all pharmacists in areas where any public health services were commissioned, rather than those known to be providing particular services. One survey involving a random sample of Scottish community pharmacists conducted in 2007 found 79% of the 223 responders agreed that public health was important to their practice [21]. Frequency of service provision was similar to previous surveys, [12,13] with smoking cessation support and supervised consumption for drug misusers being the most common public health services and emergency contraception being the most frequent supply under PGD. The lack of a relationship between self-reported service provision and PCT-reported service commissioning may be due to the lack of specificity within the NHS General Pharmaceutical reporting framework, which requires only provision of services under PGD and screening, lacking detail of which services are commissioned. This does not allow a comprehensive picture of service provision nationally. Moreover PCTs were not required to provide information about some fairly widespread services, such as weight management and vaccinations.

Interestingly, many pharmacist respondents did not view some of these services as public health, particularly some involving PGDs and screening, which were provided by relatively few pharmacists. This is somewhat surprising and may indicate that views of a service are influenced by its provision.

Over a third of the 1023 respondents to a previous large comprehensive national (Great Britain) survey felt conflicts with commercial interests were a barrier to providing public health services, and the findings indicated showed that service provision varied dependent on pharmacy ownership [13]. This study concluded that large companies held an advantageous position with regard to attracting funding for these services, with the potential that independent pharmacies may become less able to provide them. Other work, which was a pragmatic evaluation of the HLP programme, suggested that HLPs were offering more services than other pharmacies and that service uptake increased in pharmacies after becoming HLPs [16]. In contrast, our study showed no significant differences in the number of services reported as being provided, depending on either pharmacy ownership or HLP designation, however the number of HLPs was small and the categorisation of ownership limited.

Our results suggest that decisions on which services to provide frequently do not involve the pharmacists delivering them, with health organisations, such as PCTs and commercial companies/managers being most likely to decide on services. Individual pharmacists had little awareness of local documents which would inform these decisions and, while PCTs and successor organisations commissioning services are likely to base decisions on the loc al needs described in these documents, the extent to which pharmacy companies do so is not known. Our survey did not determine whether pharmacists felt constrained by their lack of involvement in decision-making, but there were a significant number who indicated a desire to provide more services than at present.

The majority of respondents expected public health services to increase in future at the expense of dispensing. However many also showed concerns for their future development, given the changes which have since taken place within primary care. This could be related to the perceptions that pharmacists working in PCTs and LPCs were key to service development, with GPs and public health directors being viewed as less supportive. Nonetheless these results must be viewed with caution, due to the low response rate. The changes implemented in April 2013 mean that GPs now have greater influence over service commissioning than at the time of this survey. There is anecdotal evidence of service commissioning bypassing LPCs and services being de-commissioned, while more recent annual NHS returns show the overall number of services provided has reduced.

4. Conclusions

The wide range of services provided and the positive expectations of pharmacists towards increased provision of public health services are important for the future development of these services. Greater involvement in decision making and awareness of local needs may enable pharmacists to tailor services more effectively. Support from both national and local organisations is needed for future commissioning and provision of pharmacy public health services.

Acknowledgements

We wish to acknowledge the support of Dalveer Singh, Mildred Mukaira, Seetay Soneji and Michael Williams with questionnaire distribution. We are also grateful to the pharmacists who agreed to interview, helped to pilot the questionnaire and all respondents. This research received no specific grant from any funding agency. It was funded by the Medway School of Pharmacy.

Author Contribution

All authors were involved in study design. Catherine Dewsbury conducted the pharmacist interviews from which the questionnaire was developed, and contributed to the questionnaire distribution. All authors contributed to questionnaire drafting and revisions, Janet Krska conducted the analysis and wrote the first draft of the paper. All authors have reviewed the paper and agree to its publication.

Conflicts of Interest

The authors declare no conflicts of interest.

References

1. Department of Health. *Saving Lives: Our Healthier Nation*; Stationery Office: London, England, 1999.
2. Department of Health. *Tackling Health Inequalities: A Programme for Action*; Department of Health (DH): London, England, 2003.
3. Department of Health. *Choosing Health through Pharmacy: A Programme for Pharmaceutical Public Health 2005–2015*; Department of Health (DH): London, England, 2005.
4. Department of Health. *Pharmacy in England: Building on Strengths—Delivering the Future*; Department of Health (DH): London, England, 2008.
5. Department of Health. *Healthy Lives, Healthy People: Our Strategy for Public Health in England*; Stationery Office: Norwich, England, 2010.
6. Clucas, K. *Pharmacy: The Report of a Committee of Inquiry Appointed by the Nuffield Foundation*; The Nuffield Foundation: London, England, 1986.
7. Royal Pharmaceutical Society of Great Britain. *Pharmacy in a New Age: Developing Strategy for the Future of Pharmacy*. Royal Pharmaceutical Society of Great Britain (RPSGB): London, England, 1995.
8. Department of Health. *Choosing Health: Making Healthy Choices Easier* Department of Health (DH): London, England, 2004.
9. Pharmaceutical Services Negotiating Committee. *The Vision for NHS Community Pharmacies: The Path to Improved Patient Care*. Pharmaceutical Services Negotiating Committee (PSNC): London, England, 2013.
10. Smith, J.; Picton, C.; Dayan, M. *Now or Never: Shaping Pharmacy for the Future*; The Report of the Commission on Future Models of Care Delivered through Pharmacy; Royal Pharmaceutical Society: London, England, 2013.
11. Blenkinsopp, A.; Bond, C.M.; Celino, G.; Inch, J.; Gray, N. *National Evaluation of the New Community Pharmacy Contract*; Pharmacy Practice Research Trust: London, England, 2007.
12. Bush, J.; Langley, C.A.; Jesson, J.K.; Wilson, K.A. Perceived barriers to the development of community pharmacy's public health function: A survey of the attitudes of directors of public health and chief pharmacists in UK Primary care organisations. *Int. J. Pharm. Pract.* **2006**, *14* (Suppl. 2), B68–B69.
13. Bush, J.; Langley, C.A.; Wilson, K.A. The corporatization of community pharmacy: Implications for service provision, the public health function, and pharmacy's claims to professional status in the United Kingdom. *Res. Soc. Admin. Pharm.* **2009**, *5*, 305–318.
14. Pharmaceutical Services Negotiating Committee. Healthy Living Pharmacies. Available online: http://psnc.org.uk/services-commissioning/locally-commissioned-services/healthy-living-pharmacies/ (accessed on 21 April 2015).

15. Brown, D.; Portlock, J.; Rutter, P.; Nazar, Z. From community pharmacy to health living pharmacy: Positive early experiences from Portsmouth, England. *Res. Soc. Admin. Pharm.* **2014**, *10*, 72–87.
16. Duggan, C.; Evans, D.; Holden, M.; Kennington, E.; Leach, R.; Root, G.; Shepherd, E. *Evaluation of the Healthy Living Pharmacy Pathfinder Work Programme 2011–2012*. Royal Pharmaceutical Society, Company Chemists' Association, Pharmaceutical Services Negotiating Committee, National Pharmacy Association: London, England, 2013.
17. NHS England. Understanding the new NHS. 2014. Available online: http://www.england.nhs.uk/wp-content/uploads/2014/06/simple-nhs-guide.pdf (accessed on 19 May 2014).
18. Eades, C.E.; Ferguson J.S.; O'Carroll, E. Public Health in community pharmacy: A systematic review of pharmacist and consumer views service. *BMC Publ. Health* **2011**, *11*, 582.
19. Anderson, C.; Blenkinsopp, A.; Armstrong, M. Pharmacists' perceptions regarding their contribution to improving the public's health: A systematic review of the United Kingdom and international literature 1990–2001. *Int. J. Pharm. Pract.* **2003**, *11*, 111–120.
20. Health and Social Care Information Centre. Available online: http://www.hscic.gov.uk (accessed on 21 April 2015).
21. Pfleger, D.E.; McHattie, L.W.; Diack, H.L.; McCaig, D.L.; Stewart, D.C. Views, attitudes and self-assessed training needs of Scottish community pharmacists to public health practice and competence. *Pharm. World Sci.* **2008**, *30*, 801–809.

16

Pharmacist and Physician Interpretation of Abbreviations for Acetaminophen Intended for Use in a Consumer Icon

Saul Shiffman [1,2,*], Helene Cotton [3], Christina Jessurun [4], Mark A. Sembower [1], Steve Pype [1] and Jerry Phillips [5]

1 Pinney Associates, 201 N. Craig Street (Suite 320), Pittsburgh, PA 15213, USA; E-Mails: msembower@pinneyassociates.com (M.S.); sype@pinneyassociates.com (S.P.)

2 Department of Psychology, University of Pittsburgh, Pittsburgh, PA 15260, USA

3 Independent market research consultant, Glenview, IL 60026, USA; E-Mail: hcotton@mac.com

4 Johnson & Johnson Consumer Inc., Skillman, NJ 08558, USA; E-Mail: CJessuru@its.jnj.com

5 Drug Safety Institute, Miami, FL 33131, USA; E-Mail: jphillips@brandinstitute.com

* Author to whom correspondence should be addressed; E-Mail: shiffman@pinneyassociates.com

Academic Editor: Keith A. Wilson

Abstract: Concomitant use of multiple acetaminophen medications is associated with overdose. To help patients identify acetaminophen medications and thus avoid concomitant use, an icon with an abbreviation for "acetaminophen" has been proposed for all acetaminophen medications. This study assessed pharmacists' and physicians' use and interpretation of abbreviations for "acetaminophen", to identify abbreviations with other meanings that might cause confusion. Physicians (n = 150) reported use and interpretation of candidate abbreviations Ac and Acm. Pharmacists (n = 150) interpretations of prescription orders using the candidate abbreviations APAP, Ac, Ace and Acm in typed, handwritten or spoken form, were judged for critical confusions likely to cause patient harm. Critical confusion was rare, except for omission by pharmacists of the acetaminophen dose for Hydrocodone/APAP prescriptions (10%). Ac was in common use to indicate "before meals", and was interpreted as such, but some physicians (8%) said they use Ac to indicate anticoagulant drugs. Most pharmacists (54%) interpreted Ace as acetaminophen, and none interpreted it as referring to ACE-inhibitors. Acm was rarely used in prescriptions, had no common interfering meanings, and was often (63%) interpreted as acetaminophen, especially when prescribed in combination with an opiate (85%). The data validated concerns about abbreviations in prescribing: all abbreviations resulted in some misinterpretations. However, Acm was rarely misinterpreted, was readily associated with "acetaminophen", and seemed appropriate for use in a graphic icon to help consumers/patients identify acetaminophen medications.

Keywords: Acetaminophen; icon; abbreviations; medication errors

1. Introduction

Acetaminophen is an analgesic and anti-pyretic in widespread use in the US, where it is estimated that 20% of adults use acetaminophen in any given week [1]. Excess intake of acetaminophen has been associated with liver injury [2], and with many emergency room visits [3]. Acetaminophen is present in both OTC and prescription medicines, often in combination with other active ingredients. Patients often do not know that acetaminophen is an active ingredient in medicines they are taking [4]. A recent study found that poor knowledge of acetaminophen as an active ingredient in medicines was associated with exceeding the recommended maximum daily dose of 4 grams [5], and that concomitant use of multiple acetaminophen medicines was also associated with overdose [5].

As a way to help users recognize which medications contain acetaminophen and avoid concomitant use, it has been suggested that an icon be placed on all acetaminophen-containing medicine containers [6]. Consistent with guidance for the design of warnings [7], icon candidates were developed through a process of iterative design, consumer feedback, and qualitative testing. The icon candidates contained letters or an abstract symbol enclosed in a hexagon (see Figure 1 for examples of OTC and prescription labels). In qualitative testing, consumers indicated that the hexagon suggested a stop sign and thus signaled caution, which was deemed an appropriate message. Consumers also indicated that abbreviations suggesting "acetaminophen" helped link the icon to the active ingredient.

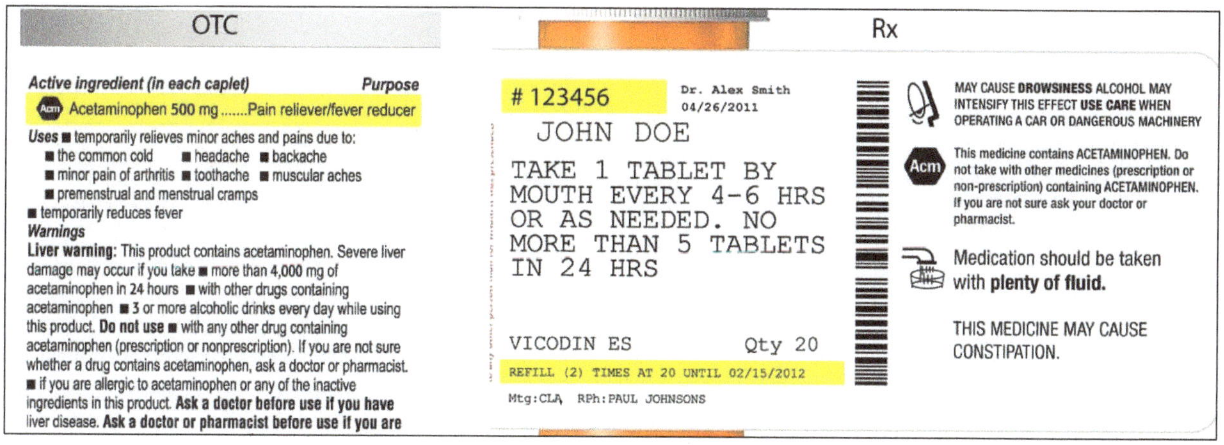

Figure 1. Sample icon-bearing Over the Counter (OTC) and Prescription (Rx) labels.

Quantitative research with consumers, the target for the icon, showed that APAP performed poorly as a symbol for acetaminophen, because consumers did not see how it was related to "acetaminophen". In contrast, icons that used letters that abbreviated of the word "acetaminophen" (Ac, Ace, Acm) effectively communicated that acetaminophen was an ingredient [8]. "Ace" was less favored, because of concern it might have promotional connotations, but Ac and Acm were regarded as particularly promising candidates.

The acetaminophen icon is intended as a communication to patients/consumers, and not for health professionals. Nevertheless, it seemed relevant to examine how it might affect prescriber and pharmacist practices if the letters incorporated in the icons were to come into use as a shorthand for "acetaminophen", much as "APAP" is already used to stand for acetaminophen. The adoption of such abbreviations is discouraged [9], but could nevertheless occur, and could potentially lead to medication errors, particularly if the abbreviations are already being used for other meanings in prescribing. For example, if AC were already being used to designate anticoagulants, or to mean before meals (ante cebum, in Latin), its use to mean "acetaminophen" could lead to medication errors that could potentially harm patients, which are designated as "critical confusions [7]". Accordingly, the study assessed how often and for what purposes Ac and Acm were already in use in prescribing.

Regardless of current use, it also seemed important to assess how prescribers and pharmacists might interpret the candidate letter combinations if they encountered them on a prescribing order. To assess this among pharmacists, we used the methods commonly used to test new proprietary drug names for confusion [10]: we presented pharmacists with prescriptions using the letters and asked them to interpret them, coding the result for correctness and also for critical confusion. The prescriptions were presented in one of three forms—typewritten, handwritten, or spoken—and both with or without "hydrocodone", the most common co-ingredient of acetaminophen in prescription medications. Pharmacists' interpretations were re-tested after the intended meaning of the icons and abbreviations was explained, mirroring the information that would accompany any introduction of the icons. Among physicians, current use of Ac and Acm in prescribing was assessed, along with their interpretation of these letters in prescribing orders.

2. Experimental Section

2.1. Methods

Participants

Pharmacists: A total of 150 pharmacists, representing community/retail (n = 93) and hospital (n = 57) practices, participated in the study. (There were no significant differences in outcomes between retail- and hospital-based pharmacists, so this distinction is not discussed further). A total of 1150 invitations were sent to pharmacists from a panel of 3226 pharmacists maintained by Brand Institute for research on medication names. To participate, pharmacists had to be licensed and practicing/dispensing at least 25% time. Data were collected in two waves, with 75 pharmacists in each (this sample size is typically used to evaluate pharmacist interpretations of proprietary drug names for potential confusion, for FDA consideration). The two waves assessed different sets of letters. The first wave assessed Ac, Ace, and APAP (as well as assessing prescriptions written for Pepcid AC). The second wave assessed Acm and APAP.

Physicians: A total of 1178 invitations were sent to physicians in a Brand Institute database of 9351 physicians, we enrolled 150 physicians engaged at least 50% time in general practice, family practice, or internal medicine in a clinical setting, with responsibility for prescribing. These specialties were targeted as the most common prescribers of acetaminophen medications. Participants were studied in two waves: the first wave was asked about Ac and the second wave about Acm.

Individuals who had participated in research in the previous 3 months and those employed by a pharmaceutical company were excluded. Table 1 shows the characteristics of the resulting pharmacist and physician samples. There were no differences between waves in pharmacists' or physicians' demographics.

Table 1. Demographics.

Pharmacists		**Physicians**	
	N = 150		*N = 150*
Gender		*Gender*	
Female	38.7%	Female	23.3%
Male	61.3%	Male	76.7%
Practice Environment		*Practice Environment*	
Hospital pharmacy	38.0%	Hospital/clinic	22.7%
Retail/community pharmacy	62.0%	Managed care/health network	5.3%
		Nursing home/long term care	0.7%
		Private practice	62.7%
		University hospital	8.7%
Years in Practice		*Years in Practice*	
Less than 2	4.0%	Less than 2	1.3%
2–10	29.3%	2–10	27.3%
11–20	33.3%	11–20	40.7%
21–30	24.7%	21–30	26.7%
More than 30	8.7%	More than 30	4.0%
Work Schedule		*Work Schedule*	
Full-Time	92.0%	Full-Time	97.3%
Part-Time	8.0%	Part-Time	2.7%
Proportion of Time Spent in Dispensing Environment		*Proportion of Time Spent in Clinical Environment*	
0%–9%	0.0%	0%–9%	0.0%
10%–24%	0.0%	10%–24%	0.0%
25%–49%	5.3%	25%–49%	0.0%
50%–74%	21.3%	50%–74%	12.0%
75%–100%	73.3%	75%–100%	88.0%

2.2. Procedures

Pharmacists: Data were collected via the web. Pharmacists were randomized (n = 50 each) to be presented with prescriptions either in typed text, handwritten text, or spoken text. The prescriptions were always presented in groups of three, with two other prescriptions for existing marketed medications serving as distractors from the relevant stimuli. Table 2 shows examples. Each prescription was presented separately when shown typewritten or handwritten; when spoken, all three prescriptions were presented (via earphones) together, as part of one order. Pharmacists responded in open-ended text boxes indicating their interpretation of product name and, separately, the signatura. Multiple responses were permitted, and "don't know" was explicitly allowed as a potential response. Respondents were also asked to state what they would do if they received such a prescription order, and their responses were coded, particularly to capture indications they would dispense a medication.

Table 2. Sample presentations of handwritten and typed prescriptions for target stimuli and distractors.

Stimulus	Typed prescriptions	Handwritten prescriptions
Target Stimulus: ACM 325mg 2 po Q4hr #20	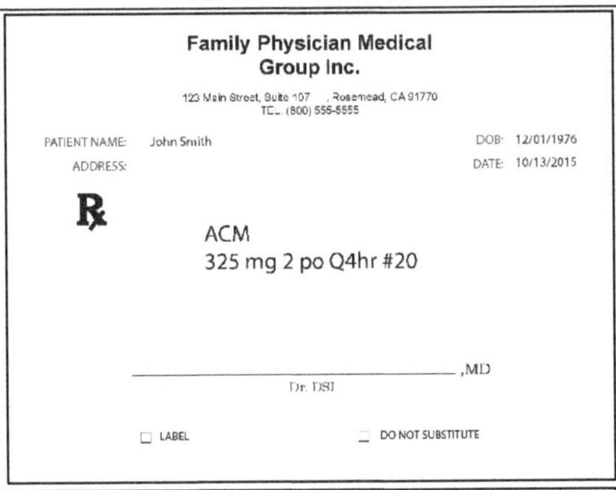	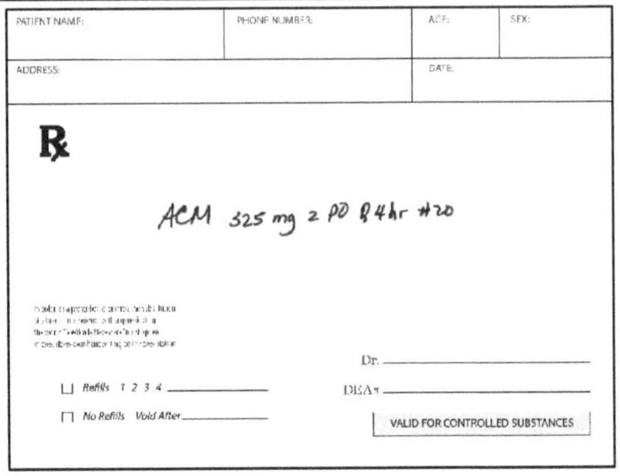
Target stimulus: Hydrocodone 5 mg/ACE 500mg, 1 po every 4–6 hours prn #30	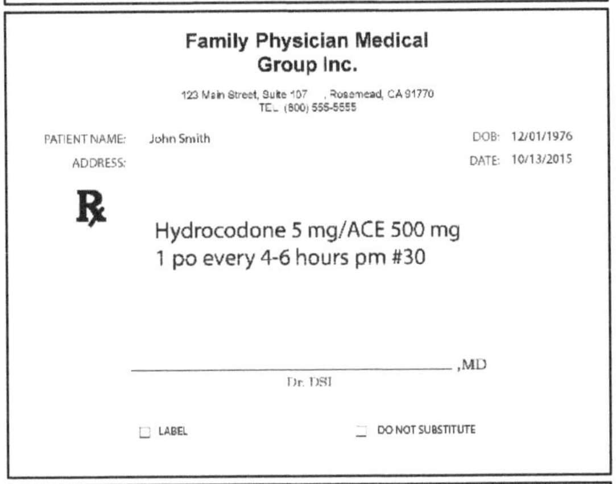	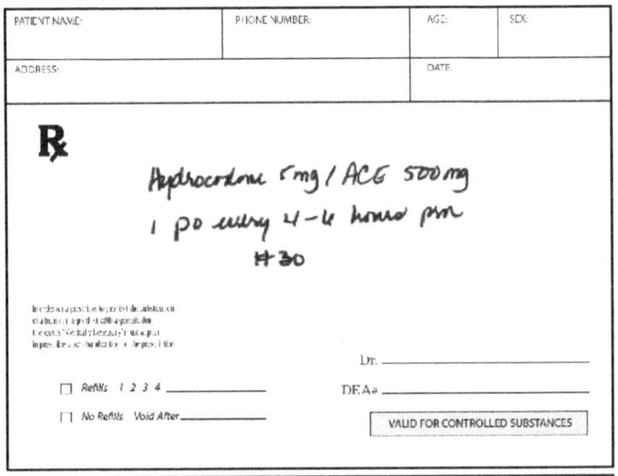
Distractor: Amaryl 2 mg PO QD #30	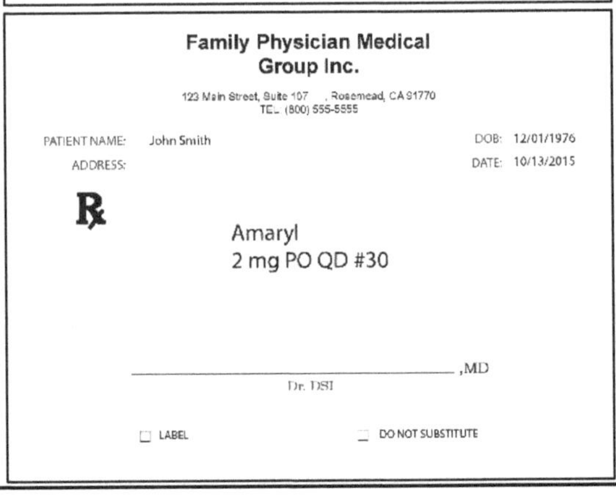	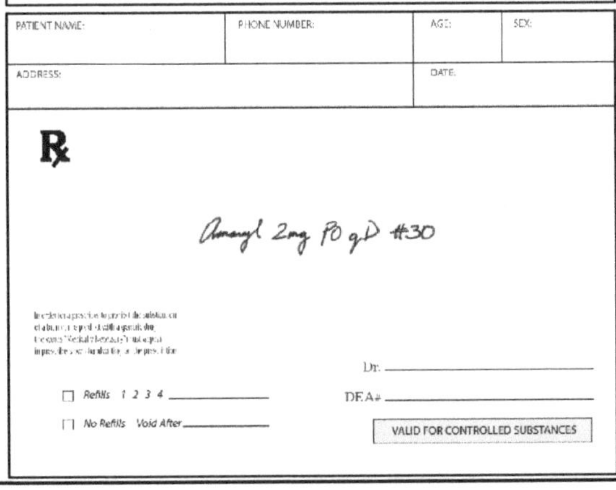

In Wave 1 pharmacists responded to three relevant prescriptions. Two were drawn randomly from Ac, Ace, and APAP; the third was always Pepcid AC. In Wave 2, pharmacists responded to two prescriptions, for Acm and APAP (in randomized order). In both waves, icon letter combinations were randomly rotated through two presentations, one that also showed the co-ingredient "hydrocodone" and one that did not. Thus, in both waves, each pharmacist saw and interpreted 2 acetaminophen-relevant prescriptions, along with several distractors. After initially responding to the test prescriptions without any information about the intended meaning of the abbreviations, pharmacists were exposed to brief text explaining their intended use as icons to mark acetaminophen medications using Ac (Wave 1) or Acm (Wave 2) as examples. (Copies of the material are available from the authors.) After this orientation, pharmacists were retested on stimulus prescriptions containing these letters.

Before being oriented to information about the icon, pharmacists were asked how often they encountered Ac (Wave 1) or Acm (Wave 2) on prescriptions, and how they interpreted these letter combinations.

Physicians: Physicians evaluated Ac in Wave 1 and Acm in Wave 2, being asked if they ever used the candidate letters in prescribing, and, if so, how often and for what purpose. In Wave 1 only, physicians were further asked, as a closed-ended yes/no question, whether they ever used Ac to stand for "anticoagulant". All physicians were subsequently asked how they would interpret the letters if they encountered them on the prescribing orders of a patient's chart or medical record, writing text responses in an open-ended text field. Multiple responses were permitted.

2.3. Measurements

Qualitative coding: Pharmacists' open-ended text interpretations of prescriptions were thematically coded by two coders, noting when the prescription was interpreted as "acetaminophen"; other interpretations (including other medications) were tallied. Additional items were also coded thematically. Percent agreement ranged from 94% to 100% across items, averaging 97%.

Adjudicated critical confusion: Three expert judges, blind to stimulus and condition, coded the pharmacists' and physicians' interpretations to identify the presence of critical confusion, defined as interpretation and behavior that was likely to expose the consumer to clinical harm - We are grateful to Louis Cantilena, MD, PhD, Jan Engle, PharmD, and Randy Juhl, PhD—all former members or chairs of the FDA's Nonprescription Drugs Advisory Committee) for their contribution in making these judgments). Pair-wise agreement among the expert judges averaged 94% for the pharmacist responses and 95% for the physician responses. Critical confusion was considered to have occurred whenever any two judges so indicated. A single judge indicated critical confusion in 8% of pharmacist responses and 5% of physician responses; this was almost all due to a particular judge assigning critical confusion to situations that the other two judges did not (e.g., failing to list the acetaminophen content of an opiate-acetaminophen medication).

2.4. Analysis

We tallied the percentage of responses considered to be critical confusion, by icon, for pharmacists and physicians. In the pharmacist data, we analyzed how often each icon was interpreted as acetaminophen, when presented with or without hydrocodone as a co-ingredient, and when presented in typed, handwritten, and spoken form. Because the comparisons involved a mix of within-subjects and between-subjects contrasts, the analysis used Generalized Estimating Equation methods [11], a form of regression analysis that accommodates this for dichotomous end-points. We also assessed whether there were any differences in response between retail- and hospital-based pharmacists. Statistical tests used a p-value of 0.05.

3. Results

3.1. Current Use and Interpretation of Ac and Acm

Pharmacists: Most (81%) pharmacists reported that they had seen the letters Ac used on prescriptions, with most of those (61%) indicating that it appeared on no more than 10% of prescriptions. Three quarters (75%) of pharmacists indicated that they would interpret Ac as "before meals" (or similar meal-related constructs), and 17% would interpret it as "acid control". Another 9% interpreted Ac as "acetaminophen". A small number of pharmacists interpreted it as other medications (Pepcid AC, 3%; codeine, 3%, ACE inhibitor, 1%; anti-coagulant, 1%). The remainder gave other, less relevant responses, or said they did not know.

In contrast, only 7% of pharmacists reported that they had ever seen the letters Acm on prescriptions. A total of 63% indicated that they would interpret it as acetaminophen. An additional 13% interpreted Acm as referring to a meal-related instruction. There were single instances of interpretations as other drugs (one each as Alclometasone, Actoplus Met, aspirin, anti-cholinergic medication, and the three-drug combination adriamycin/cyclophosphamide/methotrexate). A total of 27% provided non-drug responses, or said they did not know.

Physicians: A total of 65% of physicians said they use the letters Ac in their current prescription writing practices; 90% of these used it to refer to before meals or with meals. (The others gave non-drug responses or no response). In this open-ended query, none of the physicians said they used Ac to refer to anticoagulants. However, when specifically asked a yes/no question whether they use Ac to mean anticoagulant, 8% of the physicians indicated they did.

In contrast, only 20% of physicians said they use the letters Acm in prescriptions. Among those, reference to "before meals" and "acetaminophen" were the most common uses given (25% and 17%, respectively). Idiosyncratic responses given by one physician each included medication classes such as anticholinergic medication and anticonvulsive medication, and the three-drug combination adriamycin, cyclophosphamide, methotrexate. Other interpretations did not relate to medications.

3.2. Critical Confusion

Pharmacists: Adjudicators identified 11 pharmacist interpretations they considered to be critical confusions (*i.e.*, deemed likely to harm patients). Critical confusion was most commonly seen in interpretations of APAP: in 6 instances (of 62; 9.7%), pharmacists were presented with a prescription order for "Hydrocodone APAP, 5 mg/500 mg", but either failed to note the presence of acetaminophen or failed to note the acetaminophen dose, which judges considered to be critical confusion. An additional 4 pharmacists (of 75; 5.3%), presented with prescriptions for "Hydrocodone AC 5 mg/500mg", failed to clearly note the acetaminophen dosage. One pharmacist did not interpret Ace but simply repeated it in the response, and this was judged to be a critical confusion. No critical confusions were noted for Acm or for Pepcid AC.

Physicians: Physicians asked to interpret an entry for Ac on the prescription order page of a patient's chart or medical record made no critical confusions. Among interpretations of Acm on the prescription orders, critical confusions were judged when three physicians interpreted the orders as medical diagnoses rather than medications: one as "acute cardiomyopathy" and two as "alcoholic cardiomyopathy".

3.3. Interpretation of Abbreviations

Pharmacists: When abbreviations were not interpreted as acetaminophen (see below), respondents often simply repeated the abbreviation without interpreting it. No respondent interpreted Ace as "ACE inhibitor", and none interpreted Ac as "anti-coagulant". Pepcid AC was almost never (0.7%, 1 response) mistaken for acetaminophen, whether before or after the Ac icon for acetaminophen was explained. Altogether, among the 750 responses to hypothetical prescriptions, there was only one instance in which a pharmacist indicated he/she would dispense another drug, without checking with the prescriber—a pharmacist who interpreted Ac as aspirin and was prepared to dispense it.

As expected, given that it is an established abbreviation for "acetaminophen", APAP was fairly consistently identified as acetaminophen, whether hydrocodone was mentioned or not (Table 3). The other letter combinations have not been established as abbreviations for acetaminophen, and thus were not expected to be interpreted as such, and generally were not so interpreted, with rates lower than that for APAP. Interpretation as acetaminophen rose significantly when hydrocodone was also mentioned in the order ($p < 0.0001$). In the case of Acm/hydrocodone, this rose to 85% recognition, which approached the figure for APAP on its own (difference, $p > 0.18$).

Table 3. Pharmacist interpretation of candidate abbreviations as acetaminophen.

	Ac[1]		Acm[1]		Ace		APAP[2]		
	Alone	*Opiate*	*Alone*	*Opiate*	*Alone*	*Opiate*	*Alone*	*Opiate*	*p-value Across conditions*
Pre Orientation									
All	14.8%[a]	56.0%[b]	28.6%[a]	85.0%[c,d]	32.0%[a]	78.3%[b,c]	93.7%[d,e]	98.4%[e]	<0.0001
Overall	34.6%[a]		58.7%[b]		54.2%[b]		96.0%[c]		<0.0001
Post Orientation									
All	72.0%*	80.0%	78.7%*	81.3%					ns
Overall	76.0%*		80.0%*						ns

Different superscript letters indicate significant differences ($p < 0.05$). * Change from pre- to post-orientation, $p < 0.001$; [1] Only Ac and Acm were re-tested after orientation; [2] Combines data from Round 1 and Round 2.

Not surprisingly, interpretation of Ac and Acm as "acetaminophen" rose significantly after the intended meaning of the icon was explained (Table 3; $p < 0.0001$). These increases were more modest for prescriptions that also mentioned hydrocodone, as these were already often interpreted as acetaminophen, even before the explanation. This was especially so for Acm/hydrocodone, which was as likely to be interpreted as acetaminophen without explanation as with it.

Interpretation of letters was marginally affected by the mode of presentation ($p < 0.06$). Spoken orders for Ac, Ace, and Acm were less often interpreted as acetaminophen than typed or handwritten orders

(36.7% versus 54.4% for typed, and 60.3% for handwritten, $p < 0.02$). A similar pattern was seen for APAP (90% vs 100% and 97.6%, $p < 0.05$).

Physicians: When asked how they would interpret Ac if they saw it on a prescription order sheet in a patient's medical record (Wave 1), most physicians (75%) indicated they would interpret it as an instruction about meals, while 10% said they did not know or indicated no response. Interpretation as "acetaminophen" was rare (n = 1, 1.25%). One physician interpreted Ac as "anticoagulant" and one as "with codeine"; there were no other drug-related responses.

When interpreting Acm, when written in other physicians' prescribing orders (Wave 2), most physicians (61%) responded "don't know". Most of the remaining responses did not refer to medications or prescribing directions. Among those that did, "before meals" (11%) and acetaminophen (9%) were the most common. Some responses referred to medication classes (anticholinergic, 3%, anticonvulsants, 1%) rather than specific medications, and isolated responses referred to medication combinations (1 each albumin, calcium, magnesium and adriamycin, cyclophosphamide, methotrexate).

4. Discussion

These studies were part of a program evaluating icons that could help consumers/patients taking OTC and Rx medications recognize products containing acetaminophen. The icon is intended as a communication to the patient/consumer, and its letters are not intended for use on prescription orders, where abbreviations are discouraged [9]. Nevertheless, it was considered prudent to evaluate possible issues that could arise from use of these abbreviations in prescribing.

The study confirmed that APAP is already a well-established shorthand for acetaminophen among physicians and pharmacists. However, it resulted in the highest incidence of critical confusion, as interpreted by the expert judges, in pharmacists' interpretations of prescribing orders, primarily because pharmacists failed to note the acetaminophen dose in their interpretation. Indeed, problems with APAP are well known—it is on the Institute of Safe Medication Practices' List of Error-Prone Abbreviations that "should NEVER be used [12]". Further, APAP tested very poorly with consumers [8], the primary target audience, who did not understand how the letters could relate to "acetaminophen". This makes APAP unsuitable as the basis for a consumer-directed acetaminophen icon.

While Ac tested well with consumers, the present study showed that these letters are in widespread use to mean "before meals". Prescribers reported using it that way and pharmacists reported interpreting it that way. Additionally, some prescribers said they were using it to refer to anticoagulants. (Notably, patients taking anticoagulants showed no such confusion [8]). Reinforcing the conclusion that Ac is already in use for other meanings, a search of Davis' on-line Dictionary of Medical Abbreviations [13] found 33 cited meanings for Ac, which included "before meals", but not "acetaminophen". Thus, Ac seems a less suitable letter combination for an acetaminophen icon.

The study did not elicit competing interpretations of Ace: No pharmacist in the study interpreted Ace as "ACE inhibitor". However, searching the Medical Abbreviations dictionary [13] turns up multiple competing meanings, including several related to ACE inhibitors, suggesting Ace might not be an ideal letter set for an acetaminophen icon.

In contrast to some of the other letter combinations, Acm was not currently in common use. Few pharmacists reported seeing it used on prescriptions, and among the fraction of physicians who reported using it, it was already used to stand for acetaminophen. Although individual physicians and pharmacists occasionally interpreted Acm to refer to drug combinations, such interpretations seemed idiosyncratic, and it seems highly unlikely that such combinations would be administered to a patient based on a prescription for acetaminophen. Similarly, a few physicians said they might interpret Acm as indicating a diagnosis, even when it appeared on a prescribing order, not elsewhere in a patient's chart. These interpretations also seemed idiosyncratic: a Medical Abbreviations dictionary [13] search turned up only two established uses, which did not refer to diagnoses, medications, or prescription orders. Absent such competing meanings, Acm seemed to become readily identified with acetaminophen. Indeed, some physicians reported already using it to stand for acetaminophen, and, when the order included the term hydrocodone, Acm was interpreted as "acetaminophen" by 85% of pharmacists, even before the intended meaning was explained. Importantly, since the icon is intended as a communication to consumers, Acm was highly rated by consumers [8], suggesting Acm is a suitable candidate for inclusion in an acetaminophen icon intended for consumers and patients.

Other than the noted critical confusions involving APAP, expert judges saw scant potential for critical confusion arising from use of the studied abbreviations for acetaminophen. Indeed, in 750 dispensing decisions studied, the only instance in which a pharmacist indicated a readiness to dispense an incorrect medication was one instance in which aspirin was to be dispensed to a patient whose prescription called for acetaminophen.

Pharmacists were less likely to interpret prescription orders as acetaminophen when they were communicated orally, consistent with other findings indicating that spoken orders are more error-prone [14]. As the proposed acetaminophen icons are intended as visual cues to consumers and patients and not verbal markers for professionals, they should not be introduced into oral communication.

It is important to emphasize that the development of an icon for acetaminophen directed to consumers is not intended to encourage any use of abbreviations in prescribing. Indeed, the findings reinforce the best-practice recommendation to avoid using abbreviations [9], as even the best-established abbreviation we tested was subject to some misinterpretation. The icons being considered for acetaminophen medications are not intended as short-hand abbreviations for prescribers, but as graphic and iconic communications to patients, on patient medication containers or to consumers on OTC medication labeling, to convey the presence of acetaminophen. Research with consumers showed that the abbreviation-based icons were regarded as effective at communicating that acetaminophen was present, and were not misinterpreted in any way that could be harmful: adjudicators found no instances of critical confusion among the consumers responses [8].

Limitations

The study had some limitations. Although the study sampled both community and hospital-based pharmacists, it is not known that the sample was representative of all pharmacists. Also, larger samples may have enabled more precise inferences, but we used sample sizes often used to evaluate potential for confusion in prescription orders [10]. We studied participants' responses to an online test, and not their actual dispensing practices.

The study also had strengths. To evaluate interpretations of prescriptions, we used a test methodology that is used to test new proprietary drug names to identify potential for confusion and medication errors.

We engaged experts in internal medicine and pharmacy to judge when misinterpretations of prescriptions were likely to bring harm to patients, providing for expert judgment regarding potential problems.

5. Conclusions

Responses from both physicians and pharmacists indicated that Ac might be an unsuitable abbreviation to use inside an acetaminophen icon, because it had interfering meanings already in use among health professionals. In contrast, Acm appeared to be more easily associated with acetaminophen, and was not in common use for other meanings, making it a good candidate to be part of an icon to enable OTC consumers and Rx patients to identify medications containing acetaminophen. If testing shows that it can help consumers make appropriate medication decisions, an icon based on Acm may help avoid medication errors, acetaminophen overdose and acetaminophen toxicity. In any case, the efforts of pharmacists and prescribers will be needed to help educate patients and consumers about proper use of acetaminophen, and about the meaning and utility of an acetaminophen icon.

Acknowledgements

We are grateful to Louis Cantilena (Uniformed Services University of the Health Sciences), Jan Engle (University of Illinois at Chicago), and Randy Juhl (University of Pittsburgh), all former members or chairs of the FDA's Nonprescription Drugs Advisory Committee, for their contribution in adjudicating critical confusion. The authors are also grateful for valuable guidance from members of a board of advisors for the icon development program, including this study: Eric Brass (University of California, Los Angeles), Terry Davis (Louisiana State University Health Sciences), Dan Formosa (independent design consultant), Carol Pollack-Nelson (independent human factors consultant), and Michael Wolf (Northwestern University). The authors also acknowledge the assistance of Gina Bittner (Pinney Associates) with manuscript formatting.

Author Contributions

Saul Shiffman, Helene Cotton, and Christina Jessurun conceptualized the study. Saul Shiffman, Helene Cotton, Christina Jessurun, and Jerry Phillips designed the study, and Helene Cotton and Jerry Phillips oversaw its execution. Saul Shiffman, Mark A. Sembower, and Steve Pype conceptualized and executed the scoring and analysis of the data. Saul Shiffman drafted the manuscript, and all authors contributed substantially to the final draft.

Funding and Declaration of Interests

The project was sponsored by McNeil Consumer Healthcare, which makes acetaminophen products. The sponsor approved the design, and commented on a draft of the manuscript, but did not otherwise participate in study execution, analysis, writing, or publication. Saul Shiffman, Mark Sembower, Steve Pype, and Helene Cotton were engaged as consultants to McNeil Consumer Healthcare. Pinney Associates has provided consulting to other companies that market OTC analgesics, including Bayer, Chattem, GlaxoSmithKline Consumer Healthcare, and Pfizer Consumer Healthcare. Christina Jessurun is employed by McNeil Consumer Healthcare. Jerry Phillips heads the Drug Safety Institute, a subsidiary of Brand Institute, which was contracted by McNeil Consumer Healthcare to conduct the study.

References

1. Kaufman, D.W.; Kelly, J.P.; Rosenberg, L.; Anderson, T.E.; Mitchell, A.A. Recent patterns of medication use in the ambulatory adult population of the united states: The slone survey. *J. Amer. Med. Assoc.* **2002**, *287*, 337–344.
2. Wolf, M.S.; King, J.; Jacobson, K.; Di Francesco, L.; Bailey, S.C.; Mullen, R.; McCarthy, D.; Serper, M.; Davis, T.C.; Parker, R.M. Risk of unintentional overdose with non-prescription acetaminophen products. *J. Gen. Intern. Med.* **2012**, *27*, 1587–1593.
3. Budnitz, D.P., Pollock, D.A.; Weidenbach, K.N.; Mendelsohn, A.B.; Schroeder, T.J.; Annest, J.L. National surveillance of emergency department visits for outpatient adverse drug events. *JAMA* **2006**, *296*, 1858–1866.
4. Galson, S. Acetaminophen hepatotoxicity and nonsteroidal anti-inflammatory drug (nsaid)-related gastrointestinal and renal toxicity (Letter to the state boards of pharmacy). Available online: http://www.webcitation.org/6GGYiPt4I (accessed on 30 April 2013).
5. Kaufman, D.W.; Kelly, J.P.; Rohay, J.M.; Malone, M.K.; Weinstein, R.B.; Shiffman, S. Prevalence and correlates of exceeding the labeled maximum dose of acetaminophen among adults in a U.S.-based internet survey. *Pharmacoepidemiol Drug Saf.* **2012**, *21*, 1280–1288.
6. Suydam, L. Chpa overview and approach: Consumer healthcare products association (chpa) presentation for the 29 June 2009 joint meeting of the drug safety and risk management advisory committee with the anesthetic and life support drugs advisory committee and the nonprescription drugs advisory committee. Available online: http://www.webcitation.org/6GGfyKZxl (accessed on 30 April 2013).
7. National Electrical Manufacturers Association. Criteria for safety symbols (American national standards institute z535.3-revised). Available online: https://www.nema.org/Standards/ComplimentaryDocuments/Z535-3-Contents-and-Scope2-2.pdf (accessed on 13 October 2015).
8. Shiffman, S.; Cotton, H.; Jessurun, C.; Sembower, M.; Pype, S.; Phillips, J. Testing of candidate icons to identify acetaminophen-containing medicines, 2015, submitted.
9. National Council for Prescription Drug Programs. Ncpdp recommendations for improved prescription container labels for medicines containing acetaminophen (Version 1.1). Availeble online: http://www.webcitation.org/6GGgPV11C (accessed on 30 April 2013).
10. Food and Drug Administration. Pdufa pilot project: Proprietary name review. Availeble online: http://www.Webcitation.Org/6mopifbqx (accessed on 22 January 2014).
11. Lipsitz, S., Laird, NM.,Harrington, DP. Generalized estimating equations for correlated binary data: Using the odds ratio as a measure of association. *Biometrika* **1991**, *78*, 153–160.
12. Institute for Safe Medical Practices. Ismp's list of error-prone abbreviations, symbols, and dose designations. Availeble online: http://www.webcitation.org/6SX5oWqIL (accessed on 9 December 2014).
13. Davis, N. Medical abbreviations: 32,000 conveniences at the expense of communication and safety. Availeble online: http://www.webcitation.org/6NSM7Sdrj (accessed on 17 February 2014).

14. Committee on Identifying and Preventing Medication Errors. *Preventing Medication Errors: Quality Chasm Series*. National Academy Press: Washington, DC, USA, 2006.

Permissions

All chapters in this book were first published in Pharmacy, by MDPI; hereby published with permission under the Creative Commons Attribution License or equivalent. Every chapter published in this book has been scrutinized by our experts. Their significance has been extensively debated. The topics covered herein carry significant findings which will fuel the growth of the discipline. They may even be implemented as practical applications or may be referred to as a beginning point for another development.

The contributors of this book come from diverse backgrounds, making this book a truly international effort. This book will bring forth new frontiers with its revolutionizing research information and detailed analysis of the nascent developments around the world.

We would like to thank all the contributing authors for lending their expertise to make the book truly unique. They have played a crucial role in the development of this book. Without their invaluable contributions this book wouldn't have been possible. They have made vital efforts to compile up to date information on the varied aspects of this subject to make this book a valuable addition to the collection of many professionals and students.

This book was conceptualized with the vision of imparting up-to-date information and advanced data in this field. To ensure the same, a matchless editorial board was set up. Every individual on the board went through rigorous rounds of assessment to prove their worth. After which they invested a large part of their time researching and compiling the most relevant data for our readers.

The editorial board has been involved in producing this book since its inception. They have spent rigorous hours researching and exploring the diverse topics which have resulted in the successful publishing of this book. They have passed on their knowledge of decades through this book. To expedite this challenging task, the publisher supported the team at every step. A small team of assistant editors was also appointed to further simplify the editing procedure and attain best results for the readers.

Apart from the editorial board, the designing team has also invested a significant amount of their time in understanding the subject and creating the most relevant covers. They scrutinized every image to scout for the most suitable representation of the subject and create an appropriate cover for the book.

The publishing team has been an ardent support to the editorial, designing and production team. Their endless efforts to recruit the best for this project, has resulted in the accomplishment of this book. They are a veteran in the field of academics and their pool of knowledge is as vast as their experience in printing. Their expertise and guidance has proved useful at every step. Their uncompromising quality standards have made this book an exceptional effort. Their encouragement from time to time has been an inspiration for everyone.

The publisher and the editorial board hope that this book will prove to be a valuable piece of knowledge for researchers, students, practitioners and scholars across the globe.

List of Contributors

Deepti Vyas, Jenana Halilovic, Myo-Kyoung Kim, Marcus C. Ravnan, Edward L. Rogan and Suzanne M. Galal
University of the Pacific, Thomas J. Long School of Pharmacy and Health Sciences, 751 Brookside Road Stockton, CA 95207, USA

Jennifer W. Beall, Renee M. DeHart, Robert M. Riggs and John Hensley
McWhorter School of Pharmacy, Samford University, 800 Lakeshore Drive, Birmingham, AL 35229, USA

Katie MacLure and Derek Stewart
School of Pharmacy and Life Sciences, Robert Gordon University, Aberdeen AB10 7GJ, UK

Olufunmilola K. Odukoya and Loren J. Schleiden
Pharmacy and Therapeutics, School of Pharmacy, University of Pittsburgh, 3501 Terrace St, 720 Salk Hall, Pittsburgh, PA 15213, USA

Michelle A. Chui
Social & Administrative Sciences, School of Pharmacy, University of Wisconsin-Madison, 777 Highland Avenue, Madison, WI 53705, USA

Mona Hassan Aburahma
Department of Pharmaceutics and Industrial Pharmacy, Faculty of Pharmacy, Cairo University, Kasr El-Aini Street, Cairo 11562, Egypt

Jeffrey Atkinson
Pharmacolor Consultants Nancy (pcn-consultants), 12 rue de Versigny, 54600 Villers, France

Pat Crowley
Callum Consultancy, 571 Berwyn Baptist Road, Devon, PA 19333, USA

Kristien De Paepe
Vrije Universiteit Brussel (VUB), Laarbeeklaan 103, 1090 Brussels, Belgium

Brian Gennery and Luigi Martini
Department of Pharmacy, Waterloo Campus, King's College London, 150 Stamford Street SE1, 9NH, London, UK

Andries Koster
European Association of Faculties of Pharmacy (EAFP), Department Pharmaceutical Sciences, Utrecht University, PO Box 80082, 3508 TB Utrecht, The Netherlands

Vivien Moffat
European Federation of Pharmaceutical Industries and Associations (EFPIA), Rue du Trône, 108, 1050 Brussels, Belgium

Jane Nicholson
European Industrial Pharmacists' Group (EIPG), 4 avenue Ruysdael, Paris, France

Gunther Pauwels
Genzyme Flanders, Cipalstraat 8, 2440 Geel, Belgium

Giuseppe Ronsisvalle
Pharmacy Department, Universitá di Catania, Viale Andrea Doria 6, 95125, Catania, Italy

Vitor Sousa
Areta International, via Roberto LePetit, 21040 Gerenzano, Italy

Chris van Schravendijk
Vrije Universiteit Brussel (VUB), Laarbeeklaan 103, 1090 Brussels, Belgium

Keith Wilson
Life and Health Sciences, Aston University, Aston Triangle, B75 6D9 Birmingham, UK

Simon Leung
Memorial Regional Hospital, Hollywood, FL 33021, USA

Mara N. Poulakos
Gregory School of Pharmacy, Palm Beach Atlantic University, West Palm Beach, FL 33416; USA

Jade Machin
Boca Raton Regional Hospital, Boca Raton, FL 33486, USA

Christina H. J. Yang
Nash Drugs, Inc., Hillsdale, MI 49242, USA

Mitesh Doshi
Beaumont Health System, Royal Oak, MI 48073, USA

Nancy A. Mason
University of Michigan College of Pharmacy, 428 Church Street, Ann Arbor, MI 48109, USA

Gagandeep Kaur, Maya Saba and Bandana Saini
Faculty of Pharmacy, The University of Sydney, Camperdown, NSW 2006, Australia

Craig L. Phillips and Keith Wong
Woolcock Institute of Medical Research, Glebe, NSW 2037, Australia

Varsha Bhatt-Mehta
Department of Clinical, Social and Administrative Sciences, College of Pharmacy and Department of Pediatrics, Medical School, University of Michigan, Ann Arbor, MI, 48109, USA
Med4Kids Research Collaborative, Ltd., Edmonton, AB, T6M 2J9, Canada

Robert B. MacArthur
Clinical Development, Pharmaceutics International, Inc., Hunt Valley, MD, 21031, USA

Raimar Löbenberg
Pharmaceutical Sciences Division, Faculty of Pharmacy and Pharmaceutical Sciences, Edmonton, AB, T6G 2R3, Canada
Drug Discovery and Innovation Centre, University of Alberta, Edmonton, AB, T6G 2R3, Canada

Jeffrey J. Cies
Med4Kids Research Collaborative, Ltd., Edmonton, AB, T6M 2J9, Canada Drexel University College of Medicine, Philadelphia, PA, 19129, USA
St. Christopher's Hospital for Children, Philadelphia, PA, 19140, USA 8 Military and Veterans' Clinical Rehabilitation Research, University of Alberta, Edmonton, AB, T6G 2G4, Canada

Ibolja Cernak and Richard H. Parrish II
Med4Kids Research Collaborative, Ltd., Edmonton, AB, T6M 2J9, Canada

Maja H. Michaelsen
Pharmaceutical Care Research Group, School of Pharmacy, University College Cork, College Road, Cork, Ireland
Department of Drug Design and Pharmacology Faculty of Health and Medical Sciences, University of Copenhagen, Universitetsparken 2, DK-2100 Copenhagen, Denmark

Paul McCague
Pharmaceutical Care Research Group, School of Pharmacy, University College Cork, College Road, Cork, Ireland
Department of Drug Design and Pharmacology Faculty of Health and Medical Sciences, University of Copenhagen, Universitetsparken 2, DK-2100 Copenhagen, Denmark
School of Pharmacy, Queen's University Belfast, Lisburn Road, Belfast, UK

Colin P. Bradley
Department of General Practice, Department of General Practice,1st Floor, Brookfield Health Sciences Building, University College Cork, Cork; Ireland

Laura J. Sahm
Pharmaceutical Care Research Group, School of Pharmacy, University College Cork, College Road, Cork, Ireland
Department of Pharmacy, Mercy University Hospital, Grenville Place, Cork, Ireland

Jeffrey Atkinson
Pharmacology Department Lorraine University, Pharmacolor Consultants Nancy, 12 rue de Versigny, Villers 54600, France

Kristien De Paepe
Department of Pharmaceutical and Pharmacological Sciences, Research group of In Vitro Toxicology and Dermato-Cosmetology, Vrije Universiteit Brussel, Laarbeeklaan 103, Brussels 1090, Belgium

Antonio Sánchez Pozo
Faculty of Pharmacy, University of Granada (UGR), Campus Universitario de la Cartuja s/n, Granada 18701, Spain

Dimitrios Rekkas
School of Pharmacy, National and Kapodistrian University Athens, Panepistimiou 30, Athens 10679, Greece

Daisy Volmer
Pharmacy Faculty, University of Tartu, Nooruse 1, Tartu 50411, Estonia

Jouni Hirvonen
Pharmacy Faculty, University of Helsinki, Yliopistonkatu 4, P.O. Box 33-4, Helsinki 00014, Finland

Borut Bozic
Faculty of Pharmacy, University of Ljubljana, Askerceva cesta 7, Ljubljana 1000, Slovenia

Agnieska Skowron
Pharmacy Faculty, Jagiellonian University, UL, Golebia 24, Krakow 31-007, Poland

Constantin Mircioiu
Pharmacy Faculty, University of Medicine and Pharmacy "Carol Davila" Bucharest, Dionisie Lupu 37, Bucharest 020021, Romania

Annie Marcincal
European Association of Faculties of Pharmacy, Faculty of Pharmacy, Université de Lille 2, Lille 59000, France

Andries Koster
European Association of Faculties of Pharmacy, Department Pharmaceutical Sciences, Utrecht University, P.O. Box 80082, 3508 TB Utrecht, The Netherlands

Keith Wilson
School of Life and Health Sciences, Aston University, Birmingham B4 7ET, UK

Chris van Schravendijk
MEDINE2, Vrije Universiteit Brussel, Laarbeeklaan 103, 1090 Brussels, Belgium

Jeffrey Atkinson
Pharmacology Department, Lorraine University, 5 rue Albert Lebrun, 54000 Nancy, France
Pharmacolor Consultants Nancy, 12 rue de Versigny, Villers 54600, France

Kristien De Paepe
Department of Pharmacy, Vrije Universiteit Brussel, Laarbeeklaan 103, Brussels 1090, Belgium

Antonio Sánchez Pozo
Faculty of Pharmacy, University of Granada (UGR), Campus Universitario de la Cartuja s/n, Granada 18701, Spain

Dimitrios Rekkas
School of Pharmacy, National and Kapodistrian University Athens, Panepistimiou 30, Athens 10679, Greece

Daisy Volmer
Pharmacy Faculty, University of Tartu, Nooruse 1, Tartu 50411, Estonia

Jouni Hirvonen
Pharmacy Faculty, University of Helsinki, Yliopistonkatu 4, P.O. Box 33-4, Helsinki 00014, Finland

Borut Bozic
Faculty of Pharmacy, University of Ljubljana, Askerceva cesta 7, Ljubljana 1000, Slovenia

Agnieska Skowron
Pharmacy Faculty, Jagiellonian University, UL, Golebia 24, Krakow 31-007, Poland

Constantin Mircioiu
Pharmacy Faculty, University of Medicine and Pharmacy "Carol Davila" Bucharest, Dionisie Lupu 37, Bucharest 020021, Romania

Annie Marcincal
European Association of Faculties of Pharmacy, Faculty of Pharmacy, Université de Lille 2, Lille 59000, France

Andries Koster
European Association of Faculties of Pharmacy, Department Pharmaceutical Sciences, Utrecht University, PO Box 80082, 3508 TB Utrecht, The Netherland

Keith Wilson
School of Life and Health Sciences, Aston University, Birmingham, B4 7ET, UK

Chris van Schravendijk
Vrije Universiteit Brussel, Laarbeeklaan 103, 1090 Brussels, Belgium

Jamie Wilkinson
Pharmaceutical Group of the European Union (PGEU), Rue du Luxembourg 19, 1000 Brussels, Belgium

Catherine Dewsbury, Ruth M Rodgers and Janet Krska
Medway School of Pharmacy, The Universities of Greenwich and Kent, Central Avenue, Chatham Maritime, Kent ME4 4TB, UK

Saul Shiffman
Pinney Associates, 201 N. Craig Street (Suite 320), Pittsburgh, PA 15213, USA
Department of Psychology, University of Pittsburgh, Pittsburgh, PA 15260, USA
Independent market research consultant, Glenview, IL 60026, USA

Helene Cotton
Independent market research consultant, Glenview, IL 60026, USA

Christina Jessurun
Johnson & Johnson Consumer Inc., Skillman, NJ 08558, USA

Mark A. Sembower and Steve Pype
Pinney Associates, 201 N. Craig Street (Suite 320), Pittsburgh, PA 15213, USA

Jerry Phillips
Drug Safety Institute, Miami, FL 33131, USA